Recent Results in Cancer Research

Volume 192

Managing Editors
P. M. Schlag, Berlin, Germany
H.-J. Senn, St. Gallen, Switzerland

Associate Editors
P. Kleihues, Zürich, Switzerland
F. Stiefel, Lausanne, Switzerland
B. Groner, Frankfurt, Germany
A. Wallgren, Göteborg, Sweden

Founding Editor
P. Rentchnik, Geneva, Switzerland

For further volumes:
http://www.springer.com/series/392

Markus Joerger · Michael Gnant
Editors

Prevention of Bone Metastases

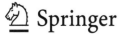 Springer

Dr. med. et phil. Markus Joerger
Department of Medical Oncology
Kantonsspital St. Gallen
Rorschacherstraße 95
9007 St. Gallen
Switzerland
e-mail: markus.joerger@gmail.com

Prof. Dr. Michael Gnant
Chirurgische Klinik
Abt. Allgemeine Chirurgie
Universitätsklinikum Wien
Währinger Gürtel 18-20
1090 Wien
Austria
e-mail: michael.gnant@meduniwien.ac.at

ISSN 0080-0015
ISBN 978-3-642-21891-0   e-ISBN 978-3-642-21892-7
DOI 10.1007/978-3-642-21892-7
Springer Heidelberg Dordrecht London New York

Library of Congress Control Number: 2011944260

© Springer-Verlag Berlin Heidelberg 2012
This work is subject to copyright. All rights are reserved, whether the whole or part of the material is concerned, specifically the rights of translation, reprinting, reuse of illustrations, recitation, broadcasting, reproduction on microfilm or in any other way, and storage in data banks. Duplication of this publication or parts thereof is permitted only under the provisions of the German Copyright Law of September 9, 1965, in its current version, and permission for use must always be obtained from Springer. Violations are liable to prosecution under the German Copyright Law.
The use of general descriptive names, registered names, trademarks, etc. in this publication does not imply, even in the absence of a specific statement, that such names are exempt from the relevant protective laws and regulations and therefore free for general use.
The publishers cannot guarantee the accuracy of any information about dosage and application contained in this book. In every individual case the user must check such information by consulting the relevant literature.

Printed on acid-free paper

Springer is part of Springer Science+Business Media (www.springer.com)

Contents

Preclinical Models that Illuminate the Bone Metastasis Cascade 1
1 The Clinical Problem of Bone Metastasis 2
2 Spontaneous Carcinogenesis in Animal Models 4
3 Chemical Induction in Cancer Animal Models 5
4 Transplantable Animal Models 5
    4.1 Orthotopic Transplantation 6
    4.2 Intra- and Supra-Osseous Implantation 8
    4.3 Humanized Transplantation Model 9
    4.4 Dorsal Skinfold Chamber Model 9
    4.5 Systemic Inoculation of Cancer Cells as a Bone
         Metastasis Model 10
5 Genetically Engineered Mouse Models 11
6 Imaging Modalities 13
    6.1 Bioluminescent Imaging 17
    6.2 Fluorescent Imaging 19
    6.3 Multimodality Imaging 21
    6.4 Functional Imaging 22
7 Future Perspectives 24
References 24

The Role of Bone Microenvironment, Vitamin D and Calcium 33
1 Bone Premetastatic Niche 34
    1.1 Starting From the Primary Tumor Site:
         The Cancer Stem Cells 35
    1.2 The Long Way to the Bone: The Importance of Chemokines ... 40
    1.3 Modification of the Bone Microenvironment:
         Premetastatic Niche Formation 45
    1.4 Osteomimicry 46
    1.5 Role of Calcium, Vitamin D and PTH in the
         Premetastatic Niche 50
References 55

Bisphosphonates: Prevention of Bone Metastases in Breast Cancer ... 65
1 Introduction 67
2 Bone-Targeted Therapies for Breast Cancer 69
3 Anticancer Effects of Oral Bisphosphonates in Early
  Breast Cancer 70
  3.1 Oral Clodronate 70
  3.2 Oral Pamidronate 71
  3.3 Anticancer Benefits of Zoledronic Acid 72
  3.4 ABCSG-12 73
  3.5 ZO-FAST 74
  3.6 AZURE 74
  3.7 Is There a Subset of Patients More Likely to Benefit
      From ZOL Anticancer Effects? 76
  3.8 Neoadjuvant Therapy 78
  3.9 Further Data From Translational Studies
      in Early Breast Cancer 78
4 Can Bisphosphonates Prevent Cancer? 79
5 Tolerability and Safety of Bisphosphonates as Adjuvant Therapy 82
6 Other Uses of Antiresorptives in Women with Early Breast Cancer ... 84
7 Conclusions 84
References 85

Bisphosphonates: Prevention of Bone Metastases in Lung Cancer 93
1 Introduction 95
2 Incidence of Bone Metastasis in Lung Cancer 95
3 Impact of Bone Metastases: The Rationale
  for Adequate Treatment 96
4 Diagnosis of Bone Metastases in Lung Cancer 97
5 Treatment of Bone Metastases in Lung Cancer:
  A Multidisciplinary Affair 99
6 Bisphosphonates in the Treatment of Bone Metastases:
  The Current Standard of Care 99
  6.1 Therapeutic Efficacy of Zoledronic Acid in Lung Cancer:
      Results From Clinical Trials 100
  6.2 Safety Issues and Recommendations for Use 101
  6.3 Biochemical Markers of Bone Turnover:
      Predictors of Clinical Outcome? 101
  6.4 Pharmaco-Economic Considerations 102
  6.5 Prevention of Bone Metastases: Under Investigation .. 103
  6.6 Evidence for Anti-Tumoral Activity in Lung Cancer? .. 104
7 Bone Metastasis Therapy in Lung Cancer:
  What the Future Might Bring 104
  7.1 Denosumab 104
  7.2 Other Small Molecules 105

8	Conclusion	105
References		106

Bisphosphonates: Prevention of Bone Metastases in Prostate Cancer 109
1 Introduction 111
   1.1 Genitourinary Malignancies: Burden of Disease and Challenges to Bone Health 111
   1.2 Hormonal Therapy for Prostate Cancer 113
2 Anticancer Activity of Antiresorptive Agents in Prostate Cancer 114
   2.1 Preclinical and Translational Data Suggesting Potential Anticancer Activity of Bone-Targeted Agents 114
   2.2 Insights From Early Bisphosphonate Trials 115
   2.3 Exploratory Analyses From Phase III, Placebo-Controlled Trials of Zoledronic Acid: Benefits in Patients with Elevated Levels of Bone Turnover Markers 115
   2.4 Ongoing Clinical Trials Evaluating the Anticancer Potential of Bone-Directed Therapies in the Prostate Cancer Setting 118
3 Anticancer Activity of Bisphosphonates in Other Genitourinary Cancers 119
   3.1 Proof-of-Principle Data From Clinical Studies 119
   3.2 Normalization of Bone Markers 120
4 Conclusions 121
References 121

Targeting Bone in Myeloma 127
1 Bone Disease in Myeloma 128
2 Mechanism of Bone Disease in Myeloma 128
3 Pathogenesis and Targeting of Bone Disease in Myeloma 130
   3.1 What is the Impact of the "Novel Therapies" on Bone Disease 131
   3.2 The Anti-Myeloma Effects of Bisphosphonates 132
   3.3 Rank/RANKL System 133
   3.4 MIP1a 133
   3.5 Anti-BAFF-Neutralizing Antibody 133
   3.6 Bone Anabolic Agents 134
4 Conclusions 136
References 137

Combinations of Bisphosphonates and Classical Anticancer Drugs: A Preclinical Perspective 145
1 Molecular Mechanism of Action of BPs 147
2 BPs-Proposed Mechanisms Behind Their Potential Antitumour Effects 148

		2.1	In Vitro Models.	148
		2.2	In Vivo Models.	148
3	BPs in Combination Therapy			149
	3.1	In Vitro Studies–The Foundation for BPs as Part of Combination Therapy.		150
	3.2	In Vivo Studies–Further Evidence of Benefits of BPs in Combination Therapy.		153
4	Combination Therapy with BPs-Effects on Tumour Growth in Bone.			153
	4.1	Summary–Effects on Tumour Growth in Bone		158
5	Combination Therapy with BPs-Effects on Peripheral Tumour Growth.			158
	5.1	Summary–Effects on Peripheral Tumour Growth.		160
6	Sequential Combination Therapy with BPs in the Clinical Setting			161
7	BPs in Combination Therapy–Effects on Normal Cells			162
	7.1	Antiangiogenic Effects of BPs as Single Agents		162
	7.2	Antiangiogenic Effects of BPs in Combination Therapy.		164
8	Conclusions			165
References.				166

Perspectives in the Elderly Patient: Benefits and Limits of Bisphosphonates and Denosumab. 171

1	Introduction	172
2	Bisphosphonates and Safety Profile: Pharmacokinetic and Pharmacodynamic Interactions	173
3	Preclinical Data on the Antitumoral Efficacy of Bisphosphonates to Prevent Bone Metastases	174
4	The Evolving Role of Zoledronic Acid in Reducing the Risk of Breast Cancer Recurrence in Elderly Patients	174
5	Bisphosphonates and the Risk of Postmenopausal Breast Cancer.	176
6	Prospective Trials of Zoledronic Acid in the Adjuvant Setting	176
7	Ongoing Adjuvant Phase III Trials	178
8	Denosumab in the Elderly: Efficacy in Metastatic Disease and New Perspectives in the Adjuvant Setting	180
9	Conclusions	182
References.		183

Denosumab: First Data and Ongoing Studies on the Prevention of Bone Metastases 187

1	Introduction		188
2	Denosumab.		189
	2.1	Current Indications and Efficacy	189
	2.2	Safety.	190

3	Denosumab: Prevention of Bone Metastases in Prostate Cancer	191
4	Denosumab: Prevention of Bone Metastases in Breast Cancer	192
5	Denosumab: Prevention of Bone Metastases in Other Tumors	194
References		195

Diagnostic and Prognostic Use of Bone Turnover Markers 197
1 Introduction 198
2 Overview on Bone Markers 199
   2.1 Bone Formation Markers 199
   2.2 Bone Resorption Markers 201
   2.3 Osteoclast Regulators: Receptor Activator of Nuclear
       Factor-κB Ligand/Osteoprotegerin 202
   2.4 Bone Sialoproteins 203
3 Prognostic Use of Bone Markers 204
   3.1 Prognostic Use of Bone Markers in Breast Cancer 208
   3.2 Prognostic Use of Bone Markers in Prostate Cancer 209
   3.3 Prognostic Use of Bone Markers in Lung Cancer 209
   3.4 Prognostic Use of Bone Markers in Multiple Myeloma .. 210
4 Diagnostic Use of Bone Markers 211
   4.1 Diagnostic Use of Bone Markers in Various Tumors 212
   4.2 Diagnostic Use of Bone Markers in Breast Cancer 213
   4.3 Diagnostic Use of Bone Markers in Prostate Cancer 214
   4.4 Diagnostic Use of Bone Markers in Lung Cancer 216
5 Conclusions 217
   5.1 Prognostic Use of Bone Turnover Markers 217
   5.2 Diagnostic Use of Bone Turnover Markers 218
References 218

**Osteolytic and Osteoblastic Bone Metastases: Two Extremes
of the Same Spectrum?** 225
1 Skeletal Responses to Tumor Invasion 226
2 Bone Remodeling in Physiological Conditions 227
3 Osteoblast-Induced Vicious Cycle: Bone Remodeling in Prostate
   Cancer Bone Metastasis 227
4 Uncoupling of Bone Turnover by Invasion of Prostate
   Cancer Cells 229
5 Osteoclast-Induced Vicious Cycle: Bone Remodeling
   in Multiple Myeloma 229
6 Osteolytic and Osteoblastic Bone Metastases: Are They Two
   Extremes of the Same Spectrum? 229
References 231

Preclinical Models that Illuminate the Bone Metastasis Cascade

Geertje van der Horst and Gabri van der Pluijm

Abstract
In this chapter currently available preclinical models of tumor progression and bone metastasis, including genetically engineered mice that develop primary and metastatic carcinomas and transplantable animal models, will be described. Understanding the multistep process of incurable bone metastasis is pivotal to the development of new therapeutic strategies. Novel technologies for imaging molecules or pathologic processes in cancers and their surrounding stroma have emerged rapidly and have greatly facilitated cancer research, in particular the cellular behavior of osteotropic tumors and their response to new and existing therapeutic agents. Optical imaging, in particular, has become an important tool in preclinical bone metastasis models, clinical trials and medical practice. Advances in experimental and clinical imaging will—in the long run—result in significant improvements in diagnosis, tumor localization, enhanced drug delivery and treatment.

Contents

1	The Clinical Problem of Bone Metastasis..	2
2	Spontaneous Carcinogenesis in Animal Models	4
3	Chemical Induction in Cancer Animal Models...	5
4	Transplantable Animal Models..	5
	4.1 Orthotopic Transplantation...	6
	4.2 Intra- and Supra-Osseous Implantation	8
	4.3 Humanized Transplantation Model..	9

G. van der Horst · G. van der Pluijm (✉)
Department of Urology, Leiden University Medical Centre, J3-100,
Albinusdreef 2, 2333 ZA, Leiden, The Netherlands
e-mail: G.van_der_Pluijm@lumc.nl

	4.4 Dorsal Skinfold Chamber Model	9
	4.5 Systemic Inoculation of Cancer Cells as a Bone Metastasis Model	10
5	Genetically Engineered Mouse Models	11
6	Imaging Modalities	13
	6.1 Bioluminescent Imaging	17
	6.2 Fluorescent Imaging	19
	6.3 Multimodality Imaging	21
	6.4 Functional Imaging	22
7	Future Perspectives	24
References		24

1 The Clinical Problem of Bone Metastasis

Bone metastases are frequent complications of cancer, occurring in up to 80% of patients with advanced breast or prostate cancer and in approximately 15–30% of patients with carcinoma of the thyroid, lung, bladder, or kidney (Coleman 1997). In addition, melanomas and multiple myeloma also readily metastasize to the skeleton. Once tumors metastasize to bone, the disease is incurable and patients may experience several skeletal-related events such as severe bone pain, hypercalcaemia, nerve compression syndromes, and pathological fractures (Mundy 2002; Roodman 2004). This severely increases morbidity and diminishes the quality of life of the patients.

Understanding the different steps of carcinogenesis and the closely linked mechanisms of invasion and metastasis is crucial for the development of new therapeutic strategies (Fig. 1). Initial stages of carcinogenesis are characterized by hyperplastic growth and neo-vascularization. In order to acquire a mesenchymal migratory phenotype, cancer cells must shed many of their epithelial characteristics and undergo oncogenic epithelial-to-mesenchymal transition (EMT) (van der Pluijm 2010).

Induction of EMT is not the only mechanism by which epithelial cells can migrate and spread. Movement of epithelial cells can also occur as a group (collective migration) in which epithelial and mesenchymal cells cooperate (reviewed in Friedl and Gilmour 2009).

It is becoming increasingly clear that the acquisition of an invasive phenotype by the cancer cells does not solely occur via somatic genetic and epigenetic mutations in the cancer cells themselves, but also via the surrounding stroma (Thiery et al. 2009; Kalluri and Weinberg 2009; Kalluri 2009). The final stages of the metastatic cascade involve intravasation, circulation in the blood flow, adhesion to the endothelium of the distant organs, extravasation, and colonization of the distant organs (Brown et al. 2011).

To study the fundamental properties of tumor growth and the metastatic cascade a number of animal model systems are currently used. However, several problems are encountered when transferring results from animal models into the clinic including differences between animal and human pathophysiology and heterogeneity. In addition, the results from one species often fails to be translated to another species. Nevertheless, animal models and real-time imaging of osteotropic cancers provide major and critical, pathogenic information about tumor progression and

Preclinical Models that Illuminate the Bone Metastasis Cascade

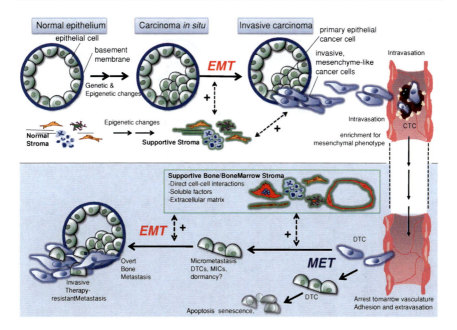

Fig. 1 Interactions between osteotropic cancer cells and their microenvironment in tumor progression and bone metastasis. Epithelial-to-mesenchyme transition (*EMT*) occurs at the primary site and allows epithelial cancer cells to invade the surrounding stroma, intravasate, circulate, and extravasate to distant sites. Upon colonization of bone marrow the cancer cells frequently can regain their original epithelial phenotype by a mesenchymal-to-epithelial transition (*MET*). Tumor-stroma interactions are critically important in the subsequent steps of the metastatic cascade. A number of growth factors, including TGFβ, PDGF, and IGFs, stimulate EMT in the primary tumor and have also been identified as stimulators of bone metastasis formation, presumably via the acquisition of an invasive phenotype of cancer cells in micrometastases. *CTCs* circulating tumor cells. *DTCs* disseminating tumor cells MIC metastasis-initiating cells (adapted from van der Pluijm 2010)

skeletal metastasis. An ideal animal model should closely mimic the clinical situation, thus facilitating the development of novel therapy for the prevention and treatment of metastatic bone disease. Clinical trials frequently fail to reproduce the highly encouraging results obtained from the preclinical models. Ideal in vivo models of human cancers that metastasize to bone would reproduce the genetic and phenotypic changes that occur at the different stages of human bone metastasis and consist of naturally occurring or chemically induced tumors. Furthermore, these preclinical models would be reproducible and should progress relatively rapidly in order to be affordable. Unfortunately the majority of spontaneously arising tumors do not metastasize, metastasize with a very long latency, or are characterized by intravascular metastases alone (Rosol et al. 2004; Pollard 1998).

Although animal models of skeletal metastasis, which mimic several aspects of human disease, have been used and refinements to the models continue to be developed, these 'ideal' preclinical models may represent an impossible objective (see Fig. 2).

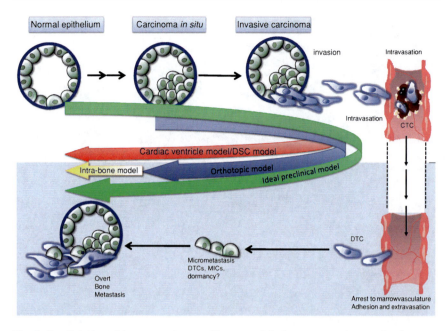

Fig. 2 Preclinical models representing specific steps of the bone metastatic cascade of events

Currently, most animal models of bone metastasis must be derived experimentally since spontaneous bone metastasis in rodents or small mammals is relatively rare. This restriction has resulted in the development of specific animal models that represent unique steps of the bone metastatic cascade of events.

In this chapter, animal models will be described that represent prostate and breast cancer in humans. Furthermore, other currently available animal models of tumor progression and metastasis, including genetically engineered mice that develop primary and metastatic carcinomas and transplantable models (xenograft or syngeneic), will be described. Subsequently, small animal imaging will be discussed, focusing on the currently available modalities including microcomputed tomography (μCT), micropositron emission tomography (μPET), single photon emission computed tomography (SPECT), magnetic resonance imaging (MRI), ultrasound imaging, and optical imaging (bioluminescence and fluorescence) (Massoud and Gambhir 2003).

2 Spontaneous Carcinogenesis in Animal Models

An impediment in the search for preclinical models of skeletal metastasis is the fact that small mammals have a very low incidence of osteotropic cancers as compared to humans.

Spontaneous prostate carcinoma occurs most commonly in dogs and is rare in rodents and other animals, including non-human primates. Some strains of rats (Lobund Wistar and ACI/Seg rats) have an increased incidence of prostate neoplasia (Pollard 1998). However, dogs can develop prostate carcinoma that eventually metastasizes to bone, with a mixture of osteoblastic and osteolytic phenotype (Rosol et al. 2004).

Rodents often develop benign as well as malignant breast cancer. However, most spontaneous breast carcinomas in rodents do not metastasize and have a low incidence of regional lymph node invasion (Rosol et al. 2004). Dogs and cats frequently develop breast carcinomas that may subsequently metastasize to the lymph nodes and lungs, but bone metastases are infrequent.

3 Chemical Induction in Cancer Animal Models

Prostate carcinomas can be induced in Noble rats by treating the rats with testosterone/estradiol or MNU/testosterone. An increased incidence of prostate carcinomas can be induced in Lobund Wistar rats administering methylnitrosourea (MNU) and testosterone (Pollard et al. 2000). However, these tumors rarely metastasize to the lymph nodes and lungs and do not metastasize to bone.

Breast carcinoma can be induced in rats by administering dimethylbenzanthracene (DMBA), MNU, and N-ethyl-N-nitrosourea (ENU) and may metastasize to the lungs (Ip 1996). The rats often develop mild hypocalcaemia, but bone metastases do not occur spontaneously (Stoica et al. 1983; Stoica et al. 1984).

4 Transplantable Animal Models

Transplantable tumor models comprise *syngeneic* models, in which the cancer cell line/tissue transplanted is of the same genetic background as the animal, and *xenograft* models referring to human cancer cell lines/tissues transplanted into immuno-compromised hosts, including BALB/c nu/nu nude and severe combined immuno-deficient (SCID) mice (Khanna and Hunter 2005). The advantage of syngeneic models is that the transplanted tissues, the microenvironment (stroma), and the host are from the same species. However, these model systems lack many of the important characteristics of human tumors. For example, they usually are derived from inbred mice and thus lack the genetic complexity of human tumors. Therefore, conclusions drawn from these models should be validated in human cancers.

Although the xenograft models have the disadvantage of an incomplete immune system, a wide range of human samples can be used to study dissemination and colonization, and most mechanistic insight into the process of metastasis is derived from xenograft studies.

Drawbacks of both transplantable animal models are that only specific stages of the metastatic cascade are represented, as well as the expansion of certain clonal constituents of polyclonal tumors due to cell culture and tissue explantation (Fig. 2).

Importantly, some crucial features of the tumor microenvironment are lost in these models. During tumorigenesis and bone metastasis, the stroma and the tumor cells closely interact (Fig. 1). Over 100 years ago, Stephen Paget emphasized the role of stroma in metastasis not only as a mechanical support but also as a fertile 'soil' for the growth of a cancer cell, the 'seed' (Paget 1889). It has become increasingly clear that primary and metastatic cancers do not exist as isolated tumor cells, but closely interact with different cell types and the extracellular matrix constituting the stroma compartment. Only recently, it has been shown that this heterogeneous and bi-directional interaction within the tumor tissue is responsible for tumor progression (Naef and Huelsken 2005). However, the molecular determinants of the stromal support have remained largely elusive. Cancer cells produce factors that can activate local stromal cells such as fibroblasts, smooth muscle cells and adipocytes, and recruit endothelial- and mesenchymal progenitors and inflammatory cells (Kim et al. 2005; Bhowmick and Moses 2005). In turn, this stromal activation leads to the secretion of additional growth factors and proteases, which further favor cancer cell proliferation and invasion (Kim et al. 2005; Bhowmick and Moses 2005; Mueller and Fusenig 2004). Moreover, the stroma may not just be an innocent bystander, but the site of primary dysfunction, which may be critical for carcinogenesis (Albini and Sporn 2007). Hence, a major drawback of most of the transplantable tumor models is that the surrounding stroma is 'normal' and not tumor-associated. As a result, the transplantable models do not necessarily recapitulate all of the interactions between the tumor and the surrounding stroma.

Cancer cells can be administered in various ways to small laboratory animals, including inoculation of the tumor cells subcutaneously, orthotopically (at the anatomical site of origin), or at the site of eventual dissemination (Figs. 2 and 3). Although subcutaneous animal models still remain a valuable approach for tumor progression and metastasis, especially for drug screening purposes, studies on tumor progression and metastasis require a more biologically relevant environment such as the tissue of origin or the tissue to which the tumor cells preferentially metastasize.

4.1 Orthotopic Transplantation

Orthotopic transplantation refers to the delivery of cancer cells to the anatomic location or tissue from which a tumor was originally derived. The use of orthotopic inoculation has resulted in tumor models that may more closely resemble human cancers including tumor histology, gene expression, responsiveness to chemotherapy, and metastatic biology (Fig. 3a). The 4T1 cell line is a transplantable murine breast cancer cell line that grows very fast at the primary site and can spontaneously form metastases in lungs, liver, bone, and brain over a period of 3–6 weeks. Because the model is syngeneic in BALB/c mice, it can be used to study the role of the immune system in tumor growth and metastasis in the 4T1 (Pulaski et al. 2001; Tao et al. 2008). Unfortunately, bone metastasis is a late event in the 4T1 model

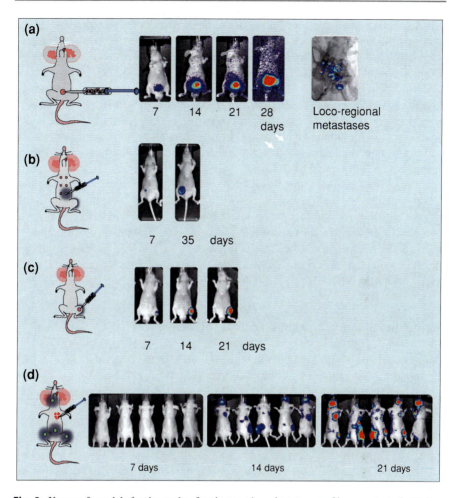

Fig. 3 Xenograft models for the study of pathogenesis and treatment of bone metastasis (Balb-c nu/nu mice). Orthotopic implantation models of human PC-3MPro4 prostate cancer cells expressing firefly luciferase implanted in the mouse prostate (**a**) and murine breast cancer cells (*KEP*) expressing firefly luciferase (**b**), **c**, Intra-osseous transplantation model. Growth of human PC-3MPro4 prostate cancer cells in the bone marrow of mouse tibia. **d** Mouse model of experimental bone metastasis. Inoculation of 100.000 human luciferase-expressing PC-3MPro4 prostate cancer cells into the left cardiac ventricle allows real-time cell racking and growth of skeletal metastasis. (Buijs et al. 2007a, b, 2010 own unpublished observations)

and as a result, the tumor load at the orthotopic site is high. Surgical removal of the orthotopically implanted, invasive 4T1 tumor cells is difficult and, as a result, the cancer often recurs. Furthermore, 4T1 cells predominantly spread to soft tissue (lungs) prior to the manifestation of bone metastasis, thus leaving a narrow time window for studying the pathogenesis or treatment of skeletal metastasis, while animals suffer from high metastatic tumor load in the lungs.

It has been shown that inoculation of PC-3MPro4 cells into the prostate results in metastasis towards the loco-regional lymph nodes (Fig. 3a). However, they have not reliably produced bone metastases (Buijs et al. 2007a; Buijs and van der Pluijm 2009; An et al. 1998). Recently, we have set up an orthotopic transplantation model using murine breast cancer (KEP) cells. KEP breast cancer cells, closely resembling invasive lobular carcinoma, were generated by somatic inactivation of E-cadherin and p53 in genetically engineered mice. Implantation of KEP cells, expressing the bioluminescence reporter firefly luciferase, into mammary glands resulted in bone metastasis with very little soft tissue involvement (Fig. 3b, see further below, Derksen et al. 2006).

Current drawbacks of the inoculation of most of the human mammary or prostate carcinoma cells into the murine mammary fat pad or the prostate, respectively, include the lack of an intact immune system and the possibility of tumor cells leaking into the peritoneum following surgery as well as the trauma of opening the mouse peritoneum itself. In order to establish a reliable orthotopic model, sensitive detection of (micro) metastatic spread by molecular imaging is a prerequisite (see Sect. 5).

4.2 Intra- and Supra-Osseous Implantation

Other models comprise the inoculation of the cells in the bone, the site to which the tumor cells preferentially metastasize (Fig. 3c). Intraosseous inoculation results in either osteolytic or osteoblastic lesions or a mixture of those, depending on the cell line used. For example, the breast cancer cell lines MDA-MB-231, MCF-7, and 4T1 as well as the prostate carcinoma lines PC-3, Du-145, and RM-1 result in osteolytic lesions. Intraosseous inoculation of human prostate cancer cell lines C4-2B, MDA-PCa-2b, LAPC-9, and LuCaP 23.1 and the breast cancer cell line ZR-75-1 results in osteoblastic lesions (Schwaninger et al. 2007; Keller and Brown 2004).

Another transplantable model of prostate and breast cancer consists of transplantation of human tumor tissue onto the surface of the calvaria (Izbicka et al. 1997). The resulting tumors are moderately differentiated prostate adenocarcinoma with osteolytic and osteoblastic changes that are similar to the histopathological features of human prostate cancer bone metastasis (Schwaninger et al. 2007; Keller and Brown 2004; Izbicka et al. 1997). In addition to prostate cancer, this model has also been applied to study the role of tumor–bone interactions in breast cancer-induced osteolysis and malignant growth in the bone microenvironment (Nannuru et al. 2009; Futakuchi et al. 2009). Limitations of these models include the lack of human tumor-to-bone metastasis and the typical location in the bone where metastatic tumors arise. However, this model has proved useful in identifying key factors driving tumor-induced osteoblastic and osteolytic changes such as MMP-7 and MMP-13 (Lynch et al. 2005; Nannuru et al. 2010).

4.3 Humanized Transplantation Model

Commonly used in vivo bone metastasis models include syngeneic rodent cancers and xenograft of human cancer in immunodeficient mice. Species-specific factors from the host (bone/bone marrow stroma) may limit the ability of human cancer cells to metastasize to rodent bones. Important improvements have been made in the generation of preclinical models of human cancer metastasis to human bone (Xia et al. 2011; Shtivelman and Namikawa 1995; Nemeth et al. 1999; Yonou et al. 2001; Kuperwasser et al. 2005). Human fetal bone and adult human rib have been implanted into non-obese diabetic/severe combined immuno-deficient (NOD/SCID) mice, a model called NOD/SCID-hu. Human prostate or breast cancer cells were administered via tail vein injections or directly introduced into the implanted bone (Shtivelman and Namikawa 1995; Nemeth et al. 1999; Yonou et al. 2001; Kuperwasser et al. 2005). The human cancer cells formed tumors only in the human bone implants and not in the mouse skeleton or in other human or mouse tissues implanted at the same ectopic site. Hence, these models enable the study of human cancer cell metastasis in a tissue-specific and species-specific manner. Recently, a model was developed based on SCID mice, called the BOM model (human Breast tissue derived Orthotopic and Metastatic model), in which human breast tissue as well as human bone was implanted into the same mouse (Wang et al. 2010; Xia et al. 2010). The human microenvironment of both the breast tissue as well as the bone tissue of this model is important, since species-specific differences may determine the interplay between the stroma and the tumor cells. Indeed, it has been shown that the behavior of breast cancer cells in the mouse model was altered in response to variations in the microenvironment (Xia et al. 2010).

4.4 Dorsal Skinfold Chamber Model

Real-time imaging of single cells in vivo can be accomplished by using the dorsal skinfold chamber model. The first transparent dorsal skinfold chambers have been used to monitor angiogenesis in vivo with high spatial resolution (Lehr et al. 1993; Sckell and Leunig 2009).

In the dorsal skinfold chamber model described by Reeves et al., a metatarsal from a newborn mouse is engrafted into a dorsal skinfold chamber implanted on a SCID mouse (Reeves et al. 2010). Subsequently, either prostate cancer (PC-3 GFP) or breast cancer (MDA-MB-231 GFP) cells are inoculated into the left cardiac ventricle to simulate micrometastatic spread (Reeves et al. 2010). The data showed that the osteotropic PC-3 and MDA cells are both capable of homing to the metatarsal within the DSC, whereas oral SSC-4 cells which are known to metastasize to lymph nodes did not. A drawback of these models is the technical skills that are required to the use of the relatively expensive multi-photon microscopy equipment. Because of these issues, it is not feasible to have high numbers of animals included into the experiments.

4.5 Systemic Inoculation of Cancer Cells as a Bone Metastasis Model

The experimental metastasis model is a widely used model and refers to systemic inoculation of the tumor cells into the left cardiac ventricle (Fig. 3d) (Arguello et al. 1988; Nakai et al. 1992; van der Pluijm et al. 2001; van der Pluijm et al. 2005; Wetterwald et al. 2002), or lateral tail vasculature (Peyruchaud et al. 2003). In our hands, inoculation of cancer cells into the cardiac ventricle (Fig. 3d) is preferred because the number of bone metastasis is higher and the distribution of the bone metastases is superior to that of the tail vasculature inoculation model. Importantly, some of the published 'tail vein papers' were abusively performed by inoculation into the tail arteries rather than the tail veins. Arguello and co-workers first described tumor cell injection into the left cardiac ventricle leading to colonization of the skeleton (Arguello et al. 1988). Depending on the inoculation site and the tropism of the tumor cells, distant metastases develop at a number of different locations in the animals (i.e., largely pulmonary metastasis when tumor cells are inoculated in the tail vasculature and predominantly bone metastasis when tumor cells are inoculated in the left cardiac ventricle). These models have been used to study the effects of drugs on bone metastases as well as the molecular biology of this process (Nakai et al. 1992; van der Pluijm et al. 2001; Wetterwald et al. 2002; Peyruchaud et al. 2003; van der Pluijm et al. 2005; Buijs et al. 2007a, b; van der Horst et al. 2011a,b). Using these model systems, the user has control over both the amount and characteristics of the cells that are inoculated in the animals.

For instance, intracardiac inoculation can be used to monitor cancer cell tropism to specific organs. The human prostate cancer cell lines PC-3MPro4 metastasizes to multiple skeletal sites and forms osteolytic tumors, whereas the human prostate cancer cell lines C4-2B and VCaP form mainly osteoblastic tumors (Thalmann et al. 2000; Korenchuk et al. 2001; Buijs et al. 2007a). The murine prostate cancer cell line RM1 has been shown to metastasize to the skeleton in over 95% of injected C57BL/6 mice. An advantage of this model is that the syngeneic RM1 tumor cells are injected into immuno-competent mice, and thus can be used to study interactions between the immune system, tumors, and bone (Power et al. 2009).

Using intracardiac inoculation, the osteotropic potential of different subpopulations of cancer cells can be investigated. For example, viable cell sorting using Aldefluor™ can be used to select for cells with high or low Aldehyde dehydrogenase activity. Using systemic inoculation, it has been shown that the subpopulation with high ALDH activity has an increased tumorigenic and metastatic potential compared to the subpopulation with low ALDH activity (van den Hoogen et al. 2010).

A potential disadvantage of these systemic inoculation models is that early steps in the metastatic cascade—i.e., carcinogenesis, invasion, and intravasation—are bypassed (Fig. 2).

5 Genetically Engineered Mouse Models

While in vitro and in vivo experimental or 'spontaneous' transplantable models have yielded many important insights into the potential molecular mechanisms of metastasis, a number of important limitations remain. For example, the introduction of cells into the circulatory system bypasses a number of important events thought to be major roadblocks in metastatic dissemination, including escape from the primary tumor, invasion into the surrounding stroma and extravasation. Ectopic or orthotopic implantation, while potentially reintroducing a more natural setting for the process, still suffers from several limitations like the lack of an intact immune system, the inability to model the premalignant neoplastic stages and the surgical procedure itself which may damage surrounding tissue and facilitate the escape of the tumor cells into the bloodstream. This may lead to distant metastasis due to the inoculation procedure instead of tumor growth at the orthotopic site.

Moreover, it has been shown that tumorigenesis and metastasis is not just the result of tumor cell characteristics, but rather is a complex interaction between tumor cells and the surrounding stroma. Transplantable models do not necessarily recapitulate all of the interactions between tumor and stroma that may play important roles in tumor dissemination (Figs. 1, 2).

Genetic engineered animal models (GEMs), which have a defined genetic background, can be used in immuno-competent hosts and usually have clinically relevant mutations (Visvader 2011). A number of genetically engineered animal models have been developed. GEMs are valuable because they allow investigators to study the contribution of particular genes to the development of metastasis. They provide flexible manipulation of gene expression at particular time points, thus supporting temporal genetic studies of tumor progression and metastasis. In spite of this, only one or two genes are altered, which is not the situation in human cancer progression. In addition, it is possible that constitutive activation or loss of genes in these models may not completely replicate spontaneous human cancer progression and metastasis. Nevertheless, transgenic mice are important models that are being used to gain insight into the development and treatment of bone metastases.

An advantage of these models is the fact that the tumors arise in their normal context and that the animals have a functional immune system. A major limitation of these models is the fact that they are labor intensive and expensive. The current generation of GEMs has a mixed and varied genetic strain background, thus, it is time- and labor-consuming to backcross these lines into a desirable, homogeneous, inbred background before being able to apply them in preclinical trials. In addition, the resources and infrastructure is lacking to consistently generate and evaluate large numbers of GEMs needed for preclinical experiments (Singh and Johnson 2006).

Recent developments in the generation of genetically engineered animal models have resulted in notable improvements in these models. GEMs can be simply classified as either *transgenic* or *endogenous*. Mutant mice that express oncogenes or dominant-negative tumor-suppressor genes under control of an *ectopic* promoter and enhancer elements are called transgenic GEMs.

Endogenous GEMs represent mutant mice that either lost the expression of genes or express dominant-negative transgenes or oncogenes from their *native* promoters (Frese and Tuveson 2007).

Transgenic GEMs overexpress a transgene being either an oncogene or a dominant-negative tumor suppressor gene using an ectopic promoter and enhancer element. Transgenic GEMs have been developed with temporal regulation of the transgene by using inducible promoters such as the TET system (doxycycline regulated transcription).

A drawback of the transgenic models is that it is difficult to obtain the control to express oncogenes at physiological levels. This is important since many overexpressed oncogenes may cause toxic effects including apoptosis and senescence (Sarkisian et al. 2007; Blakely et al. 2005).

For breast cancer, several GEMs have been developed, of which the majority overexpress oncogenes such as c-Myc, CyclinD1, Her2, and Wnt-1 via the mouse mammary tumor virus long repeat (MMTV) (reviewed in Shen and Brown 2005). This promoter has been very useful for studies of mammary gland development and tumorigenesis. However, the expression of the transgene is not homogeneous. A reverse tetracycline-dependent transcriptional activator (rtTA) system was developed with the MMTV promoter in order to obtain mammary-specific, tightly regulated, and homogeneous transgene expression in the presence of doxycycline. Using this system, the c-myc transgene was specifically induced in mammary epithelial cells (D'Cruz et al. 2001; Gunther et al. 2002). Furthermore, leukaemic HTLV-1 Tax transgenic mice (Tax$^+$ mice) develop skeletal lesions and soft tissue metastasis (Gao et al. 2004), and these transgenic mice are well suited to study the effects of anti-resorptive therapy on bone metastasis and tumor progression (Hirbe et al. 2009).

Conditional models enable site-specific recombinases such as Cre-LOX and FLP-FRT to spatio-temporal control deletion or expression of a gene in specific tissues under control of their endogenous promoter. Models include knock-out mice, in which knock-out alleles replace one or more exons with a selectable marker resulting in a null allele or knock-in models use transgenes under the control of endogenous promoter and enhancer sequences. Cre-recombinase recognizes a pair of inverted repeat DNA elements, or LoxP sites, and catalyzes recombination resulting in deletion or inversion of the intervening sequence (Lakso et al. 1992; Lewandoski 2001). The yeast FLP recombinase results in deletion of the sequences between the FRT sites (Lewandoski 2001). For instance, in a breast cancer conditional MMTV-Brca1 model, the Cre gene is under the control of the MMTV promoter. Activation of the Cre gene causes conditional deletion of the target gene Brca1. Deletion of the Brca1 gene by this system resulted in abnormal ductal development and activated apoptosis (Xu et al. 1999). Existing models of prostate carcinogenesis include the transgenic adenocarcinoma of mouse prostate model (TRAMP) and transgenic models overexpressing Myc or the SV40 large T antigen under control of prostate specific promoters. Recently, prostate-specific conditional knockouts have been generated of *NKX3.1, PTEN, P27*, and *P53* tumor suppressors that show initiation of prostatic intraepithelial neoplasia and progress into adenocarcinoma with lymph and lung metastasis (Wang et al. 2003; Gao et al. 2004; Chen et al. 2005; Kim et al. 2002; Zhou et al. 2006). Although prostate cancer progression, lymph node metastases and lung metastases can be found regularly, metastasis to the bone is rare with these models (Gingrich and Greenberg 1996; Asamoto et al. 2001; Winter et al. 2003; Tu et al. 2003).

The analysis of multiple mutations seen in human tumors is possible by interbreeding GEM to produce mutant mice with both mutations, such as the lobular breast carcinoma model (KEP model) described by Derksen and co-workers, demonstrating that somatic inactivation using Cre/loxP, keratin14 promoter Cre-mediated loss of both p53 and E-cadherin in breast epithelium resulted in spontaneous tumors resembling human invasive lobular breast carcinoma (Derksen et al. 2006, 2011).

Breast cancer metastasis was found in the gastrointestinal tract, peritoneum, lung, lymph nodes, and bone. In a ductal breast carcinoma conditional model, inactivation of only Brca2 did not result in breast cancer, whereas inactivation of both Brca2 and p53 resulted in both breast and skin tumors (Jonkers et al. 2001). After luciferase transduction of these cancer cells (KEP/luc$^+$ cells), inoculation of the cells into the left heart ventricle resulted in rapid metastatic spread throughout the whole body, especially to bone. Orthotopic implantation of KEP/luc $^+$ cells resulted in tumor growth in the mammary fat pad. After surgical removal of the orthotopic tumor, soft tissue and bone metastases were formed throughout the body (Buijs et al. 2010), (Fig. 4).

However, the results of the simultaneous mutations in the tissue may not reflect the sequential accumulation of mutations in human tumors. This can be addressed by using different site-specific recombinases (e.g., Cre-lox and FLP-FRT) in a temporal manner to produce the relevant mutations (Frese and Tuveson 2007). Another aspect is that human tumors are thought to arise from a cell containing one initial mutation, the tumor-initiating cell or cancer stem cell. The mutations in many GEMs occur in all the cells of the tissue and therefore, the tumor cells do not develop in the context of the 'normal' surrounding stroma. This can be circumvented by the use of Cre-expressing viruses at a low titer, because then the activation or silencing of genes occurs in a few cells, resulting in some mutated cells surrounded by normal cells (Frese and Tuveson 2007). This technology can also be used to introduce changes in the stroma. Recently, Kim et al. described the use of a latent, Cre-activatable c-MYC allele, which combined with a prostate-specific Cre allele (*PbCre4*) leads to focal overexpression of c-MYC in a few prostate luminal epithelial cells (Kim et al. 2011). When crossed with *Pten/p53* heterozygotic mice, the c-MYC-initiated cells progressed to prostatic intraepithelial neoplasia (mPIN) and adenocarcinoma lesions. This model is based on changes in genes that are relevant for human prostate cancer (i.e., c-MYC, PTEN and p53) and may be useful for understanding prostate cancer pathogenesis.

6 Imaging Modalities

The strength of the experimental approach is not only critically dependent on the appropriate animal model but also on the means of data acquisition and imaging.

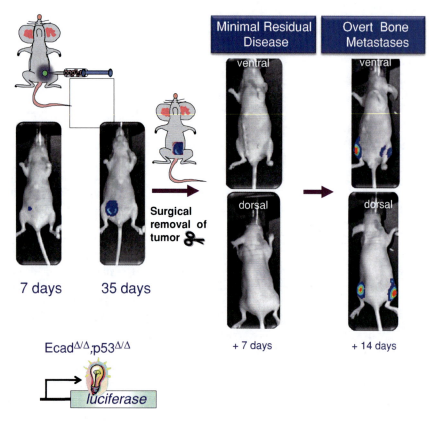

Fig. 4 a Orthotopically implanted invasive lobular breast carcinoma cells (KEP cells expressing firefly luciferase) grow readily in the mammary glands of immunodeficient mice, as detected by real-time imaging of bioluminescence. Bone metastases develop in a few weeks after surgical removal of the tumor from the mammary gland. KEP cells generate skeletal metastases with little/no lung involvement (Buijs et al. 2010). This contrasts the findings with murine 4T1 breast cancer cells that often regrow at the orthotopic site after surgical removal. Furthermore, 4T1 cells generate predominantly lung metastases, followed by bone metastases at later stage

A variety of small animal imaging technologies have been developed, such as microcomputed tomography (CT), micropositron emission tomography (PET), single photon emission computed tomography (SPECT), magnetic resonance imaging (MRI), ultrasound imaging and optical imaging, which encompass bioluminescence and fluorescence imaging (reviewed in Weissleder and Pittet 2008; Shah and Weissleder 2005; Henriquez et al. 2007 and Kaijzel et al. 2009) (Figs. 5, 6). Several imaging techniques have already been introduced in a preclinical and—occasionally—clinical setting to assess the presence, real-time growth, invasion, and metastasis of malignant tumor cells (Black et al. 2010; Buijs et al. 2007a; Kaijzel et al. 2007).

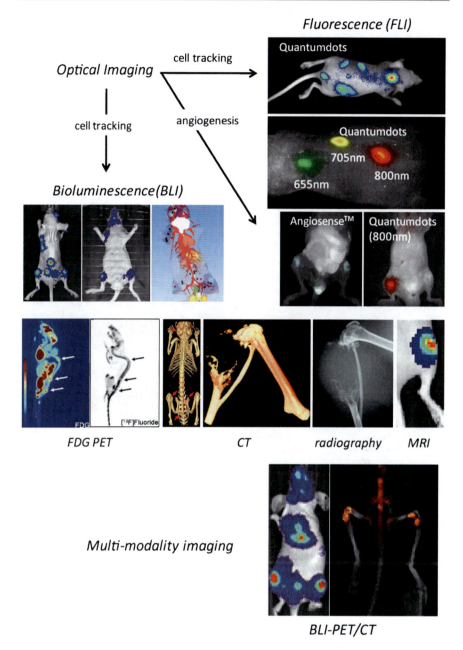

Fig. 5 Preclinical imaging modalities used for real-time imaging of skeletal metastasis and drug response. (Parts of this figure were reproduced with permission from Strube et al. 2010; Cowey et al. 2007; and Franzius et al. 2006)

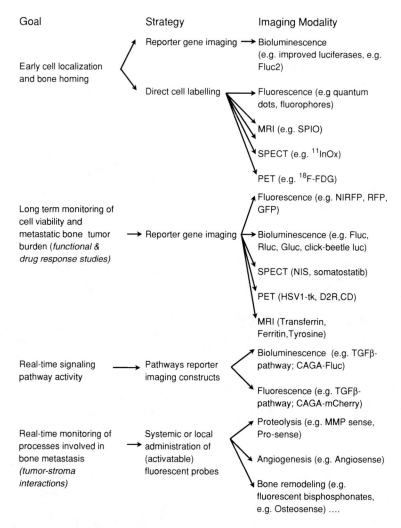

Fig. 6 Different imaging strategies for functional and drug response studies in preclinical bone metastasis models. *MRI* magnetic resonance imaging. *SPECT* single photon emission computed tomography. *PET* positron emission tomography. *NIRFP* near-infrared fluorescent protein. *RFP* red fluorescent protein. *GFP* green fluorescent protein. *Fluc* firefly luciferase *(Photonis pyralis)*. *Rluc Renilla reniformis* luciferase. *Gluc Gaussia* luciferase. *NIS* sodium iodine symporter. *HSV1-tk* herpes simplex virus type o thymidine kinase. *D2R* dopamine receptor type 2. *CD*:cytosine deaminase (adapted from Rodriguez-Porcel et al. 2009)

The ideal imaging modality is one that is quantitative, has superior spatial resolution and cell detection sensitivity, and can be used to longitudinally image cells in whole living organisms in real-time over a longer time period. Certain imaging approaches are better suited for specific applications than others (Fig. 6, Table 1). For example, CT and MRI provide a high degree of spatial resolution

Table 1 Comparison of the spatial resolution and cell detection sensitivity of the different imaging modalities on a semi-quantitative scale ranging from + to ++++ (from least to best)

Monitoring strategy	Spatial resolution	Cell detection sensitivity
Direct labeling		
Fluorescence (FMT,FRI)	++	+++
PET/SPECT	+++	+++
MRI	++++	+++
Indirect labeling (reporter constructs)		
Optical—FLI	++	+++
Optical—BLI	++	++++
PET	+++	+++
SPECT	+++	+++
MRI	++++	Unknown

FLI Fluorescence imaging. *BLI* Bioluminescence imaging. *MRI* magnetic resonance imaging. *SPECT* single photon emission computed tomography. *PET* positron emission tomography (adapted from Rodriguez-Porcel et al. 2009

that is good for showing details on anatomic structures, whereas highly sensitive methods such as PET and optical imaging are preferable for monitoring tumor cell biology as well as tumor burden, progression, and metastasis (Megason and Fraser 2007; Tsien 2003).

Noninvasive whole body optical imaging permits longitudinal and quantitative real-time gene expression, cellular localization, and drug response studies in small laboratory animals through the use of direct-targeting probes and reporter systems.

6.1 Bioluminescent Imaging

Bioluminescent imaging (BLI) is most commonly used for tracking cancer cells and studying their distribution and activity in vivo, because it is easy to use, cost-effective, and very sensitive (reviewed in O'Neill et al. 2010). BLI is ideally suited to image fundamental biological processes in vivo due to the high signal-to-noise ratio, low background, and short acquisition time.

Bioluminescence is based on the detection of photons emitted by the enzymatic reaction in which a substrate (either D-luciferin or coelenterazin) is oxidized by a luciferase. Several different luciferases exist including firefly luciferase, click beetle luciferase, *Gaussia* luciferase and *Renilla* luciferase (Henriquez et al. 2007; Kaijzel et al. 2007; Snoeks et al. 2011). Firefly luciferase (FFLuc), derived from the firefly *Photinus pyralis*, which catalyzes the substrate luciferin, is the most extensively used luciferase in cell-based bioluminescent imaging (Buijs et al. 2007a; van den Hoogen et al. 2010; Nakatsu et al. 2006; Contag et al. 1998; Rehemtulla et al. 2000). The enzymatic reaction driven by FFluc requires both

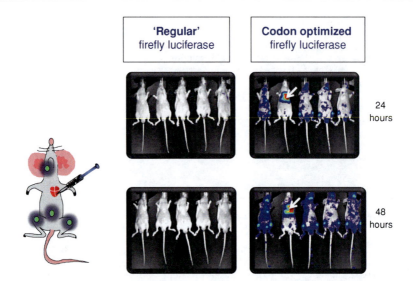

Fig. 7 Real-time imaging of skeletal metastasis after intracardiac inoculation of human prostate cancer cells, PC-3MPro4, which stably express firefly luciferase (luc) or a codon-optimized luciferase 2™ (Promega). The codon-optimized luc2 reporter construct allows superior, sensitive, real-time cancer cell tracking, bone colonization, and growth (van der Horst, manuscript in preparation). Clusters of 20–50 cells in bone can now be detected reproducibly, thus allowing the study of early steps in bone colonization and initial growth (functional and drug response studies). Furthermore, technical inoculation failures of PC-3MPro4luc2 can be visualized immediately (see *arrows*). These animals can be readily removed from the experiment leading to more reliable results

oxygen and ATP. In contrast, *Renilla* luciferase (RLuc), derived from the anthozoan sea pansy *Renilla reniformis*, catalyzes coelenterazin, a substrate distinct from luciferase and acts in an ATP-independent manner (Bhaumik and Gambhir 2002). Bioluminescent imaging of RLuc is compromised by low signal intensity, impairing imaging of cells in deeper tissues and thereby restricting imaging (Henriquez et al. 2007). The humanized Gaussia luciferase (GLuc), derived from the marine copepod *Gaussia princeps*, likewise uses coelenterazin as a substrate and does not require ATP but emits a markedly more intense signal and may therefore overcome the limitations associated with RLuc (Tannous et al. 2005). The native GLuc is secreted, allowing monitoring of tumor progression and treatment response of systemic metastases by biochemical analysis of a blood sample (Santos et al. 2009).

Especially the use of the new generation of FFLuc (the mammalian codon-optimized FFLuc2) enables extremely sensitive imaging and is very useful for monitoring cell tracking and survival in small animals (Kim et al. 2010; van der Horst et al. 2011a; Caysa et al. 2009) (Fig. 7). However, BLI provides mainly planar imaging with limited depth information and signal localization, and changes in depth of the signal can be confused with changes in cell survival. In addition,

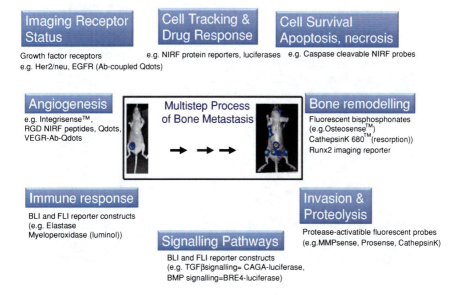

Fig. 8 Molecular imaging greatly facilitates real-time assessment of complex processes involved in the pathogenesis of skeletal metastasis

the technique is restricted to small animals and is very superficial in larger objects. However, recent developments show that BLI tomography may be able to provide 3D quantitative source information in the future (Zhang et al. 2008; Virostko and Jansen 2009).

6.2 Fluorescent Imaging

Other markers for live-cell imaging are fluorescent proteins or fluorochromes targeted to specific cell compartments or molecules. Fluorescent imaging is based on the detection of emitted light subsequent to their excitation by light of a specific wavelength (Figs. 5, 8, 9a). Fluorescent imaging can be divided into Fluorescent reflectance Imaging (FRI) and Fluorescence Molecular Tomography (FMT), the latter being able to provide 3D information (Graves et al. 2004). Some fluorescent probes can be cytotoxic (e.g., Green Fluorescent Protein, GFP), but the most recent fluorescent proteins are well tolerated by cancer cells (Tsien 2003; Schroeder 2008; Rothbauer et al. 2006; Shaner et al. 2005).

For deeper imaging of small animals, the fluorescent proteins optimally need to be in the far red or near-infrared (NIR), because then autofluorescence of the tissue is less prominent and tissue penetration is improved (Figs. 5, 9) (reviewed in Hilderbrand and Weissleder 2010). It has been shown that the red fluorescent protein DsRed-2 can be used to noninvasively follow cancer metastasis in

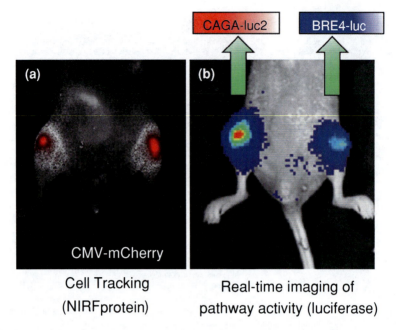

Fig. 9 Multi-modality imaging of MDA-MB-231 breast cancer cells in mouse long bones. MDA-MB-231 cells constitituvely express the fluorescent near-infrared protein mCherry for cell tracking (estimation of tumor burden, *left panel*). Simultaneous, stable expression of CAGA-luciferase and BRE-luciferase reporter construct allows real-time imaging of BMP and TGFβ pathway activity in bone metastases (*right panel*)

real-time in nude mice and transgenic GFP nude mice (Katz et al. 2003; Yang et al. 2003). Mutations in DsRed2 resulted in a series of the Living colors fruit fluorescent proteins including the red or far red proteins mCherry, mPlum and tdTomato (Shaner et al.2004, 2005).

Another far-red fluorescent protein is Katushka or mKate, bright fluorescent proteins which have high pH stability and photostability and demonstrate no toxic effects in cells (Shcherbo et al. 2007). The use of fluorescent proteins for imaging cancer dynamics in vivo at the tumor and cellular level has been reviewed by Hoffman (2009), describing for example the use of fluorescent proteins to differentially label cancer cells in the nucleus and cytoplasm to visualize the nuclear-cytoplasmic dynamics of cancer cell trafficking in both blood vessels and lymphatic vessels in small animals. In addition, to visualize tumo–stroma interactions, eNOS-GFP transgenic mice can be used. These mice possess green blood vessels; near-infrared labeled cancer cells can be inoculated in these mice and visualized by intravital microscopy (van Haperen et al. 2003).

Quantum dots (QDs) are highly fluorescent particles that can be manipulated to emit different wavelengths of light and provide brighter and more stable signals for molecular and cellular imaging (Jaiswal et al. 2003; Dubertret et al. 2002).

Nevertheless, QDs tend to aggregate in the cytoplasm, are difficult to deliver to the cells, and have nonspecific binding to multiple molecules (Fig. 5). Quantum dots and other fluorescent proteins can be coupled to antibodies and, for example, be used to monitor changes on the surface of living cells by the simultaneous detection of several cell surface markers (Jaiswal et al. 2003). However, these probes tend to have a relatively high background level due to unbound probe.

6.3 Multimodality Imaging

Taking into account that every imaging modality has its advantages and drawbacks, combining two or several imaging modalities may provide a better solution (multimodality imaging) (Fig. 5).

BLI only gives a 2D image and reveals little spatial information for cell tracking. In contrast, MRI and PET provide a higher spatial resolution and can be used in clinical imaging, but with a significantly lower detection threshold (Kraitchman et al. 2003; Hinds et al. 2003; Yaghoubi et al. 2009). For small animal imaging, several constructs have been developed. For example, a double-fusion of firefly luciferase (Fluc) and enhanced green fluorescence protein (eGFP) gene has been used in several studies, including molecular imaging of embryonic stem cells (Henriquez et al. 2007, Kaijzel et al. 2009; Snoeks et al. 2011; van der Bogt et al. 2006; Cao et al. 2007; Lee et al. 2009). Photons emitted by Fluc can be detected by sensitive CCD cameras and eGFP allows confirmation of in vivo imaging signals with traditional postmortem histology. Moreover, a triple fusion of FLuc, monomeric red fluorescent protein (mRFP), and herpes simplex virus truncated thymidine kinase (HSV-ttk) have been used by Cao et al. to monitor survival, proliferation, and migration of murine embryonic stem cells after intramyocardial transplantation (Cao et al. 2006). In this study, FLuc was used for its sensitive bioluminescent imaging, the mRFP fluorescent protein for FACS sorting and fluorescent imaging, and the HSVttk for deep tissue PET imaging with high anatomical details (Cao et al. 2006). Other multimodality studies used hybrid magnetic-fluorescent QD nanoparticles to detect tumors in mice by both MRI as well as fluorescent imaging allowing for enhanced resolution as well as anatomic information. In addition to MRI, optical imaging can also be combined with PET or CT imaging (reviewed in Hilderbrand and Weissleder 2010; McCarthy et al. 2010 and Snoeks et al. 2011).

A combination of several imaging modalities is also possible due to recent advances in data capturing and reconstruction. A combination of PET, μCT, and 3D FLI can be used to simultaneously image integrins (fluorochrome-derived RGD peptide targeting integrin (Integrisense near-infrared fluorescent probe)) in the tumor, cathepsin activity (Prosense fluorescent probe), as well as skeletal anatomical structure (PET-CT) (Nahrendorf et al. 2010).

6.4 Functional Imaging

As described above, several processes are important for the development of bone metastases, including primary tumor growth, angiogenesis, intravasation, survival in the bloodstream, extravasation, and colonization of the skeleton. In addition, for colonization of the skeleton, interactions of the tumor cells with the bone stroma are important (Figs. 1, 2). Imaging can not only be used to localize and follow the growth of the tumor cells, but also to visualize the expression and activity of specific molecules and biological processes that influence the behavior of the tumor cells (Figs. 8, 9).

Several probes have been developed to study different biological processes. For example, the skeleton can specifically be studied using bone specific probes (Fig. 8) including fluorescently labeled bisphosphonate Osteosense^{TM} (Perkin–Elmer) or the fluorescently labeled tetracycline derivative Bone Tag (LI-COR Biosciences) (Kozloff et al. 2007; Snoeks et al. 2011). These bone probes are incorporated into the bone at sites with high bone-turnover, which occurs during cancer-induced bone remodeling (van der Pluijm et al. 2005; Zaheer et al. 2001). Other interesting probes are the above described Prosense probe that can be used to visualize cathepsin K activity, which is highly present at osteolytic lesions and site of active bone resorption (Teitelbaum 2000; Drake et al. 1996; Kozloff et al. 2009). Prosense is one of the smart probes, a cleavable probe which provides information about the activity of an enzyme. The substrate of the enzymes is coupled to a fluorophore, which is quenched due to the structure and location of the fluorophore. Upon cleavage by the enzyme, the fluorophore is released and can be detected (Fig. 8).

Other smart probes were designed to visualize the matrix degradation process, which is an important process for cancer cell motility and invasiveness, such as MMPsense (Perkin-Elmer) that is activated by the matrix metalloproteases MMP2 and MMP9 (Bremer et al. 2001).

Moreover, several probes have been developed targeting $\alpha_v\beta_3$ integrin, such as Integrisense (reviewed in Snoeks et al. 2010). It has been shown that $\alpha_v\beta_3$ integrin enables tumor growth in bone (McCabe et al. 2007). In addition, α_v-integrins play a pivotal role in the supportive stroma in bone metastasis, particularly in tumor-induced osteoclastic bone resorption and angiogenesis (van der Horst et al. 2011b; Nakamura et al. 2007; Hynes 2007; Nicholson and Theodorescu 2004).

Reporter genes consist of gene regulatory elements (promoters and enhancers) that drive the expression of various luciferases or fluorescent proteins that can be used to provide functional information about gene or pathway activity (Figs. 8, 9).

For example, the transforming growth factor β (TGFβ) signaling pathway in bone metastases has been studied, sequentially over time in the same animal (Serganova et al. 2009). This simultaneous and sequential imaging of metastases in the same animals provided insight into the location and progression of metastases, and the timing and course of TGFβ signaling. In addition to the TGFβ pathway,

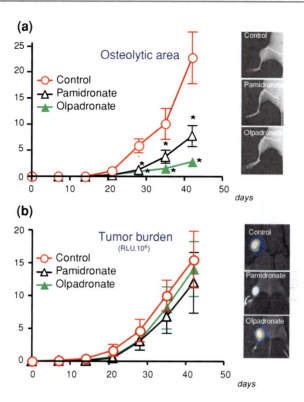

Fig. 10 Development of osteolytic lesions by MDA-MB-231 cells growing in mouse tibia. Quantifying osteolysis by radiography does not necessary correlate with tumor burden (panels A and B respectively). While bisphosphonates display strong bone-sparing effects in various in vivo models (intra-bone growth of MDA-MB-231 cells expressing luciferase, panel A) intra-bone growth of cancer cells was not significantly affected (measured by bioluminescence, panel B). Because imaging of tumor cells by bioluminescence requires ATP (and oxygen) only viable cancer cells will generate photons, thus allowing rapid assessment of drug responses (adapted from Van Der Pluijm et al. 2005)

preliminary data show that the BMP signaling pathway can be measured likewise to investigate this pathway in vivo (Fig. 9).

In addition to imaging of growth factor signaling pathways, imaging can also be used to visualize other processes important for tumor growth and metastasis such as angiogenesis. For example, a vascular endothelial growth factor receptor-2 (VEGFR2) luciferase transgenic mouse model was developed which displays VEGFR2 activity. When bound to VEGF (a pro-angiogenic ligand), VEGFR2 induces angiogenesis by stimulating vascular endothelial cell growth (Zhang et al. 2004).

7 Future Perspectives

Better understanding of the processes involved in skeletal metastasis and the development of new therapies requires noninvasive high-resolution in vivo imaging. Ideal preclinical models of bone metastasis mimic the genetic and phenotypic changes that occur in human cancers, including all the steps in the metastatic cascade. In addition, such models are reproducible and progress rapidly to enable cost-effective investigations. Finally, the ideal model should be able to predict human response to therapy.

In this chapter, several preclinical models of bone metastasis have been discussed with their advantages, limitations, and pitfalls (Fig. 10). Transplantation models (either xenograft or syngeneic), and especially the humanized models, will continue to be indispensable to investigate the pathogenesis of bone metastasis in vivo as well as to conduct preclinical studies on chemotherapeutics and new therapeutics. Given the complexity of bone metastasis, many genes are expected to be involved in the pathogenesis and few are likely to be indispensable. Transgenic models of several target genes continue to be refined and eventually will mirror human disease more closely enabling the identification of key targets for therapeutic intervention. In addition to the tumor, the tumor-associated stroma plays a pivotal role in the process of bone metastasis, and studying the role of the stroma will definitely identify key targets for therapeutic intervention.

Further refinements of the preclinical models also include the refinement of the imaging techniques used to monitor the preclinical models. Small animal optical imaging is a cost-effective and attractive tool to study the multi-step process of bone metastasis. Near-infrared emitting molecular imaging agents have recently been introduced to in vivo bone metastasis models.

In particular, the combination of optical imaging agents and techniques with anatomical data from other imaging modalities (e.g., CT or MRI) will certainly aid in the understanding of the pathological process of bone metastasis. These innovations will improve drug development and eventually also clinical application, by supporting the diagnostic process, the detection of minimal residual disease, and by enabling image-guided surgery.

Acknowledgments The authors wish to thank Mr. Henry Cheung (Leiden Univ. Med. Ctr., dept. Urology, Leiden, the Netherlands) and Mr. Ivo Que (Leiden Univ. Med. Ctr., Dept. Endocrinology, Leiden, the Netherlands) for real-time optical imaging of osteotropic cancer cells in vivo.

References

Albini A, Sporn MB (2007) The tumour microenvironment as a target for chemoprevention. Nat Rev Cancer 7:139–147

An Z, Wang X, Geller J, Moossa AR, Hoffman RM (1998) Surgical orthotopic implantation allows high lung and lymph node metastatic expression of human prostate carcinoma cell line PC-3 in nude mice. Prostate 34:169–174

Arguello F, Baggs RB, Frantz CN (1988) A murine model of experimental metastasis to bone and bone marrow. Cancer Res 48:6876–6881

Asamoto M, Hokaiwado N, Cho YM, Takahashi S, Ikeda Y, Imaida K et al (2001) Prostate carcinomas developing in transgenic rats with SV40 T antigen expression under probasin promoter control are strictly androgen dependent. Cancer Res 61:4693–4700

Bhaumik S, Gambhir SS (2002) Optical imaging of Renilla luciferase reporter gene expression in living mice. Proc Natl Acad Sci USA 99:377–382

Bhowmick NA, Moses HL (2005) Tumor-stroma interactions. Curr Opin Genet Dev 15:97–101

Black PC, Shetty A, Brown GA, Esparza-Coss E, Metwalli AR, Agarwal PK et al (2010) Validating bladder cancer xenograft bioluminescence with magnetic resonance imaging: the significance of hypoxia and necrosis. BJU Int 106:1799–1804

Blakely CM, Sintasath L, D'Cruz CM, Hahn KT, Dugan KD, Belka GK et al (2005) Developmental stage determines the effects of MYC in the mammary epithelium. Development 132:1147–1160

Bremer C, Tung CH, Weissleder R (2001) In vivo molecular target assessment of matrix metalloproteinase inhibition. Nat Med 7:743–748

Brown RL, Reinke LM, Damerow MS, Perez D, Chodosh LA, Yang J et al (2011) CD44 splice isoform switching in human and mouse epithelium is essential for epithelial-mesenchymal transition and breast cancer progression. J Clin Invest 121:1064–1074

Buijs JT, van der Pluijm G (2009) Osteotropic cancers: from primary tumor to bone. Cancer Lett 273:177–193

Buijs JT, Rentsch CA, van der Horst G, van Overveld PG, Wetterwald A, Schwaninger R et al (2007a) BMP7, a putative regulator of epithelial homeostasis in the human prostate, is a potent inhibitor of prostate cancer bone metastasis in vivo. Am J Pathol 171:1047–1057

Buijs JT, Henriquez NV, van Overveld PG, van der Horst G, Que I, Schwaninger R et al (2007b) Bone morphogenetic protein 7 in the development and treatment of bone metastases from breast cancer. Cancer Res 67:8742–8751

Buijs JT, Cheung H, Doumont G, Derksen PW, Jonkers J, van der Pluijm G (2010) A new mouse model of invasive lobular carcinoma of the breast representative of the multi-step process of bone metastasis and minimal residual disease micrometastasis. Bone 47:S282

Cao F, Lin S, Xie X, Ray P, Patel M, Zhang X et al (2006) In vivo visualization of embryonic stem cell survival, proliferation, and migration after cardiac delivery. Circulation 113:1005–1014

Cao F, Drukker M, Lin S, Sheikh AY, Xie X, Li Z et al (2007) Molecular imaging of embryonic stem cell misbehavior and suicide gene ablation. Cloning Stem Cells 9:107–117

Caysa H, Jacob R, Muther N, Branchini B, Messerle M, Soling A (2009) A redshifted codon-optimized firefly luciferase is a sensitive reporter for bioluminescence imaging. Photochem Photobiol Sci 8:52–56

Chen Z, Trotman LC, Shaffer D, Lin HK, Dotan ZA, Niki M et al (2005) Crucial role of p53-dependent cellular senescence in suppression of Pten-deficient tumorigenesis. Nature 436:725–730

Coleman RE (1997) Skeletal complications of malignancy. Cancer 80:1588–1594

Contag PR, Olomu IN, Stevenson DK, Contag CH (1998) Bioluminescent indicators in living mammals. Nat Med 4:245–247

Cowey S, Szafran AA, Kappes J, Zinn KR, Siegal GP, Desmond RA et al (2007) Breast cancer metastasis to bone: evaluation of bioluminescent imaging and microSPECT/CT for detecting bone metastasis in immunodeficient mice. Clin Exp Metastasis 24(5):389–401

D'Cruz CM, Gunther EJ, Boxer RB, Hartman JL, Sintasath L, Moody SE et al (2001) c-MYC induces mammary tumorigenesis by means of a preferred pathway involving spontaneous Kras2 mutations. Nat Med 7:235–239

Derksen PW, Liu X, Saridin F, van der Gulden H, Zevenhoven J, Evers B, van Beijnum JR, Griffioen AW, Vink J, Krimpenfort P, Peterse JL, Cardiff RD, Berns A, Jonkers J (2006) Somatic inactivation of E-cadherin and p53 in mice leads to metastatic lobular mammary carcinoma through induction of anoikis resistance and angiogenesis. Cancer Cell 105:437–449

Derksen PW, Braumuller TM, van der Burg E, Hornsveld M, Mesman E, Wesseling J et al (2011) Mammary-specific inactivation of E-cadherin and p53 impairs functional gland development and leads to pleomorphic invasive lobular carcinoma in mice. Dis Model Mech 4:347–358

Drake FH, Dodds RA, James IE, Connor JR, Debouck C, Richardson S et al (1996) Cathepsin K, but not cathepsins B, L, or S, is abundantly expressed in human osteoclasts. J Biol Chem 271:12511–12516

Dubertret B, Skourides P, Norris DJ, Noireaux V, Brivanlou AH, Libchaber A (2002) In vivo imaging of quantum dots encapsulated in phospholipid micelles. Science 298:1759–1762

Franzius C, Hotfilder M, Poremba C, Hermann S, Schäfers K, Gabbert HE, Jürgens H, Schober O, Schäfers M, Vormoor J (2006) Successful high-resolution animal positron emission tomography of human Ewing tumours and their metastases in a murine xenograft model. Eur J Nucl Med Mol Imaging 33(12):1432–1441

Frese KK, Tuveson DA (2007) Maximizing mouse cancer models. Nat Rev Cancer 7:645–658

Friedl P, Gilmour D (2009) Collective cell migration in morphogenesis, regeneration and cancer. Nat Rev Mol Cell Biol 10:445–457

Futakuchi M, Nannuru KC, Varney ML, Sadanandam A, Nakao K, Asai K et al (2009) Transforming growth factor-beta signaling at the tumor-bone interface promotes mammary tumor growth and osteoclast activation. Cancer Sci 100:71–81

Gao H, Ouyang X, Banach-Petrosky W, Borowsky AD, Lin Y, Kim M et al (2004) A critical role for p27kip1 gene dosage in a mouse model of prostate carcinogenesis. Proc Natl Acad Sci USA 101:17204–17209

Gingrich JR, Greenberg NM (1996) A transgenic mouse prostate cancer model. Toxicol Pathol 24:502–504

Graves EE, Weissleder R, Ntziachristos V (2004) Fluorescence molecular imaging of small animal tumor models. Curr Mol Med 4:419–430

Gunther EJ, Belka GK, Wertheim GB, Wang J, Hartman JL, Boxer RB et al (2002) A novel doxycycline-inducible system for the transgenic analysis of mammary gland biology. FASEB J 16:283–292

Henriquez NV, van Overveld PG, Que I, Buijs JT, Bachelier R, Kaijzel EL et al (2007) Advances in optical imaging and novel model systems for cancer metastasis research. Clin Exp Metastasis 24:699–705

Hilderbrand SA, Weissleder R (2010) Near-infrared fluorescence: application to in vivo molecular imaging. Curr Opin Chem Biol 14:71–79

Hinds KA, Hill JM, Shapiro EM, Laukkanen MO, Silva AC, Combs CA et al (2003) Highly efficient endosomal labeling of progenitor and stem cells with large magnetic particles allows magnetic resonance imaging of single cells. Blood 102:867–872

Hirbe AC, Roelofs AJ, Floyd DH, Deng H, Becker SN, Lanigan LG et al (2009) The bisphosphonate zoledronic acid decreases tumor growth in bone in mice with defective osteoclasts. Bone 44(5):908–916

Hoffman RM (2009) Imaging cancer dynamics in vivo at the tumor and cellular level with fluorescent proteins. Clin Exp Metastasis 26:345–355

Hynes RO (2007) Cell-matrix adhesion in vascular development. J Thromb Haemost 5(suppl 1):32–40

Ip C (1996) Mammary tumorigenesis and chemoprevention studies in carcinogen-treated rats. J Mammary Gland Biol Neoplasia 1:37–47

Izbicka E, Dunstan CR, Horn D, Harris M, Harris S, Adams R, Mundy GR (1997) Effects of human tumor cell lines on local new bone formation in vivo. Calcif Tissue Int 602:210–215

Jaiswal JK, Mattoussi H, Mauro JM, Simon SM (2003) Long-term multiple color imaging of live cells using quantum dot bioconjugates. Nat Biotechnol 21:47–51

Jonkers J, Meuwissen R, van der Gulden H, Peterse H, van der Valk M, Berns A (2001) Synergistic tumor suppressor activity of BRCA2 and p53 in a conditional mouse model for breast cancer. Nat Genet 29:418–425

Kalluri R (2009) EMT: when epithelial cells decide to become mesenchymal-like cells. J Clin Invest 119:1417–1419

Kalluri R, Weinberg RA (2009) The basics of epithelial-mesenchymal transition. J Clin Invest 119:1420–1428

Kaijzel EL, van der Pluijm G, Lowik CW (2007) Whole-body optical imaging in animal models to assess cancer development and progression. Clin Cancer Res 13:3490–3497

Kaijzel EL, Snoeks TJ, Buijs JT, van der Pluijm G, Lowik CW (2009) Multimodal imaging and treatment of bone metastasis. Clin Exp Metastasis 26:371–379

Katz MH, Takimoto S, Spivack D, Moossa AR, Hoffman RM, Bouvet M (2003) A novel red fluorescent protein orthotopic pancreatic cancer model for the preclinical evaluation of chemotherapeutics. J Surg Res 113:151–160

Keller ET, Brown J (2004) Prostate cancer bone metastases promote both osteolytic and osteoblastic activity. J Cell Biochem 91:718–729

Khanna C, Hunter K (2005) Modeling metastasis in vivo. Carcinogenesis 26:513–523

Kim MJ, Cardiff RD, Desai N, Banach-Petrosky WA, Parsons R, Shen MM et al (2002) Cooperativity of Nkx3.1 and Pten loss of function in a mouse model of prostate carcinogenesis. Proc Natl Acad Sci USA 99:2884–2889

Kim JB, Stein R, O'Hare MJ (2005) Tumour-stromal interactions in breast cancer: the role of stroma in tumourigenesis. Tumour Biol 26:173–185

Kim JB, Urban K, Cochran E, Lee S, Ang A, Rice B, et al (2010) Non-invasive detection of a small number of bioluminescent cancer cells in vivo. PLoS One 5:e9364

Kim J, Roh M, Doubinskaia I, Algarroba GN, Eltoum IE, Abdulkadir SA (2011) A mouse model of heterogeneous, c-MYC-initiated prostate cancer with loss of Pten and p53. Oncogene 20:1–11

Korenchuk S, Lehr JE, MClean L, Lee YG, Whitney S, Vessella R et al (2001) VCaP, a cell-based model system of human prostate cancer. In Vivo 15:163–168

Kozloff KM, Weissleder R, Mahmood U (2007) Noninvasive optical detection of bone mineral. J Bone Miner Res 22:1208–1216

Kozloff KM, Quinti L, Patntirapong S, Hauschka PV, Tung CH, Weissleder R et al (2009) Non-invasive optical detection of cathepsin K-mediated fluorescence reveals osteoclast activity in vitro and in vivo. Bone 44:190–198

Kraitchman DL, Heldman AW, Atalar E, Amado LC, Martin BJ, Pittenger MF et al (2003) In vivo magnetic resonance imaging of mesenchymal stem cells in myocardial infarction. Circulation 107:2290–2293

Kuperwasser C, Dessain S, Bierbaum BE, Garnet D, Sperandio K, Gauvin GP et al (2005) A mouse model of human breast cancer metastasis to human bone. Cancer Res 65:6130–6138

Lakso M, Sauer B, Mosinger B Jr, Lee EJ, Manning RW, Yu SH et al (1992) Targeted oncogene activation by site-specific recombination in transgenic mice. Proc Natl Acad Sci USA 89:6232–6236

Lee AS, Tang C, Cao F, Xie X, van der Bogt K, Hwang A et al (2009) Effects of cell number on teratoma formation by human embryonic stem cells. Cell Cycle 8:2608–2612

Lehr HA, Leunig M, Menger MD, Nolte D, Messmer K (1993) Dorsal skinfold chamber technique for intravital microscopy in nude mice. Am J Pathol 143:1055–1062

Lewandoski M (2001) Conditional control of gene expression in the mouse. Nat Rev Genet 2:743–755

Lynch CC, Hikosaka A, Acuff HB, Martin MD, Kawai N, Singh RK et al (2005) MMP-7 promotes prostate cancer-induced osteolysis via the solubilization of RANKL. Cancer Cell 7:485–496

Massoud TF, Gambhir SS (2003) Molecular imaging in living subjects: seeing fundamental biological processes in a new light. Genes Dev 17:545–580

McCabe NP, De S, Vasanji A, Brainard J, Byzova TV (2007) Prostate cancer specific integrin alphavbeta3 modulates bone metastatic growth and tissue remodeling. Oncogene 26:6238–6243

McCarthy JR, Bhaumik J, Karver MR, Sibel ES, Weissleder R (2010) Targeted nanoagents for the detection of cancers. Mol Oncol 4:511–528

Megason SG, Fraser SE (2007) Imaging in systems biology. Cell 130:784–795

Mueller MM, Fusenig NE (2004) Friends or foes—bipolar effects of the tumour stroma in cancer. Nat Rev Cancer 4:839–849

Mundy GR (2002) Metastasis to bone: causes, consequences and therapeutic opportunities. Nat Rev Cancer 2:584–593

Naef F, Huelsken J (2005) Cell-type-specific transcriptomics in chimeric models using transcriptome-based masks. Nucl Acids Res 19:e111

Nahrendorf M, Keliher E, Marinelli B, Waterman P, Feruglio PF, Fexon L et al (2010) Hybrid PET-optical imaging using targeted probes. Proc Natl Acad Sci USA 107:7910–7915

Nakai M, Mundy GR, Williams PJ, Boyce B, Yoneda T (1992) A synthetic antagonist to laminin inhibits the formation of osteolytic metastases by human melanoma cells in nude mice. Cancer Res 52(19):5395–5399

Nakamura I, Duong lT, Rodan SB, Rodan GA (2007) Involvement of alphav)beta3 integrins in osteoclast function. J Bone Miner Metab 25:337–344

Nakatsu T, Ichiyama S, Hiratake J, Saldanha A, Kobashi N, Sakata K et al (2006) Structural basis for the spectral difference in luciferase bioluminescence. Nature 440:372–376

Nannuru KC, Futakuchi M, Sadanandam A, Wilson TJ, Varney ML, Myers KJ et al (2009) Enhanced expression and shedding of receptor activator of NF-kappaB ligand during tumor-bone interaction potentiates mammary tumor-induced osteolysis. Clin Exp Metastasis 26:797–808

Nannuru KC, Futakuchi M, Varney ML, Vincent TM, Marcusson EG, Singh RK (2010) Matrix metalloproteinase MMP-13 regulates mammary tumor-induced osteolysis by activating MMP9 and transforming growth factor-beta signaling at the tumor-bone interface. Cancer Res 70:3494–3504

Nemeth JA, Harb JF, Barroso U Jr, He Z, Grignon DJ, Cher ML (1999) Severe combined immunodeficient-hu model of human prostate cancer metastasis to human bone. Cancer Res 59:1987–1993

Nicholson B, Theodorescu D (2004) Angiogenesis and prostate cancer tumor growth. J Cell Biochem 91:125–150

O'Neill K, Lyons SK, Gallagher WM, Curran KM, Byrne AT (2010) Bioluminescent imaging: a critical tool in pre-clinical oncology research. J Pathol 220:317–327

Paget S (1889) The distribution of secondary growths in cancer of the breast. 1889. Cancer Metastasis Rev 8:98–101

Peyruchaud O, Serre CM, NicAmhlaoibh R, Fournier P, Clezardin P (2003) Angiostatin inhibits bone metastasis formation in nude mice through a direct anti-osteoclastic activity. J Biol Chem 278:45826–45832

Pollard M (1998) Lobund-Wistar rat model of prostate cancer in man. Prostate 37:1–4

Pollard M, Wolter WR, Sun L (2000) Prostate-seminal vesicle cancers induced in noble rats. Prostate 43:71–74

Power CA, Pwint H, Chan J, Cho J, Yu Y, Walsh W et al (2009) A novel model of bone-metastatic prostate cancer in immunocompetent mice. Prostate 69:1613–1623

Pulaski BA, Ostrand-Rosenberg S (2001) Mouse 4T1 breast tumor model. Curr Protoc Immunol Chap. 20:Unit 20.2

Reeves K, van der Pluijm G, Cecchini MG, Eaton CL, Hamdy FC, Brown ND (2010) A new in vivo model of prostate cancer metastasis to bone. Bone. 47:S282

Rehemtulla A, Stegman LD, Cardozo SJ, Gupta S, Hall DE, Contag CH et al (2000) Rapid and quantitative assessment of cancer treatment response using in vivo bioluminescence imaging. Neoplasia 2:491–495

Rodriguez-Porcel M, Wu, JC, Gambhir, SS (2009) Molecular imaging of stem cells (July 30, 2009). Stembook (ed) The stem cell research community, stembook. doi:10.3824/stembook. 1.49.1, http://www.stembook.org

Roodman GD (2004) Mechanisms of bone metastasis. N Engl J Med 350:1655–1664

Rosol TJ, Tannehill-Gregg SH, Corn S, Schneider A, McCauley LK (2004) Animal models of bone metastasis. Cancer Treat Res 18:47–81

Rothbauer U, Zolghadr K, Tillib S, Nowak D, Schermelleh L, Gahl A et al (2006) Targeting and tracing antigens in live cells with fluorescent nanobodies. Nat Methods 3:887–889

Santos EB, Yeh R, Lee J, Nikhamin Y, Punzalan B, Punzalan B et al (2009) Sensitive in vivo imaging of T cells using a membrane-bound Gaussia princeps luciferase. Nat Med 15:338–344

Sarkisian CJ, Keister BA, Stairs DB, Boxer RB, Moody SE, Chodosh LA (2007) Dose-dependent oncogene-induced senescence in vivo and its evasion during mammary tumorigenesis. Nat Cell Biol 9:493–505

Schroeder T (2008) Imaging stem-cell-driven regeneration in mammals. Nature 453:345–351

Sckell A, Leunig M (2009) The dorsal skinfold chamber: studying angiogenesis by intravital microscopy. Methods Mol Biol 467:305–317

Schwaninger R, Rentsch CA, Wetterwald A, van der Horst G, van Bezooijen RL, van der Pluijm G et al (2007) Lack of noggin expression by cancer cells is a determinant of the osteoblast response in bone metastases. Am J Pathol 170:160–175

Serganova I, Moroz E, Vider J, Gogiberidze G, Moroz M, Pillarsetty N et al (2009) Multimodality imaging of TGFbeta signaling in breast cancer metastases. FASEB J 23: 2662–2672

Shah K, Weissleder R (2005) Molecular optical imaging: applications leading to the development of present day therapeutics. NeuroRx 2:215–225

Shaner NC, Campbell RE, Steinbach PA, Giepmans BN, Palmer AE, Tsien RY (2004) Improved monomeric red, orange and yellow fluorescent proteins derived from Discosoma sp red fluorescent protein. Nat Biotechnol 22:1567–1572

Shaner NC, Steinbach PA, Tsien RY (2005) A guide to choosing fluorescent proteins. Nat Methods 2:905–909

Shcherbo D, Merzlyak EM, Chepurnykh TV, Fradkov AF, Ermakova GV, Solovieva EA et al (2007) Bright far-red fluorescent protein for whole-body imaging. Nat Methods 4:741–746

Shen Q, Brown PH (2005) Transgenic mouse models for the prevention of breast cancer. Mutat Res 576:93–110

Shtivelman E, Namikawa R (1995) Species-specific metastasis of human tumor cells in the severe combined immunodeficiency mouse engrafted with human tissue. Proc Natl Acad Sci USA 92:4661–4665

Singh M, Johnson L (2006) Using genetically engineered mouse models of cancer to aid drug development: an industry perspective. Clin Cancer Res 12:5312–5328

Snoeks TJ, Lowik CW, Kaijzel EL (2010) 'In vivo' optical approaches to angiogenesis imaging. Angiogenesis 13:135–147

Snoeks TJ, Khmelinskii A, Lelieveldt BP, Kaijzel EL, Lowik CW (2011) Optical advances in skeletal imaging applied to bone metastases. Bone 48:106–114

Stoica G, Koestner A, Capen CC (1983) Characterization of N-ethyl-N-nitrosourea–induced mammary tumors in the rat. Am J Pathol 110:161–169

Stoica G, Koestner A, Capen CC (1984) Neoplasms induced with high single doses of N-ethyl-N-nitrosourea in 30-day-old Sprague-Dawley rats, with special emphasis on mammary neoplasia. Anticancer Res 4:5–12

Strube A, Stepina E, Mumberg D, Scholz A, Hauff P, Käkönen SM (2010) Characterization of a new renal cell carcinoma bone metastasis mouse model. Clin Exp Metastasis 27(5):319–330

Tannous BA, Kim DE, Fernandez JL, Weissleder R, Breakefield XO (2005) Codon-optimized Gaussia luciferase cDNA for mammalian gene expression in culture and in vivo. Mol Ther 11:435–443

Tao K, Fang M, Alroy J, Sahagian GG (2008) Imagable 4T1 model for the study of late stage breast cancer. BMC Cancer 8:228

Teitelbaum SL (2000) Bone resorption by osteoclasts. Science 289:1504–1508

Thalmann GN, Sikes RA, Wu TT, Degeorges A, Chang SM, Ozen M et al (2000) LNCaP progression model of human prostate cancer: androgen-independence and osseous metastasis. Prostate 44:91–103

Thiery JP, Acloque H, Huang RY, Nieto MA (2009) Epithelial-mesenchymal transitions in development and disease. Cell 139:871–890

Tsien RY (2003) Imagining imaging's future. Nat Rev Mol Cell Biol Suppl:SS16–SS21

Tu WH, Thomas TZ, Masumori N, Bhowmick NA, Gorska AE, Shyr Y et al (2003) The loss of TGF-beta signaling promotes prostate cancer metastasis. Neoplasia 5:267–277

van der Bogt KE, Swijnenburg RJ, Cao F, Wu JC (2006) Molecular imaging of human embryonic stem cells: keeping an eye on differentiation, tumorigenicity and immunogenicity. Cell Cycle 5:2748–2752

van Haperen R, Cheng C, Mees BM, van DE, de Waard M, van Damme LC et al (2003) Functional expression of endothelial nitric oxide synthase fused to green fluorescent protein in transgenic mice. Am J Pathol 163:1677–1686

van den Hoogen C, van der Horst G, Cheung H, Buijs JT, Lippitt JM, Guzman-Ramirez N et al (2010) High aldehyde dehydrogenase activity identifies tumor-initiating and metastasis-initiating cells in human prostate cancer. Cancer Res 70:5163–5173

van der Horst G, van Asten JJ, Figdor A, van den Hoogen C, Cheung H, Bevers RF et al (2011a) Real-time cancer cell tracking by bioluminescence in a preclinical model of human bladder cancer growth and metastasis. Eur Urol 60:337–343

van der Horst G, van den Hoogen C, Buijs JT, Cheung H, Bloys H, Pelger RC et al (2011b) Targeting of alphav)-integrins in stem/progenitor cells and supportive microenvironment impairs bone metastasis in human prostate cancer. Neoplasia 13:516–525

van der Pluijm G (2010) Epithelial plasticity, cancer stem cells and bone metastasis formation. Bone 48:37–43

van der Pluijm G, Sijmons B, Vloedgraven H, Deckers M, Papapoulos S, Lowik C (2001) Monitoring metastatic behavior of human tumor cells in mice with species-specific polymerase chain reaction: elevated expression of angiogenesis and bone resorption stimulators by breast cancer in bone metastases. J Bone Miner Res 16:1077–1091

van der Pluijm G, Que I, Sijmons B, Buijs JT, Lowik CW, Wetterwald A et al (2005) Interference with the microenvironmental support impairs the de novo formation of bone metastases in vivo. Cancer Res 65:7682–7690

Virostko J, Jansen ED (2009) Validation of bioluminescent imaging techniques. Methods Mol Biol 574:15–23

Visvader JE (2011) Cells of origin in cancer. Nature 20:314–322

Wang S, Gao J, Lei Q, Rozengurt N, Pritchard C, Jiao J et al (2003) Prostate-specific deletion of the murine Pten tumor suppressor gene leads to metastatic prostate cancer. Cancer Cell 4: 209–221

Wang J, Xia TS, Liu XA, Ding Q, Du Q, Yin H et al (2010) A novel orthotopic and metastatic mouse model of breast cancer in human mammary microenvironment. Breast Cancer Res Treat 120:337–344

Weissleder R, Pittet MJ (2008) Imaging in the era of molecular oncology. Nature 452:580–589

Wetterwald A, van der Pluijm G, Que I, Sijmons B, Buijs J, Karperien M et al (2002) Optical imaging of cancer metastasis to bone marrow: a mouse model of minimal residual disease. Am J Pathol 160(3):1143–1153

Winter SF, Cooper AB, Greenberg NM (2003) Models of metastatic prostate cancer: a transgenic perspective. Prostate Cancer Prostatic Dis 6:204–211

Xia TS, Wang J, Yin H, Ding Q, Zhang YF, Yang HW et al (2010) Human tissue-specific microenvironment: an essential requirement for mouse models of breast cancer. Oncol Rep 24:203–211

Xia TS, Wang GZ, Ding Q, Liu XA, Zhou WB, Zhang YF et al (2011) Bone metastasis in a novel breast cancer mouse model containing human breast and human bone. Breast Cancer Res Treat. 3 Jan 2011 [Epub ahead of print]

Xu X, Weaver Z, Linke SP, Li C, Gotay J, Wang XW et al (1999) Centrosome amplification and a defective G2-M cell cycle checkpoint induce genetic instability in BRCA1 exon 11 isoform-deficient cells. Mol Cell 3:389–395

Yaghoubi SS, Jensen MC, Satyamurthy N, Budhiraja S, Paik D, Czernin J et al (2009) Noninvasive detection of therapeutic cytolytic T cells with 18F-FHBG PET in a patient with glioma. Nat Clin Pract Oncol 6:53–58

Yang M, Li L, Jiang P, Moossa AR, Penman S, Hoffman RM (2003) Dual-color fluorescence imaging distinguishes tumor cells from induced host angiogenic vessels and stromal cells. Proc Natl Acad Sci USA 100:14259–14262

Yonou H, Yokose T, Kamijo T, Kanomata N, Hasebe T, Nagai K et al (2001) Establishment of a novel species- and tissue-specific metastasis model of human prostate cancer in humanized non-obese diabetic/severe combined immunodeficient mice engrafted with human adult lung and bone. Cancer Res 61:2177–2182

Zaheer A, Lenkinski RE, Mahmood A, Jones AG, Cantley LC, Frangioni JV (2001) In vivo near-infrared fluorescence imaging of osteoblastic activity. Nat Biotechnol 19:1148–1154

Zhang N, Fang Z, Contag PR, Purchio AF, West DB (2004) Tracking angiogenesis induced by skin wounding and contact hypersensitivity using a Vegfr2-luciferase transgenic mouse. Blood 103:617–626

Zhang Q, Yin L, Tan Y, Yuan Z, Jiang H (2008) Quantitative bioluminescence tomography guided by diffuse optical tomography. Opt Express 16:1481–1486

Zhou Z, Flesken-Nikitin A, Corney DC, Wang W, Goodrich DW, Roy-Burman P et al (2006) Synergy of p53 and Rb deficiency in a conditional mouse model for metastatic prostate cancer. Cancer Res 66:7889–7898

The Role of Bone Microenvironment, Vitamin D and Calcium

Daniele Santini, Francesco Pantano, Bruno Vincenzi,
Giuseppe Tonini and Francesco Bertoldo

Abstract
Starting first from Paget's "seed and soil" to the latest hypothesis about metastatic process involving the concept of a premetastatic niche, a large amount of data suggested the idea that metastatization is a multistep coordinated process with a high degree of efficiency. A specific subpopulation of cells with tumor-initiating and migratory capacity can selectively migrate toward sites that are able to promote survival, and/or proliferation of metastatic tumor cells through a microenvironment modification. Bone plays a pivotal role in this process, acting not only as a preferential site for cancer cells' homing and proliferation, due to a complex interplay between different cellular phenotypes such as osteoblasts and osteoclasts, but also as a source of bone marrow precursors that are able to facilitate the metastatic process in extraskeletal disease. Moreover, bone microenvironment has the unique capacity to retain cancer stem cells in a quiescent status, acting as a reservoir that is able to cause a metastatic spread also many years after the resection of the primary tumor. To add a further level of complexity, these mechanisms are strictly regulated through the signalling through several soluble factors including PTH, vitamin D or calcium concentration. Understanding this complexity represents a major challenge in anti-cancer research and a mandatory step towards the development of new drugs potentially able not only to reduce the consequences

---

D. Santini (✉) · F. Pantano · B. Vincenzi · G. Tonini
Medical Oncology, University Campus Bio-Medico,
Via Alvaro del Portillo, 200, 00128 Rome, Italy
e-mail: d.santini@unicampus.it

F. Bertoldo
Dipartimento di Medicina, Sezione di Medicina Interna D,
Università di Verona, Verona, Italy

of bone lesions but also to target the metastatization process from the "bone pre-neoplastic niche" to "visceral pre-neoplastic niches".

Contents

1	Bone Premetastatic Niche	34
	1.1 Starting From the Primary Tumor Site: The Cancer Stem Cells	35
	1.2 The Long Way to the Bone: The Importance of Chemokines	40
	1.3 Modification of the Bone Microenvironment: Premetastatic Niche Formation	45
	1.4 Osteomimicry	46
	1.5 Role of Calcium, Vitamin D and PTH in the Premetastatic Niche	50
References		55

1 Bone Premetastatic Niche

Paget's "seed and soil" theory postulated that cancer cells "colonize" the organs whose microenvironment is advantageous. Starting from this theory, we can say that metastasis is a remarkably efficient, multistep process. The determinants of 'successful metastatic growth in a given organ are poorly understood, but there is substantial evidence to suggest that tumor cells and host tissue both play important roles in metastasis. This hypothesis started from a new model of metastasis formation. This 'early metastasis model' suggests that tumor cells leave the primary site much earlier in tumourigenesis (Pardal et al. 2003). The model is based on experimental data about cancer stem-like cells (CSC), a population of cells, within tumor mass, able to navigate in the bloodstream and to localize new metastatic sites (Pardal et al. 2003; Al-Hajj et al. 2003).

Populations of cells with tumor-initiating capacity have been shown to exist in human acute myeloid leukaemia (Lapidot et al. 1994; Bonnet and Dick 1997) and in several solid malignancies, such as breast (Al-Hajj et al. 2003) and colon cancer (O'Brien et al. 2007). Accordingly, "premetastatic niches" can be defined as a localized microenvironment that is being formed in metastatic target organs, prior to the arrival of metastatic tumor cells. Moreover, premetastatic niches consist of a collection of specific proteins and Bone Marrow Derived Cells (BMDCs). In fact, during the early development of primary tumors, neovascularization is guaranteed by VEGF-receptor 1+ (VEGFR1+), hematopoietic progenitor cells (HPC) which support the recruitment and incorporation of bone marrow-derived VEGF receptor 2+ (VEGFR2+) endothelial progenitors cells (EPC). These bone marrow-derived cells are also able to form clusters of cells in the tissue parenchyma at common sites of metastasis before actual tumor cell seeding. At these sites, bone marrow-derived cells express VEGFR1, CD11b, c-kit and other markers of their progenitor cell status within the tissue parenchyma of the premetastatic niche. Then, in response to the primary tumor chemokine secretion and other events, the VEGFR1+ HPCs proliferate and circulate in the bloodstream, but also preferentially localize to areas of increased fibronectin, newly synthesized by resident fibroblasts and fibroblast-like cells. The VEGFR1+ HPCs express integrin VLA-4 (or $\alpha 4\beta 1$), allowing them to adhere specifically to the newly synthesized fibronectin for the initiation of cellular cluster formation. Other mediators such as metalloprotease 9 (MMP-9) allow extravasation of VEGFR1+ HPC. The VEGFR1+ HPCs, along with fibronectin and associated stromal cells, cause modifications of the local microenvironment, which leads to the activation of other integrins and chemokines such as SDF-1. SDF-1 itself promotes attachment, survival and growth of tumor cells.

Therefore, premetastatic niches are thought to be fertile regions of tissue that facilitate the invasion, survival and/or proliferation of metastatic tumor cells, providing a highly novel mechanism for the promotion of metastasis (Kaplan et al. 2005). Furthermore, some tissues are more receptive to a given metastasizing tumor cell type, which can explain the tendency of tumor cells to metastasize to some organs more often than other organs in a way that cannot be explained by differences in blood flow. In addition to target organ-specific growth of metastases, metastatic tumor foci seem to grow preferentially in specific areas of some tissues. So, we can postulate that cross-talking between bone microenvironment and cancer cells facilitates bone tropism of cancer cells. Moreover, there is some evidence that a specific subpopulation of cancer cells forming primary tumor sites can circulate as stem cells do.

1.1 Starting From the Primary Tumor Site: The Cancer Stem Cells

1.1.1 Cancer Stem Cell Characteristics

Stem cells are defined by their ability for self-renewal, differentiation into adult tissue and migration. Cancer stem-like cells are defined as cells capable of giving rise to a new tumor, and are thought to be the root cause of cancer. While still controversial, the Cancer Stem-like Cell (CSC) hypothesis may be directly relevant to metastatic theory, as such cells are good candidates for the acquisition of migratory capabilities and propagation of heterogeneous tumor cell populations at distant sites. Cancer stem-like cells may show some similarities to normal stem cells, but there appear to be differences too. While normal stem cells are present in tissues in relatively low numbers, the proportion of cells with specific CSC surface markers residing in a given tumor seems to vary greatly, up to 24.5% in colon cancer or 12–60% in breast cancer. In addition, putative breast cancer stem-like cells expressing CD44 (an adhesion molecule that binds hyaluronate) and lacking CD24 (an adhesion molecule that binds P-selectin) have been shown to switch to a more differentiated CD24-positive phenotype in distant metastases with loss of CD44, which can even progress to initiate further metastases (Shipitsin et al. 2007). As tumors progress through clonal selection of more malignant and less differentiated cells, differentiation between putative highly successful cancer stem-like cells and the rest of the tumor cells is difficult (Shipitsin and Polyak 2008). Another CSCs surface marker is CD133, which has been shown to be expressed in several solid malignancies such as

Table 1 Signaling pathway involved in stem-cells renewal

Pathway	Normal function	Function in tumorigenesis
WNT	WNT are secreted proteins that bind Frizzled receptors, causing a chain of reactions with final induction of cell proliferation	It activates the overexpression of target genes promoting cancer cell proliferation
PTEN	It plays an important role in self-renewal and activation of hematopoietic stem cells	It forms a complex signaling network and maintains the cancer stem cell population
NOTCH	It plays a role in the normal development of many tissues and cell types through diverse effects on cell fate decision, stem cell renewal, differentiation, survival and proliferation	Its upregulation is involved in tumor metastatization
SHH	It promotes osteoblast differentiation in multipotent mesenchymal cells by upregulating the expression and function of RUNX2	Abnormal activation of the pathway leads to development of disease through transformation of adult stem cells into cancer stem cells

intestine, brain, lung and prostate (Sing 2003; Collins et al. 2005; Shmelkov et al. 2008; Bertolini et al. 2009). However, it was demonstrated that CD133 is expressed in differentiated epithelium cells. Moreover, both CD133-positive and CD133-negative metastatic cells were able to start tumorigenesis. These findings raised the question of whether the CD133-negative cells have represented a largely non-epithelial population of stromal and inflammatory cells.

1.1.2 The Acquisition of Self-Renewal and Migration Ability (The Epithelial Mesenchymal Transition)

Many signaling pathways involved in stem-cells renewal cause neoplastic proliferation and migration when dysregulated by mutations. The most studied pathways are WNT, sonic hedgehog (SHH), NOTCH and PTEN.

The features of these pathways in normal and neoplastic cells are summarized in Table 1.

WNT Pathway

WNTs are secreted proteins which bind Frizzled receptors. This link activates Dishevelled (DSH) which disrupts the complex of glycogen synthase kinase 3β (GSK3β), Casein Kynase 1 (CK1), axin and adenomatosis polyposis coli (APC). This disruption inhibits interaction with APC-β-catenin and allows β-catenin to accumulate and translocate to the nucleus, binding LEF\TCF transcription factors and activating the expression of target genes promoting cellular proliferation. Mutations of this pathway have been implicated in many types of cancers (Polakis

1999; Zhu and Watt 1999). Expression of stabilized β-catenin promotes the self-renewal of many types of stem cells. WNT signaling activates the same pathway in colorectal cancer cells (Chenn and Walsh 2002). Mutations that activate WNT signaling cause the hyperproliferation of crypt progenitors, generating benign polyps (Powell et al. 1992). So, tumorigenesis in the intestinal epithelium seems to be caused by the hyper-self-renewal of intestinal-crypt stem cells, followed by the accumulation of additional mutations (Kinzler and Vogelstein 1996).

PTEN Pathway

PTEN plays an important role not only in self-renewal and activation of hematopoietic stem cells but also in the prevention of leukemogenesis (Zhang et al. 2006). It is quite likely that PTEN also plays an important role in breast cancer stem cells by negatively regulating PI3K/mTOR/STAT3 signaling. Some in vitro studies showed that overexpression of PTEN decreased cancer cell tumorigenicity (Cheney et al. 1998; Zhou et al. 2007). PTEN/PI3K/mTOR/STAT3 signaling forms a complex signaling network that is able to maintain the cancer stem cell population within the whole cell population (Zhou et al. 2007).

Notch Signaling System

Notch plays a key role in the normal development of many tissues and cell types through diverse effects on stem cell renewal, cellular differentiation, survival and proliferation (Artavanis-Tsakonas et al. 1999). The Notch signaling system includes Notch ligands (Jagged 1), receptors, negative and positive modifiers and Notch target transcription factors. One of the most important functions of the Notch pathway is expansion of the hematopoietic stem cell compartment during bone development, and participation in osteoblast differentiation (Nobta et al. 2005). Moreover, this signaling system is aberrantly activated in a variety of human cancers, including T-cell acute lymphoblastic leukemia and carcinomas of the lung, colorectum, prostate and the breast (Radtke and Raj 2003; Kunnimalaiyaan and Chen 2007; Proweller et al. 2006). Notch upregulation is involved in tumor metastatization, and its inhibition impairs tumor spreading (Hughes 2009). Osteoblasts within the bone marrow are identified as the niche for supporting long-term hematopoietic stem cells, providing the Notch ligand Jagged1 and other factors under regulation by bone morphogenetic protein (BMP) and PTH/PTHrP signaling (Calvi et al. 2003). Increasing evidence suggests that the osteoblast niche inhibits drug-induced apoptosis and confers de novo drug resistance in myeloma cells (Nefedova et al. 2004). This type of paracrine Notch signaling in metastatic cancer cells could explain their predisposition to bone metastasis. Moreover, cross-talk occurs between TGF-β and the Notch pathway. TGF-β increases the expression of Hes-1, a direct target of Notch, in several cell types (Blokzijl et al. 2003). TGF-β induces the interaction of the intracellular domain of Notch1 with Smad3. TGF-β-induced EMT is blocked by RNA silencing of the Notch target gene Hey-1 and the Notch ligand Jagged1, and by chemical inactivation of Notch (Zavadil et al. 2004).

SHH Pathway

Sonic hedgehog (SHH) ligands have an autocrine and paracrine action. When SHH reaches its target cell, it binds to the Patched-1 (PTCH1) and −2 (PTCH2) receptors. These in turn relieve the Smoothened (SMO) inhibition, leading to activation of the GLI (GLI 1, GLI 2, GLI 3) transcription factors. Abnormal activation of the pathway probably results in early carcinogenesis through transformation of adult stem cells into cancer stem cells (Dahmane et al. 1997; Ruiz i Altaba et al. 2002). In vitro models showed that cancer cells overexpressing SHH upregulated the expression of SHH-responsive target genes GLI1 and PTCH1 in pre-osteoblasts cells, leading to the induction of early phase osteoblast differentiation. Cancer cells that metastasize to bone are in close physical contact with bone stromal cells including bone cells and their osteoblast progenitors, fibroblasts, hematopoetic cells and multipotent mesenchymal stem cells, and the SHH pathway induces bone modification in order to create the conditions for the premetastatic niche. In fact, downstream mechanism through which SHH-signaling induces osteoblast differentiation is not fully understood. A recent study has demonstrated that SHH promotes osteoblast differentiation in multipotent mesenchymal cells by upregulating the expression and function of RUNX2 (Shimoyama et al. 2007; Spinella-Jaegle et al. 2001). Other data suggest that in cells that are already committed to the osteoblast lineage and express endogenous levels of RUNX2, the induction of osteoblast differentiation by SHH occurs through a mechanism that does not require further transcriptional upregulation of RUNX2 (Zunich et al. 2009).

These and other pathways enable cancer cells to acquire stem cell-like characteristics. Furthermore, the acquisition of mesenchymal markers such as fibronectin, and progressive loss of E-cadherin in tumor cells with nuclear β-catenin accumulation, suggest that they have undergone an epithelial–mesenchymal transition (EMT) or transdifferentiation. This process of EMT can be described by the chronological sequence of five morphogenetic events:

1. Disassembly of tight junctions, which results in the redistribution of Zonula Occludens (ZO) proteins, claudins and occludins.
2. Disruption of the polarity complex.
3. Initiation of cytoskeleton reorganization (through actin reorganization).
4. Metalloprotease upregulation.
5. Increased deposition of extracellular matrix proteins.

In vitro and in vivo experiments showed that EMT is also promoted by Tumor Growth Factor β (TGF-β) (Miettinen et al. 1994; Piek et al. 1999; Derynck et al. 2001; Hugo et al. 2007). In fact, its related proteins cause transcription of different mesenchymal genes and repression of epithelial genes (Xu et al. 2009). These phenotypic changes finally promote cell mobility and migration to the premetastatic niche (bone microenvironment), and eventually cellular differentiation into distinct cell types (acquisition of the osteomimetic phenotype, osteomimicry). EMT is initiated by external signals, the extracellular matrix and soluble factors such as those of the TGF-β superfamily. These signaling pathways are thought to control the invasive behavior of solid cancers.

1.1.3 Tumor-Associated Macrophages

Solid tumors are not only composed of malignant cells, but they are also complex organ-like structures comprising many cell types, including a wide variety of migratory hematopoietic and resident stromal cells. Migration of these cell types into tumors has been interpreted as evidence for an immunological response of the host against any growing tumor. However, it is now acknowledged that tumors are largely recognized as self and lack efficient antigens. Instead, they appear to have been selected to escape the host immune system, to prevent rejection and facilitate tumor growth and spreading. This led to the proposal that infiltrates of hematopoietic cells have a causal role in carcinogenesis. Clinical data collected from a wide range of solid tumors underscore these findings, showing high densities of leukocytic infiltrations—mostly macrophages—correlating with a poor prognosis. Tumor-Associated Macrophages (TAM) originate from circulating monocytes and are activated macrophages of the polarized type II (M2 macrophages or activated macrophages), mainly induced by IL-4, IL-10, IL-13 and corticosteroids. Differential cytokine and chemokine production, and coordinated temporal and spatial activities of these cells in the tumor stroma are key features of polarized macrophages, which promote tumor angiogenesis and growth (Pollard 2009). These data suggest the new hypothesis that tumors can modify the behavior of macrophages from a potentially hostile antitumor phenotype to one that promotes malignancy. But what is the precise nature and function of these tumor-promoting macrophages? Can they participate in the building of a premetastatic niche? Increasing data support the identifying of a specific subpopulation of macrophages which:

1. Express the endothelial-cell marker TIE2 receptor (also known as TEK); their importance is shown by their ablation that blocks angiogenesis in xenograft tumors (De Palma et al. 2007).
2. Secrete VEGF through the HIF pathway (Murdoch et al. 2008).
3. Facilitate tumor cell motility; moreover, intravasation of tumor cells also occurs next to clusters of macrophages on the vessel surface (Wyckoff 2007).
4. Secrete MMP leading to ECM degradation (Hagemann 2005).
5. Secrete TNF, and activates the wNT-β-catenin pathway (Pukrop et al. 2006).

Moreover, TAM produce TGF-β which is involved in the process of EMT (Mantovani et al. 2006; Pollard 2009; Kagan and Li 2003). By doing so, macrophages may participate in the building of a premetastatic niche. M2 macrophages are known as differentiated cells in response to parasitic infection, allergic conditions and during tissue repair. IL-13 and IL-4 are the most important cytokines supporting the process of EMT. In the tumor microenvironment however, macrophages develop in the presence of growth factors such as CSF1, or in response to molecules that signal through nuclear factor-κB (NF-κB), becoming non-immunogenic and trophic (Pollard 2009). Overall, these data suggest macrophages to substantially participate in the building of the premetastatic niche.

1.1.4 Lysyl Oxidase

Lysyl Oxidase (LOX) is produced by fibrogenic cells. The main activity of LOX is thought to be oxidation of specific lysine residues of collagen (Kagan and Li 2003). Increased expression of LOX has been found in metastatic and/or invasive breast cancer cell lines and is associated with higher stages of disease in patients with renal cell carcinoma (Kirschmann et al. 2002). Hypoxic tumor cells often have increased LOX expression and secretion, enabling cell movement to more oxygenated and nutrient-rich areas. Then, LOX increases cell invasion and migration through regulation of cell–matrix adhesion. In addition, matrix remodeling by invasive tumor cells provides a more ideal soil for any succeeding tumor cells, building a kind of "highway to metastasis". LOX may be involved in tumor interactions with the cell–matrix required for intravasation and extravasation. Then, LOX is required for the formation of a mature ExtraCellular Matrix (ECM) at the secondary site, allowing tumor cell survival and possibly BMDC recruitment (Erler and Giaccia 2006). LOX secreted by hypoxic tumor cells accumulates at premetastatic sites, crosslinks collagen IV in the basement membrane and is essential for myeloid cell recruitment. Finally, tumor cells adhere to crosslinked collagen IV and produce matrix metalloproteinase-2, which cleaves collagen, enhancing the invasion and recruitment of BMDCs and metastasizing tumor cells (Erler et al. 2009).

1.2 The Long Way to the Bone: The Importance of Chemokines

Chemokines are small chemoattractant cytokines that bind to specific G-protein-coupled transmembrane receptors present on the plasma membranes of target cells. These molecules can guide circulating cancer cells to the bone.

1.2.1 CXCR4\SDF-1 Pathway

The chemokine receptor CXCR4 (or CD184) is an alpha-chemokine receptor for stromal-derived-factor-1 (SDF-1 or CXCL12) alpha or beta. SDF-1 and CXCR4 are a relatively 'monogamous' ligand-receptor pair (in contrast to other chemokines that bind several chemokine receptors in a more 'promiscuous' manner) (Arya et al. 2007). In the normal bone marrow, SDF-1 is produced by osteoblasts, fibroblasts and endothelial cells. Parathyroid hormone (PTH), PDGF (platelet-derived growth factor), interleukin-1 (IL-1), vascular endothelial growth factor (VEGF) and tumor necrosis factor alpha (TNF-α all induce SDF-1 production by osteoblasts (Jung et al. 2006). SDF-1 is important in hematopoietic stem cell homing to the bone marrow and in hematopoietic stem cell quiescence. It has been demonstrated that by blocking the CXCR4 receptor, hematopoietic stem cells mobilize into the bloodstream as peripheral blood stem cells. Moreover, it has been demonstrated that SDF-1 production can induce all of the following:

1. Osteoclast precursor recruitment by promoting chemotaxis, proteinase activity and collagen transmigration (Yu et al. 2003a, b).

2. Angiogenesis by recruiting endothelial progenitor cells (EPC) from the bone marrow via CXCR4-dependent mechanisms (Zheng et al. 2007).
3. Lymphocyte chemotaxis (Bleul et al. 1996; Ma et al. 1998).

There are many experimental data concerning the importance of the CXCR4\SDF-1 pathway for neovascularisation and metastatic spreading to SDF-1-expressing tissues, especially the bones:

1. Cancer cells in some organs such as lung, liver and bone produce large quantities of SDF-1 (Muller et al. 2001).
2. SDF-1 mRNA expression is observed in the metaphysis of the long bones, near the endosteal surfaces covered by osteoblastics (Sun et al. 2005). In an experimental animal model of breast cancer bone metastasis, it has been demonstrated that single tumor cells are homing to the metaphyses of the long bones after systemic inoculation. Furthermore, they were mostly located in close proximity to osteoblasts and lining cells (Phadke et al. 2006).
3. A gradient of chemokine expression was found between peripheral blood and bone marrow, with an increased expression of SDF-1 in the bone marrow along with lower concentrations of SDF-1 in serum, while increased expression of CXCR4 is found in peripheral blood with lower expression in bone marrow. This gradient promotes cancer cell migration into the bone marrow and prevents further trafficking of cancer cells (Hofbauer et al. 2008).
4. There is some evidence that activation of the SDF-1/CXCR4 pathway not only regulates migration and homing of cancer cells to the bone but also regulates adhesion, invasion and cytoskeletal rearrangement of cancer cells (Gerritsen et al. 2002).
5. Blocking CXCR4 with antibodies reduces the formation of experimental bone metastases induced by CXCR4-expressing breast or prostate cancer cells (Liang et al. 2004).

1.2.2 RANK\RANK-L Pathway

The RANK\RANK-L pathway is involved in tumor-induced osteoclastogenesis and osteolysis. RANK-L is physiologically produced by osteoblasts and stimulates osteoclast precursor recruitment and maturation. Then, mature osteoclasts cause bone reabsortion (Lacey et al. 1998). Normal glandular epithelial cells express RANK, and the RANK–RANKL pathway is involved in normal development of lactating mammary glands (Fata et al. 2000). It has been demonstrated that RANK expression facilitates cancer cell migration into the bones. Recent in vivo studies demonstrated the association between RANK expression and cancer cell osteotropism (Jones et al. 2006). In fact, it has been found that RANK is expressed by solid tumors, with a high concordance of the expression profile between bone metastases and corresponding primary tumors (Santini et al. 2010a, b). Moreover, RANK is clearly associated with early bone metastasis formation in breast cancer (Santini et al. 2010a, b) and, consistent with those data, it has been demonstrated that osteoprotegerin (OPG), a natural RANK-inhibitor, blocks cancer cell osteotropism (Dougall and Chaisson 2006).

1.2.3 The Integrin System

The study by Kaplan et al. (2005) showed that VLA4 or anti-VEGFR1 antibodies inhibit the proliferation and binding affinity of tumor cells to VEGFR1-positive HPCs, demonstrating their direct role in adhesion and growth of tumor cells. Moreover, other integrins are critical for cancer cell homing in other target organs. In fact, breast cancer cells expressing $\alpha v \beta 3$-integrin and prostate cancer cells expressing $\alpha v \beta 2$-integrin, which bind many bone matrix components, have a higher propensity for spreading to the bones (Pecheur et al. 2002). Additionally, proto-oncogenic tyrosine kinase c-SRC is similarly involved in the integrin's pathway, and has an important role in cancer cell osteotropism. SRC binds to activated RANK, thereby recruiting TRAF6 and Grb2-associated binder 2 (Gab2), followed by phosphorylation of IκBα and JNK, which ultimately leads to activation of the transcription factors NF-κB and AP-1.

There are clinical and experimental data suggesting that SRC expression:
1. Increases the survival of tumor cells in the bone microenvironment, leading to the establishment of bone metastases (latent phase of bone metastasis).
2. Increases cell mobility (Zhang et al. 2009).
3. Increases osteotropism of tumor cells (Rucci et al. 2006; Boyce et al. 2003).

Moreover, expression of SRC is involved in bone marrow seeding and sustains the outgrowth of indolent cancer cells in the bone marrow microenvironment. Activated SRC plays a critical role in the initiation and maintenance of a tumor cell response to bone-derived factors CXCL12/SDF and TRAIL. Latency status is maintained until overt progression to the phase of osteolytic outgrowth.

1.2.4 The BMP Receptor Axis

Bone morphogenetic proteins (BMP) are members of the TGF-β (transforming growth factor-β) family. So far, three BMP receptors have been characterized: BMP-R Ia, Ib and II (van Dijke et al. 1994). It has been shown that prostate, breast and lung cancer cells express BMP-2 mRNA and its protein. Moreover, BMP receptors are expressed in prostate cancer cell lines (Schwalbe et al. 2003). The most important functions of BMP-2 in cancer cells are:
1. Promotion of cancer cell migration to the bones (Ite et al. 1997).
2. Modulation of cancer cell migration through the integrins axis.

In fact, breast cancer cell lines upregulate bone sialoprotein (BSP) expression in pre-osteoblasts (Bunyaratavej et al. 2000), and in vivo inhibition of BMP in osteoinductive prostate cancer cells inhibits the osteoblastic response in bone (Schwaninger et al. 2007). Moreover, BMP has been shown to reverse TGF-β-induced EMT by decreasing vimentin expression and increasing E-cadherin expression in breast cancer cells and in normal mouse mammary epithelial cells (Zeisberg et al. 2003; Valcourt et al. 2005).

The role of the cited chemokine network is summarized in Table 2.

Table 2 The importance of chemokines

Pathway	Normal function	Function in tumorigenesis
CXCR4/SDF-1	Osteoclastic precursor recruitment, endothelial progenitor cell recruitment, lymphocyte chemotaxis	It is linked to the neovascularisation and metastatic spreading to tissues releasing the ligands such as bone
RANK/RANKL	Osteoclast precursor recruitment and maturation	It is involved in tumor-induced osteoclastogenesis and osteolysis
Integrin system (avb3 e avb2)	Integrins are expressed by normal osteoclasts and interact with components of the bone matrix, contributing to bone resorption	Tumor cells expressing these integrins, which bind many bone matrix components, have higher incidence of bone metastases
BMPs/BMP	Bone morphogenetic proteins (BMP) are a group of growth factors able to induce the formation of bone and cartilage. They have an important role during embryonic development and on early skeletal formation	It has two important functions: promotion of migration of cancer cells to the bone, and modulation of migration of cancer cells through the integrin axis
VCAM-1/ICAM-1	Allows the adhesion and transmigration of hematopoietic and lymphoid cells	The cancer cells migrate through the vasculature using a process of attachment–detachment through a cell adhesion mechanism mediated by these molecules
OPN	Promotes the adherence of osteoclasts and hematopoietic stem cells to the bone matrix	Is involved in bone metastatic spread of breast, prostate and lung cancer, and OPN expression confers migratory abiliy and invasive phenotype in human mammary cells
Endothelin-1	Stimulates mitogenesis in osteoblasts	Induces expression and activation of the tumor proteases that degrade the tissue matrix to permit local invasion and formation of metastases

1.2.5 Other Adhesion Molecules

Osteopontin
Osteopontin (OPN) is a glycophosphoprotein and is one of the major components of non-collagenous bone matrix. OPN is expressed in osteoblasts and osteocyctes (bone-forming cells) as well as osteoclasts (bone-resorbing cells).

Osteopontin promotes the adherence of osteoclasts and hematopoietic stem cells to the bone matrix (Asou et al. 2001). Hypocalcemia and hypophosphatemia both stimulate kidney proximal tubule cells to produce calcitriol (1α,25-dihydroxyvitamin D3) that stimulates OPN gene translation via the VDRE (vitamin D response element) in the OPN promoter region (Prince and Butler 1987; Yucha and Guthrie 2003). OPN expression is also regulated by exposure of cells to various factors and metabolic settings, including tumor necrosis factor α, infterleukin-1β, angiotensin II, transforming growth factor β (TGFβ) and parathyroid hormone (PTH), hyperglycemia and hypoxia (Noda and Rodan 1989; Hullinger et al. 2001). Finally, it has been shown that OPN is involved in bone metastatic spread of breast, prostate and lung cancer cells (Wai and Kuo 2004), and OPN expression confers migratory ability and invasive phenotype in human mammary cells (Tuck et al. 2003).

Sinusoidal Endothelial Cell Adhesion Molecules

Cancer cells usually settle in bone metaphysis that is rich in sinusoidal microvasculature, rather than bone diaphysis. This is mainly caused by:
1. Hemodynamic properties of the sinusoidal vascular bed, with 90% of the blood circulating through metaphyseal sinusoids.
2. Characteristics of the sinusoidal endothelia, allowing adhesion and transmigration of hematopoietic and lymphoid cells.

In a model studying the kinetics of metastatic breast cancer cell trafficking in bone, it has been shown that the majority of cancer cells tended to settle in the endosteal marrow, rather than in the centrum of the marrow and that primary tumor cells most often locate in close proximity to osteoblasts and bone lining cells.

However, migration to the sinusoids of the bone marrow is not sufficient to ensure colonization by cancer cells. Moreover, cancer cells migrate through the vasculature using a process of attachment–detachment through cell adhesion mediated by several adhesion molecules such as E-selectin, N-cadherin, intracellular adhesion molecule (ICAM-1) and vascular cell adhesion molecule (VCAM-1) (Makuch et al. 2006). VCAM-1, a member of the immunoglobulin family of cell adhesion molecules, has ICAM-1 and VLA-4 as its main receptors, with the latter being constitutively activated in osteoclasts and are also found on many cancer cells. Inflammatory cytokines produced by osteoblasts in the presence of breast cancer cells may cause endothelial activation, expression of adhesion molecules and cancer cell invasion (Glinsky et al. 2001).

Endothelin 1 and ET Receptors

Endothelin-1 (ET-1) has been detected in osteocytes, osteoblasts, osteoclasts and vascular endothelial cells (Sasaki and Hong 1993). Endothelin-1 stimulates mitogenesis in osteoblasts (Stern et al. 1995). Moreover, ET-1 enhances the effect of other osteoblast-stimulatory factors, such as BMP-7, to induce bone formation (Nelson et al. 1995; Kitten et al. 1997).

Additionally, ET-1 stimulates the expression of osteopontin and osteocalcin in rat osteosarcoma cells (Shioide and Noda 1993), and mineralization of the bone matrix also depends on the ET-1 receptor pathway. Other studies of ET-1 null mice showed that ET-1 may regulate proliferation and migration of osteogenic cells rather than modulating the expression of bone matrix proteins (Kitano et al. 1998).

Nevertheless, the role of the ET-1 pathway in bone metastasis is not clear. Malignant tumors of the breast and prostate are typically associated with osteoblastic bone metastases, and both tumors express ET-1 and its receptors. Importantly, paracrine effects of ET-1 on bone cells may provide a favorable growth environment for tumor cells in bone. Endothelin-1 is found in normal prostate epithelium, throughout the entire gland. Addition of exogenous ET-1 increases the proliferation of prostate cancer cells and enhances the mitogenic effects of IGF-1, IGF-2, PDGF, epidermal growth factor (EGF) and FGF-2 on cancer cells. Moreover, ET-1 concentrations were significantly higher in men with advanced, hormone-refractory prostate cancer with established metastases to the bones as compared to patients with early-stage disease (Nelson et al. 1995). Increased ET-1 production has been described in prostate cancer cells through contact with bone (Chiao et al. 2000). Tumor-derived ET-1 stimulates new bone formation via ETA receptors on the surface of osteoblasts. Subsequently, growth factors produced by osteoblasts are incorporated into the new bone matrix as well as the local microenvironment. Interestingly, ET-1 mediates vasoconstriction of distal blood vessels, but not of those vessels directly supplying the tumor bed. This 'vascular steal phenomenon' improves local blood supply to the tumor and thereby improves oxygenation of tumor cells. Activation of endothelial cells by ET-1 stimulates the production of vascular endothelial growth factor (VEGF) by increasing the levels of hypoxia-inducible factor-1α (HIF-1α). Endothelin-1, acting through ETA, also induces the expression and activation of tumor-associated proteases, matrix metalloproteinases (MMPs) and urokinase plasminogen activator (uPA) (Spinella et al. 2003). Metalloproteinases degrade the local tissue matrix to permit local tumor invasion and formation of metastases. Urokinase plasminogen activator in turn converts plasminogen into plasmin, which degrades the tumor stroma, allowing the tumor to invade the surrounding tissue and prepare metastatic spread. Urokinase plasminogen activator might also activate MMP. Taken together, these factors have the potential to stimulate tumor growth as well as further increase tumor production of ET-1 (Guise et al. 2003).

1.3 Modification of the Bone Microenvironment: Premetastatic Niche Formation

Many data suggest the hypothesis that growth of macrometastases starts from the interaction between the target organ (e.g. bone) and the primary tumor that builds the premetastatic niche. In fact, studies in breast cancer demonstrated that although about 30% of patients may have micrometastatic disease in their bone marrow at the time of presentation, only 50% of these patients develop overt bone metastatic disease after 5 years. Furthermore, many patients with breast and prostate cancer do not develop bone metastases until many years after the surgical removal of the primary cancer. The Paget's "seed and soil theory" hypothesizes that metastatic cells can enter into the bone marrow and remain in a quiescent status for many years. However, molecular mechanisms and signaling pathways that promote the switch to a premetastatic bone microenvironment are not well understood. We can postulate that cancer stem cells, like physiologic haematopoietic stem cells, can establish a relationship with bone marrow stroma in order to mantain their survival. Physiologically, two fundamental niches exist in the bone marrow:

1. *Endosteal Niche.* Stem cells are closely associated with spindle-shaped N-cadherin positive osteoblasts (SNO). Moreover, these osteoblasts are involved in the maintenance of stem cell quiescence. The same osteoblasts might also bind cancer stem cells, thereby maintaining their dormancy (Yin et al. 2006).
2. *Vascular Niche.* More differentiated cells are generally located in central parts of the bone marrow.

It is well understood that circulating cancer cells arrive in the endosteal niche and are kept in a dormancy status via the link with SNO and the release of inhibitory molecules by stromal cells (such as fibronectin). RANK\RANK-L is also involved in cancer cell reactivation via osteoclast activation and the consequent release of growth factors such as TGF-β, BMPs, PTH-related protein (Oh et al. 2004). These factors are typically involved in the process of epithelial–mesenchymal transition, and likely activate dormant metastatic cancer cells. Activated osteoclasts may directly induce hematopoietic stem cells, and probably metastatic cancer cells, to separate from the endosteal niche through increasing proteolytic activity of MMP-9 and cathepsin K, which clive and inactivate SDF-1, osteopontin and other niche factors (Kollett et al. 2006). Moreover, stromal cells secrete inactive metalloprotease-2, which is activated by cancer cells increasing their migratory capacity (Harada and Rodan 2003). At the time of bone marrow colonization, when pathologic bone lesions are still not evident, cancer cells acquire a bone-like phenotype, and this process is known as osteomimicry (Knerr et al. 2004).

1.4 Osteomimicry

We still do not know whether cancer cells already possess the osteomimetic phenotype when they detach from their primary tumor, or whether these characteristics are acquired when they colonize the bone niche. There is some evidence though that at least some cancer cells do need a biological signature to invade osseous structures (Ramaswamy et al. 2003).

As shown in Table 3, many molecules are produced from cancer cells invading bone marrow.

Table 3 Molecules produced from cancer cells invading the bone marrow (osteomimicry)

Molecules	Function when expressed by normal cells	Function when expressed by cancer cells
PTHrP	Homolog of PTH that has a direct action on the PTH receptor, stimulating bone resorption and renal tubular calcium resorption	It causes bone microenvironment modification that facilitates the establishment of circulating cancer cells, the release of bone-derived growth factors and the formation of the premetastatic bone niche
RANKL/OPG/TRAIL	RANKL induces osteoclast activation, OPG binds RANKL thys inhibiting osteoclast development, TRAIL is an anticancer cytokine which binds OPG	The RANK expression status determines the predominant migration into bone, where RANKL is abundantly expressed
VEGF	Induces angiogenesis	It drives bone marrow-derived cells to neoangiogenetic sites in the tumor
C-KIT/SCF		Both ligand (SCF) and receptor (C-KIT) are expressed by cancer cells for intraosseous development, indicating the existence of an autocrine loop
IGF system	Stimulates osteoblast differentiation, increases bone matrix apposition and decreases collagen degradation	It increases prostate cancer cell proliferation and chemotaxis
RUNX	Essential for osteoblastic differentiation and skeletal morphogenesis	It promotes transcription of genes involved in the acquisition of migration and invasiveness
Calcium sensing receptor	Implicated in the regulation of ion and water transport, proliferation, differentiation and apoptosis	Its activation leads to increased PTHrP secretion which drives osteolysis by osteoclasts leading to release of growth factors and calcium from the bone matrix and further stimulation of tumoral cell proliferation

1.4.1 PTHRP

The parathyroid hormone-related protein is a homolog of PTH and has a direct action on PTH receptors, stimulating bone resorption and renal tubular calcium resorption (Yates et al. 1988). PTHRP is released by cancer cells of many solid tumors (Moseley et al. 1987; Burtis et al. 1987; Strewler et al. 1987), and contributes to metastatic spreading. It has been demonstrated that PTHRP is abundant in tumors with osteoclastic and osteoblastic bone metastases. In fact, breast carcinomas metastatic to the bones express PTHRP in >90% of the cases, compared with only 17% of metastases to extraosseous sites (Southby et al. 1990; Grill et al. 1991; Powell et al. 1991; Vargas et al. 1992). Furthermore, growth factors such as TGF-β or IGF, which are abundant in mineralized bone matrix (Hauschka et al. 1986), are released and activated by osteoclastic bone resorption (Pfeilschifter and Mundy 1987) and may enhance PTHRP secretion from cancer cells (Zakalik et al. 1992; Merryman et al. 1994). Finally, other studies have shown that PTHRP, secreted by prostate cancer cells, stimulates ostoblastogenesis and osteoblast differentiation (Liao et al. 2008). Accordingly, it was postulated that PTHRP causes bone microenvironment modification in order to facilitate the establishment of circulating cancer cells, the release of bone-derived growth factors and the formation of the premetastatic bone niche.

1.4.2 RANKL\OPG\TRAIL

RANKL is produced by osteoblasts and stromal cells for inducing osteoclast activation and bone resorption. It was demonstrated that many types of solid tumors produce RANKL, both at the primary site and in metastatic bone lesions (Brown et al. 2001a, b; Chen et al. 2006; Sasaki et al. 2007). OPG is a soluble decoy-receptor of RANKL, which is expressed by various cell types, including osteoblasts and tumor-associated stromal cells. OPG binds RANKL and prevents RANK–RANKL association, inhibiting osteoclast development (Cross et al. 2006). It was observed that many tumor cell lines produce OPG (Holen et al. 2005; Holen et al. 2002). High serum levels of OPG were found in patients with advanced-stage prostate cancer (Brown et al. 2001a, b). Furthermore, inhibition of RANKL results in inhibition of malignant bone lesions and tumor growth in bone (Canon et al. 2008; Kostenuik et al. 2009), while OPG inhibits cancer-induced osteoclastogenesis (Zhang et al. 2001) and increases bone density. Moreover, OPG shares some sequence homology with Endothelin-1 (ET-1), and was shown to stimulate bone formation through ET-A receptor activation (Nelson et al. 1999). OPG also binds tumor necrosis factor (TNF)-related apoptosis-inducing ligand (TRAIL) (Emery et al. 1998), the latter being an anticancer cytokine. Finally, based on high constitutive RANK expression in breast cancer cell lines, recent data actually indicate that RANK expression by cancer cells determines whether tumors predominantly migrate into bone, where the corresponding ligand RANKL is abundantly expressed (Jones et al. 2006). In murine animal models, the correlation between high expression of RANK and osteotropism has been demonstrated across different tumor types, including breast cancer and melanoma.

1.4.3 VEGF

Tumor induces angiogenesis through VEGF signaling (Ferrara 2009). Moreover, VEGF secretion attracts bone marrow-derived cells such as VEGFR1-positive HPC and VEGFR2-positive EPC to neoangiogenic sites in the tumor (Lyden et al. 1999). VEGF is closely associated with the early phases of bone remodeling and induces osteoblast chemotaxis and differentiation (Tombran-Tink and Barnstable 2004; Li et al. 2005). VEGF also upregulates RANK on endothelial cells, resulting in the amplification of the angiogenic response in the presence of RANKL (Min et al. 2003). In effect, VEGF mediates both a direct and an indirect effect on bone growth by activating osteoblasts and promoting angiogenesis in metastatic sites with high concentrations of RANKL (Street et al. 2002). For these reasons, the localized production of VEGF, such as that observed in metastatic tissue, is likely to contribute to osteolysis and local tumor progression (Aldridge et al. 2005).

1.4.4 C-KIT\SCF

C-kit (or CD 117) is a tyrosine kinase receptor of the Stem Cell Factor (SCF). In vitro models demonstrated that prostate cancer cells in bone express high levels of c-kit, while prostate cancer cells from extraosseous sites are c-kit negative. Additionally, SCF was found to be overexpressed in bone metastases from prostate cancer (Wiesner et al. 2008). In vivo models showed that prostate cancer cells preferentially metastasize to regions of the bone marrow where SCF was expressed by stromal cells (BMS) interacting with c-kit expressed on the surface of bone marrow progenitor cells (Heissig et al. 2002). There is an association between coexpression of SCF and c-kit in prostate cancer cells and bone metastases, suggesting that both ligand and receptor should be expressed by prostate cancer cells for intraosseous development, also suggesting some autocrine loops. The increased expression of c-kit in bone metastases from prostate cancer might be the result of a selective dissemination and/or growth into the bone of c-kit-positive cells already present in primary tumors of the prostate, which are known to be heterogeneous (Patrawala et al. 2006). These c-kit-positive cancer cells could also represent cancer stem cells which were reported to be present in some metastatic lesions from human carcinomas (Kleeberger et al. 2007; Wiesner et al. 2008).

1.4.5 IGF

The Insulin-Like Growth Factors (IGF) comprise 3 receptors, 3 ligands and 6 binding proteins (IGFBP). IGF-I and IGF-II are known to induce osteoblast differentiation, increase bone matrix apposition and decrease collagen degradation (Koch et al. 2005). IGF are abundant in the bone microenvironment, and in vitro studies showed that they increase prostate cells proliferation and chemotaxis. Moreover, the IGF-I pathway is upregulated in prostate cancer cells localized in the bones (Ritchie et al. 1997a, b; Rubin et al. 2004). However, IGF-I is neither necessary nor sufficient for an adequate osteoblast response to prostate cancer metastases (Rubin et al. 2004).

In addition, tumor cells invading the bone express several transcription factors that are involved in the acquisition of the osteomimetic phenotype, among other RUNX.

1.4.6 RUNX

RUNX is a family of transcription factors (RUNX2 and RUNX1 and RUNX3). It was demonstrated that RUNX2 is essential for the differentiation of osteoblasts and skeletal morphogenesis (Li et al. 2008). RUNX2 is overexpressed in metastatic breast cancers cells, promotes transcription of genes involved in the acquisition of migration and invasiveness, including MMP and VEGF among others. Importantly, inhibition of Runx2 function in metastatic breast cancer cells transplanted to bone results in prevention of tumorigenesis and osteolysis (Javed et al. 2005).

These data indicate that a multigenic program facilitates the acquisition of osteomimetic properties by certain cancer cells, improving their chance for survival, adaptation to the bone environment and the development of bone metastases.

1.4.7 The Role of the Calcium Sensing Receptor in Bone Marrow Homing

The calcium sensor (CaSR) is also expressed in several cell types in the kidney, osteoblasts, a variety of hematopoietic cells in the bone marrow, the gastrointestinal mucosa and squamous epithelial cells of the esophagus. At these sites, the CaSR has been implicated in the regulation of a number of cellular processes, such as ion and water transport, proliferation, differentiation and apoptosis. Moreover, human breast cancer cell lines express CaSR and its activation leads to increased PTHrP secretion from these cells. The secretion of PTHrP by tumoral cells drives osteoclast-mediated osteolysis, leading to the release of growth factors and calcium from the bone matrix, and further stimulation of cell proliferation (Coyle et al. 2006). Additionally, the loss of CaSR expression in the transition from normal colonic epithelial cells to malignant adenocarcinoma cells is associated with a low potential of colonic carcinomas to generate bone metastases (Rodland 2004).

1.5 Role of Calcium, Vitamin D and PTH in the Premetastatic Niche

1.5.1 Vitamin D

Serum concentrations of calcium are closely regulated by a close interplay between 25(OH)D levels and PTH levels. The precision of this integrated control is such that in normal individuals, serum ionized calcium fluctuates by no more than 0.1 mg/dl in either direction from its physiological set-point throughout the day. Interestingly, PTH gene expression is not only regulated through serum calcium concentrations by the CaSR but also independently through vitamin D metabolites, principally 25(OH)D, regardless of both 1,25(OH)D and calcium. (Pepe et al. 2006). 25(OH)D and 1,25 (OH)D control PTH gene expression, CaSR and VDR gene expression, and the proliferation of parathyroid cells. Therefore, low serum calcium concentrations and/or low vitamin D levels increase PTH secretion, in turn increasing distal tubular calcium reabsorption, intestinal 1,25(OH)D-mediated calcium absorption and osteoclast-medicated bone resorption to normalize serum calcium concentrations.

1.5.2 Antineoplastic Effect of Vitamin D

Vitamin D depletion (and secondary hyperparathyroidism) has been reported as a very common condition worldwide both in men and women, with many implications for general health conditions (Holick and Chen 2008). Very recently, it has been documented that low serum vitamin D levels are similarly prevalent in young individuals (Adami et al. 2009; Crew et al. 2009). Biological and epidemiological data suggest vitamin D levels to influence cancer development (IARC Working Group Reports 2008), but data are not consistent. For breast and prostate cancer, case-control studies suggest an inverse association between serum 25(OH)D concentration and the prevalence of these diseases, but this finding was not confirmed by prospective studies that analyzed 25(OH)D years before the diagnosis of cancer (Yin and Grandi 2010; Trump et al. 2009; Tretli et al. 2009; Yin et al. 2009; Chlebowski et al. 2008; Lappe et al. 2007). This might indicate that low 25(OH)D concentrations in serum are rather a consequence of the malignant disease than causing cancer. Also, studies on intake/supplementation of vitamin D in breast or prostate cancer patients showed conflicting results (Trump et al. 2006; Flaig and Barqawi 2006; Chan and Beer 2008; Attia et al. 2008). Many molecular pathways mediate the anticancer effects of calcitriol. The active form of vitamin D, 1,25(OH)D has been established as an antiproliferative and pro-differentiation agent. More recent work showed calcitriol to be a proapoptotic agent and an inhibitor of cell migration and angiogenesis, supporting its potential in cancer prevention and cure (Peterlik and Grant 2009; Matthews et al. 2010). Among the breast cancer cell lines that do respond to 1,25(OH)D, a range of phenotype alterations have been reported, emphasizing that the mechanistic basis for the differentiating effects of 1,25(OH)D in cellular systems of breast cancer is very complex. (Gocek and Studzinski 2009). An interesting link to differentiation in 1,25(OH)D-treated breast cancer cells is the fact that vitamin D receptor (VDR) and Estrogen Receptor (ER) pathways converge to regulate BRCA-1, thus controlling the balance between cellular differentiation and proliferation (Campbell et al. 2000). In the prostate cancer cell line LNCaP, 1,25(OH)D up-regulates the expression of the insuline-like factor binding protein 3 (IGFBP-3) that functions to inhibit cell proliferation and up-regulates the expression and activity of the androgen receptor (AR) and the AR-mediated androgenic differentiation (Gocek and Studzinski 2009). The receptor of vitamin D (VDR) has been described in many types of cancer cells, including tumors of the breast, prostate, colon, bladder, skin, pancreas, leukaemia and lymphoma cells (Bouilon et al. 2006). In Caucasians, polymorphisms of VDR (VDR FokI and BsmI) migh modulate the risk of malignant tumors of the breast, skin and prostate, and possibly affect cancer risk also at other sites (Raimondi et al. 2009).

1.5.3 Inhibition of NFkB Activation, Angiogenesis, Invasion and Metastasis

Angiogenic factors such as IL8 and VEGF are crucial for the promotion of the premetastatic niche, and are similarly important for continued tumor growth and disease progression. NFkB plays a major role in the control of immune responses and inflammation, and promotes malignant behaviour by increasing the transcription of the antiapoptotic gene BCL-2, proteolytic enzymes such as matrix metalloproteinase 9 (MMP-9), urokinase-type plasminogen activator and angiogenic factors such as IL-8 and VEGF (Catz and Johnoston 2001). Calcitriol is known to directly modulate basal and cytokine-induced NFkB activity in many cells, including lymphocytes, monocytes, fibroblasts, osteoblasts and in cancer cells. In addition to the direct inhibition of NFkB, 1,25(OH)D indirectly inhibits NFkB-signaling by up-regulating the expression of other proteins that interfere with NFkB activation such as IGFBP-3 and Clusterin (CLU) (Folkman 1995). Early studies indicate that calcitriol is a potent inhibitor of tumor cell-induced angiogenesis by inhibiting VEGF-induced endothelial cell tube formation in vitro, decreasing tumor vascularization in mice and inhibiting angiogenesis through IL-8 in a NFkB-dependent manner (Bao et al. 2006). Furthermore, calcitriol directly inhibits the proliferation of endothelial cells (Chung et al. 2009). MMP in turn promote angiogenesis by mediating the degradation of the basement membrane of the vascular epithelium and the extracellular matrix. In human prostate cancer cells, calcitriol decreases the expression of MMP-9 by increasing the activity of TIMP-1 (tissue inhibitor of MMP-1) (Bao et al. 2006). Finally, it has been demonstrated that calcitriol reduces the invasive and metastatic potential of many malignant cells. In prostate cancer, calcitriol increase E-cadherin, a tumor suppressor gene, whose expression is inversely correlated with metastatic potential (Campbell et al. 1997).

1.5.4 Calcium

Inadequate calcium intake, low serum calcium (through CaSR) together with low vitamin D levels may directly or indirectly (through PTH) impact cell proliferation, differentiation and function. The CaSR, VDR and PTH-1R are expressed both in normal and malignant breast cells, and their expression is correlated with the occurrence of skeletal metastases. Interestingly, signaling pathways that are initiated via VDR and CaSR converge on the same downstream elements, e.g. the canonical Wnt pathway. Increasing extracellular calcium levels increases cellular differentiation in experimental models, decreases proliferation, induces apoptosis and down-modulates invasion, all of which seem to have tumor-protective effects (McGrath et al. 1984). Several studies have suggested an inverse association between dietary calcium intake and serum calcium levels with breast cancer risk in pre- and post-menopausal women (Almquist et al. 2007; Cui and Rohan 2006). However, the relationship between serum calcium concentrations and cancer risk is not consistent and complex, also because of the reciprocal effects of PTH and vitamin D levels. High serum calcium concentrations could indicate high bone turnover, which in turn suggests a bone microenvironment rich in chemotactic, adhesive and neoangiogenic factors that might promote the homing of cancer cells and the development of metastases (Schnieder et al. 2005). On the other hand, low serum calcium concentrations are generally associated with low 25(OH)D levels and high PTH levels that both promote cancer progression and bone metastases. Very likely, calcium concentrations play a crucial role in cellular signaling in bones in general and in the premetastatic niche in particular. The bone microenvironment is enriched in calcium during osteoclast-mediated bone resorption, reaching high local concentrations up to 40 mmol/L. Serum calcium homeostasis is closely regulated by the calcium sensing receptor (CaSR) expressed on parathyroid cells, modulating PTH secretion. However, CaSR is also expressed at high levels in breast cancer cells from patients with bone metastases and in prostate cancer cells (Mihai 2008). Activation of the CaSR by high calcium concentrations induces PTHrP expression, but may also attract breast and prostate cancer cells in areas of increased bone remodeling, thereby facilitating migration of cancer cells into the bones. Furthermore, high concentrations of calcium enhanced proliferation of prostate cancer cell lines and the proliferative response is associated with CaSR overexpression (Casimiro et al. 2009). Notably, CaSR is essential for stem cell migration and the settlement of HSC in the endosteal niche, suggesting preferential localization of these cells expressing CaSR in close proximity to calcium-releasing osteoclasts (Adams 2005).

1.5.5 PTH

PTH and Factors Involved in the Premetastatic Niche

Primary and secondary hyperparathyroidism is associated with a poor prognosis in patients with cancer (Schwartz 2008). PTH and PTHrP are immunologically distinct proteins that bind to the PTH-1R with equal affinity (Bryden et al. 2002). Many cancer cell types express PTHrP and its receptor PTH-1R, and PTHrP acts as an autocrine growth factor promoting proliferation, migration and disease progression (Deftos et al. 2005; Henderson et al. 2006). PTH could play a crucial role in promoting the homing of cancer cells in the bone environment, the persistence of the cancer stem cell niche, and the development of cancer metastases (Ritchie et al. 1997a, b). PTH and PTHrP both induce the activation of chemokines through PTH-1R, further inducing SDF-1 expression in the bone marrow. Major sources of SDF-1 in the marrow are cells of the osteoblastic lineage, mainly osteoblasts lining the bone endosteum (Ponomariov et al. 2000). The SDF-1/CXCR4 axis is known for regulating many aspects of stem cell functioning, including stem cell trafficking and development. It has been demonstrated that transgenic animals expressing constitutively active PTH/PTHrP receptors have increased numbers of hematopoietic stem cells recovered from the animals' bone marrow (Calvi et al. 2003). Intersingly, PTH increased the expression of SDF-1 in the local marrow environment in animal models, along with decreased SDF-1 in serum, creating a homing gradient for hematopoietic stem cells towards the bone marrow (Jung et al. 2006). There are many parallels between the metastasis of circulating carcinoma cells and the homing behavior of hematopoietic cells (Sun et al. 2003). Therefore, high circulating PTH levels in cancer patients could prime the marrow for metastatic spread by altering the SDF-1 axis. Physiologic bone remodeling takes place in specialized vascular structures called bone remodeling compartments (BRC), and PTH induces high bone turnover with subsequent expansion of the BRC space (Eriksen et al. 2007) Angiogenesis is closely associated with bone turnover, and angiogenic factors such as VEGF and endothelin are important regulators of both osteoclast and osteoblast activity. In addition, it has recently been demonstrated that PTH induces osteoclast formation in cooperation with RANKL, osteoclast activity through KDR/Flk-1 and/or Flt-1 receptors expressed in mature osteoclast, and survival involving beta-3-integrin-mediated attachment of osteoclasts to the extracellular matrix (Nakagawa et al. 2000). PTH/PTHrp induces PKC, ERK, MAPK and p38, with the MAPK pathway ultimately resulting in VEGF gene expression in osteoblasts and in epithelial cells of normal rat renal tubules (Esbrit et al. 2000; Alonso et al. 2008). VEGF expression was specifically observed in PTH1R-positive cancer cells after invasion of the bone marrow, using in vivo and in vitro models (Isowa et al. 2010). Finally, VEGF has been reported to increase SDF-1 expression in endothelial cells and in several prostate cancer cell lines (Dai et al. 2004).

PTH and the Hematopoietic Stem Cell Niche

The endosteal surface is rich in vasculature with close approximation of osteoblasts and vessel walls. Within the bone marrow, cells of the osteoblast lineage have unequivocally been shown to constitute a niche for Hematopoietic Stem Cells (HSC) (Xie et al. 2009). Cells derived from osteoprogenitors provide distinct niches for hematopoietic cells. Terminally differentiated osteoblasts along the endosteal surface could serve as a niche for HSC in their most quiescent stage, whereas the stromal reticular cell fraction including osteoprogenitors located in the bone marrow induce proliferation and differentiation of hematopoietic cells (Wu et al. 2009). It is widely known that stem cells are usually in the quiescent state or G0 phase, and this prevents stem cells from entering into the cell cycle and undergoing differentiation. CXCL12/CXCR4-mediated chemokine signaling plays an essential role in maintaining the quiescent pool of HSC (Sugiyama et al. 2006). Osteopontin (OP) and Angiopoietin-1 expressed by osteoblasts interact with Tie-2 expressed in HSC, activating N-cadherin and integrin (Arai et al. 2004). These interactions enhance the adhesion between the hematopoietic stem-cell niche and the stem cell, contributing to the maintenance of HCS quiescence. The bone morphogenetic protein (BMP) signaling pathway, which acts through BMP receptor type IA expressed in osteoblast, controls the number of HSC by regulating the size of the niche and is involved in maintaining quiescence and supressing proliferation. Different signaling pathways such as Wnt/cathenin and Notch/Jagged 1 promote self-renewal, proliferation and differentiation of HSC (Iwasaki and Suda 2009). Therefore, osteoblasts clearly have a role in the establishment and mainteinance of the HSC niche that could be modulated through PTH and other molecular mechanisms that are incompletely defined so far. Osteoblasts are the main targets of PTH/PTHrP, and PTH/PTHrp also has some modulating potential on HSC via osteoblasts. PTH may increase the proportion of bone marrow-derived stromal cells (BMC) that commit to the osteoblastic lineage both in vitro and in vivo, thus expanding the osteoblast pool. Furthermore, PTH induces osteoblasts to express BMP, SDF-1, VEGF, osteopontin and activate signaling pathways involved in the HSC niche. It has been demonstrated that PTH expands the HSC pool through activation of the PTH-1R on osteoblasts. The Jagged1/Notch signaling pathway is implicated in the control of stem cell self-renewal in several organs, and is necessary for PTH-dependent HCS expansion (Calvi 2006). PPR activation by the Notch ligand Jagged-1 in osteoblasts is associated with an increase in the number of HSC, and this increase can be stopped by administration of a secretase inhibitor. The same effects can be achieved by using exogenous PTH (Calvi 2006). Furthermore, PTH (as well as other stress conditions including inflammation, injury or chemotherapy) could result in a destabilization of HSC with induction of massive stem mobilization. Accordingly, osteoclast activity has been demonstrated to promote the proliferation and mobilization of hematopoietic progenitors from HCS. Bone resorbing osteoclasts secrete enzymes, including MMP-9 and cathepsin K that give them SDF-1 and osteopontin degradation capacity (Kollt et al. 2006). Therefore, PTH could impact both bone turnover and the bone marrow niche through modulation of osteoblast and osteoclast activity, resulting in improved engraftment both of HSC and cancer stem cells. It is notable that the majority of the signaling pathways involved in the interaction between normal stem cells and their niche are also involved in the interaction between cancer stem cells and their niche.

References

Adami S, Bertoldo F, Braga S et al (2009) 25-hydroxy vitamin D levels in healthy premenopausal women: association with bone turnover markers and bone mineral density. Bone 45:423–426

Adams GB (2005) Stem cell engraftment at the endosteal niche is specified by the Calcium sensing receptor. Nature 439:599–603

Aldridge SE, Lennard TW, Williams JR et al (2005) Vascular endothelial growth factor acts as an osteolytic factor in breast cancer metastases to bone. Br J Cancer 92:1531–1537

Al-Hajj M, Wicha MS, Benito-Hernandez A et al (2003) Prospective identification of tumorigenic breast cancer cells. Proc Natl Acad Sci USA 100:3983–3988

Almquist M, Manjer J, Bondenson L et al (2007) Serum calcium and breast cancer risk: results from a prospective cohort study of 7, 847 women. Cancer Cause Control 18:595–602

Alonso V, deGortazar AR, Ardura JA (2008) Parathyroid hormone related protein increases human osteoblastic cell survival by activation of vascular endothelial factor receptor-2. J Cell Physiol 217:717–727

Arai F, Hirao A, Ohmura M et al (2004) Tie2/angiopoietin -1 signaling regulates hematopoietic stem cell quiescence in the bone marrow niche. Cell 18:149–161

Artavanis-Tsakonas S, Rand MD, Lake RJ (1999) Notch signaling: cell fate control and signal integration in development. Science 284:770–776

Arya M, Ahmed H, Silhi N et al (2007) Clinical importance and therapeutic implications of the pivotal CXCL12-CXCR4 (chemokine ligand-receptor) interaction in cancer cell migration. Tumour Biol 28(3):123–131

Asou Y, Rittling SR, Yoshitake H et al (2001) Osteopontin facilitates angiogenesis, accumulation of osteoclasts, and resorption in ectopic bone. Endocrinology 142:969–973

Attia S, Eickhoff J, Wilding G et al (2008) Randomized double blinded phase II evaluation of docetaxel with or without doxecalciferol in patients with metastatic androgen independent prostate cancer. Clin Canc Res 14:2437–2443

Bao BY, Yao J, Lee YF (2006) Alpha 25hydroxyvitamin D3 suppresses interleukin-8-mediated prostate cancer cell angiogenesis. Carcinogenesis 247:122–129

Bertolini G, Roz L, Perego P (2009) Highly tumorigenic lung cancer CD133+ cells display stem-like features and are spared by cisplatin treatment. Proc Natl Acad Sci USA 106(38):16281–16286

Bleul CC, Fuhlbrigge RC, Casasnovas JM (1996) A highly efficacious lymphocyte chemoattractant, stromal cell-derived factor 1 (SDF-1). J Exp Med 184(3):1101–1109

Blokzijl A, Dahlqvist C, Reissmann E (2003) Cross-talk between the Notch and TGF-beta signaling pathways mediated by interaction of the Notch intracellular domain with Smad3. J Cell Biol 163(4):723–728

Bonnet D, Dick JE (1997) Human acute myeloid leukaemia is organised as a hierarchy that originates from a primitive hematopoietic cell. Nat Med 3:730–737

Bouilon E et al (2006) Vitamin D and cancer. J Steroid Biochem Mol Biol 102:156–162

Boyce BF, Xing L, Shakespeare W et al (2003) Regulation of bone remodelling and emerging breakthrough drugs for osteoporosis and osteolytic bone metastases. Kidney Int Suppl 85:S2–S5

Brown J, Corey E, Lee Z et al (2001a) Osteoprotegerin and rank ligand expression in prostate cancer. Urology 57:611–616

Brown JM, Vessella RL, Kostenuik PJ et al (2001b) Serum osteoprotegerin levels are increased in patients with advanced prostate cancer. Clin Cancer Res 7(10):2977–2983

Bryden AAG, Hoyland JA, Freemong AJ et al (2002) Parathyroid hormone relate peptide and receptor expression in paired primary prostate cancer and bone metastases. Br J Cancer 86:322–325

Bunyaratavej P, Hullinger TG, Somerman MJ (2000) Bone morphogenetic proteins secreted by breast cancer cells upregulate bone sialoprotein expression in preosteoblast cells. Exp Cell Res 260:324–333

Burtis WJ, Wu T, Bunch C, Wysolmerski J et al (1987) Identification of a novel 17,000-dalton parathyroid hormone-like adenylate cyclase-stimulating protein from a tumor associated with humoral hypercalcemia of malignancy. J Biol Chem 262(15):7151–7156

Calvi L (2006) Osteoblastic activation in the hematopoietic stem cell niche. Ann NY Acad 1068:477–488

Calvi LM, Adams GB, Weibrecht KW et al (2003) Osteoblastic cells regulate the hematopoietic stem cell niche. Nature 425:841–846

Campbell MJ, Elstner E, Holden S et al (1997) Inhibition of proliferation of prostate cancer cells by a 19-norhexafluoride vitamin D 3 analogue involves the induction of p21 waf1p27 kip 1 and E-cadherin. J Mol Endocrinol 19:15–27

Campbell MJ, Gombart AF, Kwok SH et al (2000) The antiproliferative effects of 1alpha 25(OH)D on breast and prostate cancer cell are associated with induction of BRCA1 gene expression. Oncogene 19:5091–5097

Canon JR, Roudier M, Bryant R et al (2008) Inhibition of RANKL blocks skeletal tumor progression and improves survival in a mouse model of breast cancer bone metastasis. Clin Exp Metastasis 25(2):119–129

Casimiro S, Guise A, Chirgwin J (2009) The critical role of bone microenvironment in cancer metastasis. Mol Cell Endocrinol 310:71–81

Catz SD, Johnoston JL (2001) Transcriptional regulation of BCL-2 by nuclear factor kappa and its significance in prostate cancer. Oncogene 41:3283–3294

Chan JS, Beer TM, Quin DI et al (2008) A phase II study of high dose calcitriol combined with mitoxantrone and prednisone for androgen.indipendent prostate cancer. BJU Int 102:1601–1606

Chen G, Sircar K, Aprikian A et al (2006) Expression of RANKL/RANK/OPG in primary and metastatic human prostate cancer as markers of disease stage and functional regulation. Cancer 107:289–298

Cheney IW, Johnson DE, Vaillancourt MT et al (1998) Suppression of tumorigenicity of glioblastoma cells by adenovirus-mediated MMAC1/PTEN gene transfer. Cancer Res 58(11):2331–2334

Chenn A, Walsh CA (2002) Regulation of cerebral cortical size by control of cell cycle exit in neural precursors. Science 297:365–369

Chiao JW, Moonga BS, Yang YM et al (2000) Endothelin-1 from prostate cancer cells is enhanced by bone contact which blocks osteoclastic bone resorption. Br J Cancer 83:360–365

Chlebowski RT, Jhonson KC, Kooperberger C et al (2008) Calcium plus vitamin D supplementation and the risk of breast cancer. J Natl Cancer Inst 100:1581–1591

Chung I, Han G, Seshadri M et al (2009) Role of vitamin D receptor in the proliferative effects of cacitriol in tumor derived endothelial cells and tumor angiogenesis in vivo. Cancer Res 69:967–975

Collins AT, Berry PA, Hyde C et al (2005) Prospective identification of tumorigenic prostate cancer stem cells. Cancer Res 65:10946–10951

Coyle D, McNeill RE, Hennessy E (2006) Calcium sensing receptor gene expression and breast to bone metastases. Br J Surg 93:898

Crew KD, Shane E, Cremers S et al (2009) High prevalence of vitamin D deficiency despite supplementation in premenopausal women with breast cancer undergoing adjuvant chemotherapy. J Clin Oncol 27:2151–2156

Cross SS, Harrison RF, Balasubramanian SP et al (2006) Expression of receptor activator of nuclear factor kappabeta ligand (RANKL) and tumour necrosis factor related, apoptosis inducing ligand (TRAIL) in breast cancer, and their relations with osteoprotegerin, oestrogen receptor, and clinicopathological variables. J Clin Pathol 59(7):716–720

Cui Y, Rohan TE (2006) Vitamin D, calcium and breast cancer risk: a review. Canc Epidemiol Biomarkers Prev 15:1427–1437

Dahmane N, Lee J, Robins P et al (1997) Activation of the transcription factor Gli1 and the Sonic hedgehog signalling pathway in skin tumours. Nature 389(6653):876–881

Dai J, Kitagawa Y, Zhang J et al (2004) Vascular endothelial growth factors contributes to the prostate cancer-induced osteoblast differentiation mediated by bone morphogentic protein. Cancer Res 64:994–999

De Palma M, Murdoch C, Venneri MA et al (2007) Tie2-expressing monocytes: regulation of tumor angiogenesis and therapeutic implications. Trends Immunol 28:519–524

Deftos LJ, Barken I, Burton DW (2005) Direct evidences that PTHrp expression promotes prostate cancer progression in bone. Biochem Biophys Res Commun 327:468–472

Derynck R, Akhurst RJ, Balmain A (2001) TGF-b signaling in tumor suppression and cancer progression. Nat Genet 29:117–129

Dougall WC, Chaisson M (2006) The RANK/RANKL/OPG triad in cancer-induced bone diseases. Cancer Metastasis Rev 25:541–549

Emery JG, McDonnell P, Burke MB et al (1998) Osteoprotegerin is a receptor for the cytotoxic ligand TRAIL. J Biol Chem 273:14363–14367

Eriksen EF, Eghbali-Fatourechi GZ, Klosha S (2007) Remodeling and vascular space in bone. J Bone Miner Res 22:1–6

Erler JT, Giaccia AJ (2006) Lysyl oxidase mediates hypoxic control of metastasis. Cancer Res 66(21):10238–10241

Erler JT, Bennewith KL, Cox TR et al (2009) Hypoxia-induced lysyl oxidase is a critical mediator of bone marrow cell recruitment to form the premetastatic niche. Cancer Cell 15:35–44

Esbrit P, Alvarez-Arroyo MV, DeMiguel F et al (2000) C-terminal parathyroid hormone-related protein increases vascular endothelial growth factor in human osteoblastci cell. J Am Soc Nephrol 11:1085–1092

Fata JE, Kong YY, Li J et al (2000) The osteoclast differentiation factor osteoprotegerin ligand is essential for mammary gland development. Cell 103:41–50

Ferrara N (2009) Vascular endothelial growth factor. Arterioscler Thromb Vasc Biol 29(6): 789–791

Flaig TW, Barqawi A, Miller G et al (2006) A phase II trail of dexamethasone, vitamin D, and carboplatin in patients with hormone refractory prostate cancer. Cancer 107:266–274

Folkman J (1995) Angiogenesis in cancer, vascular, rheumatoid and other disease. Nat Med 1:27–31

Gerritsen ME, Peale FV, Wu T (2002) Gene expression profiling in silico: relative expression of candidate angiogenesis associated genes in renal cell carcinomas. Exp Nephrol 10:114–119

Glinsky VV, Glinsky GV, Rittenhouse-Olson K et al (2001) The role Thomsen-Friedenreich antigen in adhesion of human breast and prostate cancer cells to the endothelium. Cancer Res 61:4851–4857

Gocek E, Studzinski GP (2009) Vitamin D and differentiation in cancer. Crit Rev Clin Lab Sci 46:190. doi:10.1080/10408360902982128

Grill V, Ho P, Body JJ et al (1991) Parathyroid hormone-relate protein: elevated levels in both humoral hypercalcemia and hypercalcemia complicating metastatic breast cancer. J Clin Endocrinol Metab 73:1309–1315

Guise TA, Yin JJ, Mohammad KS (2003) Role of endothelin-1 in osteoblastic bone metastases. Cancer 97(3):779–784

Hagemann T (2005) Macrophages induce invasiveness of epithelial cancer cells via NF-κB and JNK. J Immunol 175:1197–1205

Harada S, Rodan GA (2003) Control of osteoblast function and regulation of bone mass. Nature 423:349–355

Hauschka PV, Mavrakos AE, Iafrati MD et al (1986) Growth factors in bone matrix. J Biol Chem 261:12665–12674

Heissig B, Hattori K, Dias S et al (2002) Recruitment of stem and progenitor cells from the bone marrow niche requires MMP-9 mediated release of kit-ligand. Cell 109:625–637

Henderson MA, Danks JA, Slavin JL et al (2006) Parathyroid hormone-related protein localization in breast cancers predict improved prognosis. Cancer Res 66:7402–7411

Hofbauer L, Rachner T, Singh S (2008) Fatal attraction: why breast cancer cells home to bone. Breast Cancer Res 10:101

Holen I, Croucher PI, Hamdy FC et al (2002) Osteoprotegerin is a survival factor for human prostate cancer cells. Cancer Res 62:1619–1623

Holen I, Cross SS, Neville-Webbe HL et al (2005) Osteoprotegerin expression by breast cancer cells in vitro and breast tumours in vivo—a role in tumour cell survival? Breast Cancer Res Treat 92:207–215

Holick MF, Chen TC (2008) Vitamin D deficiency: a world wide problem with health consequences. Am J Clin Nutr 87:1080S–1086S

Hughes DP (2009) How the NOTCH pathway contributes to the ability of osteosarcoma cells to metastasize. Cancer Treat Res 152:479–496

Hugo H, Ackland ML, Blick T et al (2007) Epithelial-mesenchymal and mesenchymal-epithelial transitions in carcinoma progression. J Cell Physiol 213:374–383

Hullinger TG, Pan Q, Viswanathan HL (2001) TGFbeta and BMP-2 activation of the OPN promoter: roles of smad- and hox-binding elements. Exp Cell Res 262(1):69–74

Isowa A, Shimo T, Ibaragi S et al (2010) PTHrP regulates angiogenesis and bone resorption via VEGF expression. Anticancer Res 30:2755–2768

Ite H, Yoshida T, Matsumoto N, Aoki K, Osada Y, Sugimura T, Terada M (1997) Growth regulation of human prostate cancer cells by bone morphogenetic protein-2. Cancer Res 57:5022–5027

Iwasaki H, Suda T (2009) Cancer stem cell and their niche. Cancer Sci 100:1166–1172

Javed A, Barnes GL, Pratap J et al (2005) Impaired intranuclear trafficking of Runx2 (AML3/CBFA1) transcription factors in breast cancer cells inhibits osteolysis in vivo. Proc Natl Acad Sci USA 102:1454–1459

Jones DH, Nakashima T, Sanchez OH et al (2006) Regulation of cancer cell migration and bone metastasis by RANKL. Nature 440:692–696

Jung Y, Wang J, Schneider A (2006) Regulation of SDF-1 (CXCL12) production by osteoblasts a possible mechanism for stem cell homing. Bone 38:497

Kagan HM, Li W (2003) Lysyl oxidase: properties, specificity, and biological roles inside and outside of the cell. J Cell Biochem 88:660–672

Kaplan RN, Riba RD, Zacharoulis S et al (2005) VEGFR1-positive haematopoietic bone marrow progenitors initiate the pre-metastatic niche. Nature 438(7069):820–827

Kinzler KW, Vogelstein B (1996) Lessons from hereditary colorectal cancer. Cell 87:159–170

Kirschmann DA, Seftor EA, Fong SF et al (2002) A molecular role for lysyl oxidase in breast cancer invasion. Cancer Res 62:4478–4483

Kitano Y, Kurihara H, Kurihara Y et al (1998) Gene expression of bone matrix proteins and endothelin receptors in endothelin-1-deficient mice revealed by in situ hybridization. J Bone Miner Res 13:237–244

Kitten AM, Harvey SA, Criscimagna N et al (1997) Osteogenic protein-1 downregulates endothelin A receptors in primary rat osteoblasts. Am J Physiol 272((6 Pt 1)):E967–E975

Kleeberger W, Bova GS, Nielsen ME, Epstein JI, Berman DM et al (2007) Roles for the stem cell associated intermediate filament Nestin in prostate cancer migration and metastasis. Cancer Res 67:9199–9206

Knerr K, Ackermann K, Neidhart T et al (2004) Bone metastasis: osteoblasts affect growth and adhesion regulons in prostate tumor cells and provoke osteomimicry. Int J Cancer 11:152–159

Koch H, Jadlowiec JA, Campbell PG (2005) Insulin-like growth factor-I induces early osteoblast gene expression in human mesenchymal stem cells. Stem Cells Dev 14:621–631

Kollett O, Dar A, Schvtiel S et al (2006) Osteoclasts degrade endosteal components and promote mobilization of hematopoietic progenitor cells. Nat Med 12:657–664

Kollt O, Dar A, Shivtiel S et al (2006) Osteoclasts degradate endosteal components and promote mobilization of hematopoietic progenitor cells. Nature Med 12:657–664

Kostenuik PJ, Nguyen HQ, McCabe J et al (2009) Denosumab, a fully human monoclonal antibody to RANKL, inhibits bone resorption and increases BMD in knock-in mice that express chimeric (murine/human) RANKL. J Bone Miner Res 24:182–195

Kunnimalaiyaan M, Chen H (2007) Tumor suppressor role of Notch-1 signaling in neuroendocrine tumors. Oncologist 12:535–542

Lacey DL, Timms E, Tan HL et al (1998) Osteoprotegerin ligand is a cytokine that regulates osteoclast differentiation and activation. Cell 93:165–176

Lapidot T, Sirard C, Vormoor J et al (1994) A cell initiating human acute myeloid leukaemia after transplantation into SCID mice. Nature 367:645–648

Lappe JM, Travers-Gustafson D, Davies KM et al (2007) Vitamin D and calcium supplementation reduces cancer risk:results of a randomized trial. Am J Clin Nutr 85:1586–1591

Li G, Cui Y, McIlmmuray L et al (2005) rhBMP2, rhVEGF (165), rhPTN and thrombin related peptide, TP 508 induce chemotaxis of human osteoblasts and microvascular endothelial cells. J Ortop Res 23:680–685

Li X, Huang M, Zheng H, Wang Y (2008) CHIP promotes Runx2 degradation and negatively regulates osteoblast differentiation. J Cell Biol 181(6):959–972

Liang Z, Wu T, Lou H et al (2004) Inhibition of breast cancer metastasis by selective synthetic polypeptide against CXCR4. Cancer Res 64:4302–4308

Liao J, Li X, Koh AJ et al (2008) Tumor expressed PTHrP facilitates prostate cancer-induced osteoblastic lesions. Int J Cancer 123(10):2267–2278

Lyden D, Young AZ, Zagzag D et al (1999) Id1 and Id3 are required for neurogenesis, angiogenesis and vascularization of tumour xenografts. Nature 401:670–677

Ma Q, Jones D, Borghesani PR et al (1998) Impaired B-lymphopoiesis, myelopoiesis, and derailed cerebellar neuron migration in CXCR4- and SDF-1-deficient mice. Proc Natl Acad Sci USA 95(16):9448–9453

Makuch LA, Sosnoski DM, Gay CV (2006) Osteoblast-conditioned media influence the expression of E-selectin on bone-derived vascular endothelial cells. J Cell Biochem 98:1221–1229

Mantovani A, Schioppa T, Porta C et al (2006) Role of tumor-associated macrophages in tumor progression and invasion. Cancer Metastasis Rev 25(3):315–322

Matthews D, LaPorta E, Zinser GM et al (2010) Genomic vitamin D signalling in breast cancer: insights from animal models and human cells. J Steroid Biochem Mol Biol 121:36–367

McGrath CM, Soule HD et al (1984) Calcium regulation of normal human mammary epithelial cell growth in culture. In Vitro 20:625–662

Merryman JI, DeWille JW, Werkmeister JR et al (1994) Effects of transforming growth factor-β on parathyroid hormone-related protein production and ribonucleic acid expression by a squamous carcinoma cell line in vitro. Endocrinology 134:2424–2430

Miettinen PJ, Ebner R, Lopez AR, Derynck R (1994) TGF-b induced transdifferentiation of mammary epithelial cells to mesenchymal cells: involvement of type I receptors. J Cell Biol 127:2021–2036

Mihai M (2008) The calcium sensing receptor: from understanding parathyroid calcium homeostasis to bone metastasis. Ann R Coll Sur Engl 90:271–277

Min JK, Kim JM et al (2003) Vascular endothelial growth factor up-regulates expression of receptor activator of NF-kappaB (RANK) in endothelial cells. Concomitant increase of angiogenic response to RANK ligand. J Biol Chem 278:39548–39557

Moseley JM, Kubota M, Diefenbach-Jagger H et al (1987) Parathyroid hormone-related protein purified from a human lung cancer cell line. Proc Natl Acad Sci USA 84:5048–5052

Muller A, Homey B, Soto H et al (2001) Involvement of chemokine receptors in breast cancer metastasis. Nature 410:50–56

Murdoch C, Muthana M, Coffelt SB et al (2008) The role of myeloid cells in the promotion of tumour angiogenesis. Nature Rev Cancer 8:618–631

Nakagawa M, Kaneda T, Arakawa T et al (2000) Vascular endothelial growth factor (VEF^GF) directly enhances osteoclastic bone resorption and survival of mature osteoclast. FEBS Lett 473:161–164

Nefedova Y, Cheng P, Alsina M (2004) Involvement of Notch-1 signaling in bone marrow stroma-mediated de novo drug resistance of myeloma and other malignant lymphoid cell lines. Blood 103(9):3503–3510

Nelson JB, Hedican SP, George DJ et al (1995) Identification of endothelin-1 in the pathophysiology of metastatic adenocarcinoma of the prostate. Nat Med 1:944–949

Nelson JB, Nguyen SH, Wu-Wong JR et al (1999) New bone formation in an osteoblastic tumor model is increased by endothelin-1 overexpression and decreased by endothelin A receptor blockade. Urology 53(5):1063–1069

Nobta M, Tsukazaki T, Shibata Y et al (2005) Critical regulation of bone morphogenetic protein-induced osteoblastic differentiation by Delta1/Jagged1-activated notch1 signaling. J Biol Chem 280(16):15842–15848

Noda M, Rodan GA (1989) Transcriptional regulation of osteopontin production in rat osteoblast-like cells by parathyroid hormone. J Cell Biol 08(1):713–718

O'Brien CA, Pollet A, Gallinger S et al (2007) A human colon cancer cell capable of initiating tumour growth in immunodeficient mice. Nature 445:106–110

Oh HS, Moharita A, Potian JG et al (2004) Bone marrow stroma influences tranforming growth factor-beta production production in breast cancer cells to regulate c-myc activation of the preprotachykinin-I gene in breast cancer cells. Cancer Res 64:6327–6336

Pardal R, Clark MF, Morrison SJ (2003) Applying the principals of stem-cell biology to cancer. Nat Rev Cancer 3:895–902

Patrawala L, Calhoun T, Schneider-Broussard R et al (2006) Highly purified CD44+ prostate cancer cells from xenograft human tumors are enriched in tumorigenic and metastatic progenitor cells. Oncogene 25:1696–1708

Pecheur I, Peyruchaud O, Serre CM et al (2002) Integrin $\alpha v \beta 3$ expression confers on tumor cells a greater propensity to metastasixe to bone. FASEB J 16:1266–1268

Pepe J, Romagnoli E, Nofroni I et al (2006) Vitamin D status as the major factor determining the circulating levels of parathyroid hormone: a study in normal subjects. Osteopor Int 16:805–812

Peterlik M, Grant WB, Cross HS (2009) Calcium, vitamin D and cancer. Anticancer Res 29:3687–3698

Pfeilschifter J, Mundy GR (1987) Modulation of transforming growth factor β activity in bone cultures by osteotropic hormones. Proc Natl Acad Sci USA 84:2024–2028

Phadke PA, Mercer R, Harms JF (2006) Kinetics of metastatic breast cancer cell trafficking bone. Clin Cancer Res 12(5):1431–1440

Piek E, Moustakas A, Kurisaki A et al (1999) TGF-b type I receptor/ALK-5 and Smad proteins mediate epithelial to mesenchymal transdifferentiation in NMuMG breast epithelial cells. J Cell Sci 112:4557–4568

Polakis P (1999) The oncogenic activation of β-catenin. Curr Opin Genet Dev 9:15–21

Pollard JW (2009) Trophic macrophages in development and disease. Nat Rev Immunol 9(4):259–270

Ponomariov T, Peled A, Petit I et al (2000) Induction of the chemokines stromal-derived factor-1 following DNA damage improves human stem cell functions. J Clin Invest 106:1331–1339

Powell GJ, Southby J, Danks JA et al (1991) Localization of parathyroid hormone-related protein in breast cancer metastasis: increased incidence in bone compared with other sites. Cancer Res 51:3059–3061

Powell SM, Zilz N, Beazer-Barclay Y et al (1992) APC mutations occur early during colorectal tumorigenesis. Nature 359:235–237

Prince CW, Butler WT (1987) 1, 25-Dihydroxyvitamin D3 regulates the biosintheis of osteopontin, a bone-derived cell attachment protein, in clonal osteoblast-like osteosarcoma cells. Coll Relat Res 7:305–313

Proweller A, Tu L, Lepore JJ et al (2006) Impaired notch signaling promotes de novo squamous cell carcinoma formation. Cancer Res 66:7438–7444

Pukrop T, Klemm F, Hagemann TH et al (2006) Wnt 5a signaling is critical for macrophage-induced invasion of breast cancer cell lines. Proc Natl Acad Sci USA 103:5454–5459

Radtke F, Raj K (2003) The role of Notch in tumorigenesis: oncogene or tumour suppressor? Nat Rev Cancer 3:756–767

Raimondi S, Johansson H, Maisonneuve P et al (2009) Review and meta-analysis on vitamin D receptor polymorphisms and cancer risk. Carcinogenesis 30:1170–1180

Ramaswamy S, Ross KN, Lander ES et al (2003) A molecular signature of metastasis in primary solid tumors. Nat Genet 33:49–54

IARC Working Group Reports (2008) IARC vitamin D and cancer, vol 5. International Agency for Research on Cancer

Ritchie CK, Andrews LR, Thomas KG et al (1997a) The effects of growth factors associated with osteoblasts on prostate carcinoma proliferation and chemotaxis: implications for the development of metastatic disease. Endocrinology 138:1145–1150

Ritchie CK, Thomas KG, Andrews LR et al (1997b) Effects of the calciotrophic peptides calcitonin and PTH on prostate growth and chemotaxis. Prostate 30:183–187

Rodland KD (2004) The role of the calcium-sensing receptor in cancer. Cell Calcium 35(3):291–295

Rubin J, Chung LW, Fan X et al (2004) Prostate carcinoma cells that have resided in bone have an upregulated IGF-I axis. Prostate 58:41–49

Rucci N, Recchia I, Angelucci A et al (2006) Inhibition of protein kinase c-Src reduces the incidence of breast cancer metastases and increases survival in mice: implication for therapy. J Pharmacol Exp Ther 318:161–172

Ruiz i Altaba A, Sánchez P, Dahmane N (2002) Gli and hedgehog in cancer: tumours, embryos and stem cells. Nat Rev Cancer 2(5):361–372

Santini D, Perrone G, Roato I et al (2010a) Expression pattern of receptor activator of NFκB (RANK) in a series of primary solid tumors and related bone metastases. J Cell Physiol 226:780–784

Santini D, Vincenzi B, Russo A et al. (2010b) Association of receptor activator of NF-kb (RANK) expression with bone metastasis in breast carcinomas. ASCO 2010 abstract 1053

Sasaki T, Hong MH (1993) Endothelin-1 localization in bone cells and vascular endothelial cells in rat bone marrow. Anat Rec 237:332–337

Sasaki A, Ishikawa K, Haraguchi N et al (2007) Receptor activator of nuclear factor-kappaB ligand (RANKL) expression in hepatocellular carcinoma with bone metastasis. Ann Surg Oncol 14(3):1191–1199

Schnieder A, Kalikin LM, Mattos AC (2005) Bone turnover mediates preferential localization of prostate cancer in the skeleton. Endocrinology 146:1727–1736

Schwalbe M, Sanger J, Eggers R et al (2003) Differential expression and regulation of bone morphogenetic protein 7 in breast cancer. Int J Oncol 23:89–95

Schwaninger R, Rentsch CA, Wetterwald A, van der Horst G, van Bezooijen RL, van der Pluijm G, Lowik CW, Ackermann K, Pyerin W, Hamdy FC et al (2007) Lack of noggin expression by cancer cells is a determinant of the osteoblast response in bone metastases. Am J Pathol 170:160–175

Schwartz GG (2008) Prostate cancer, serum parathyroid hormone and the progression of skeletal metastases. Canc Epidemiol Biomarkers Prev 17:478–483

Shimoyama A, Wada M, Ikeda F et al (2007) Ihh/Gli2 signaling promotes osteoblast differentiation by regulating Runx2 expression and function. Mol Biol Cell 18:2411–2418

Shioide M, Noda M (1993) Endothelin modulates osteopontin and osteocalcin messenger ribonucleic acid expression in rat osteoblastic osteosarcoma cells. J Cell Biochem 53:176–180

Shipitsin M, Polyak K (2008) The cancer stem cell hypothesis: in search of definitions, markers and relevance. Lab Invest 88:459–463

Shipitsin M, Campbell LL, Argani P et al (2007) Molecular definition of breast tumor heterogeneity. Cancer Cell 11:69–82

Shmelkov SV, Butler JM, Hooper AT et al (2008) CD133 expression is not restricted to stem cells, and both CD133+ and CD133− metastatic colon cancer cells initiate tumors. J Clin Invest 118:2111–2120

Sing SK (2003) Identification of a cancer stem cell in human brain tumours. Cancer Res 63: 5821–5828

Southby J, Kissin MW, Danks JA et al (1990) Immunohistochemical localization of parathyroid hormone-related protein in breast cancer. Cancer Res 50:7710–7716

Spinella F, Rosanò L, Di Castro V et al (2003) Endothelin-1 decreases gap junctional intercellular communication by inducing phosphorylation of connexin 43 in human ovarian carcinoma cells. J Biol Chem 278(42):41294–41301

Spinella-Jaegle S, Rawadi G, Kawai S et al (2001) Sonic hedgehog increases the commitment of pluripotent mesenchymal cells into the osteoblastic lineage and abolishes adipocytic differentiation. J Cell Sci 114:2085–2094

Stern PH, Tatrai A, Semler DE et al (1995) Endothelin receptors, second messengers, and actions in bone. J Nutr 125(Suppl):2028S–2032S

Street J, Bao M, deGuzman L et al (2002) Vascular endothelial growth factor stimulates bone repair by promoting angiogenesis and bone turnover. Proc Natl Acad Sci USA 99:9656–9661

Strewler GJ, Stern P, Jacobs J, Eveloff J, Klein RF, Leung SC et al (1987) Parathyroid hormone-like protein from human renal carcinoma cells structural and functional homology with parathyroid hormone. J Clin Invest 80:1803–1807

Sugiyama T, Kohara H, Noda M et al (2006) Maintainance of the hematopoietic stem cell pool by CXCL12-CXCR4 chemokine signalling in bone marrow stromal cell niches. Immunity 25:977–988

Sun YX, Shelburne CE, Lopatin DE et al (2003) The expression of CXCR4 and CXCL12 (SDF-1) in human prostate camncers in vivo. J Cell Biochem 89:462–473

Sun YX, Schneider A, Jung Y et al (2005) Skeletal localization and neutralization of the SDF1 (CXCL12)/CXCR4 axis blocks prostate cancer metastasis and growth in osseus sites in vivo. J Bone Miner Res 20:318–329

Tombran-Tink J, Barnstable CJ (2004) Osteoblasts and osteoclasts express PEDF, VEGF-A isoforms, and VEGF receptors: possible mediators of angiogenesis and matrix remodelling in the bone. Biochem Biophys Res Commun 316:573–579

Tretli S, Hernes E, Berg JP (2009) Association between serum 25(OH)D and death from prostate cancer. Br J Canc 100:450–454

Trump DL, Potter DM, Muindi J et al (2006) Phase II trial of high dose intermittent calcitriol and dexamethasone in androgen independent prostate cancer. Cancer 106:2136–2142

Trump DL, Chadha MK, Sunga AY et al (2009) Vitamin D deficiency and insufficiency among patients with prostate cancer. BJU Int 104:909–914

Tuck AB, Hota C, Wilson SM et al (2003) Osteopontin-induced migration of human mammary epithelial cells involves activation of EGF receptor and multiple signal transduction pathways. Oncogene 22:1198–1205

Valcourt U, Kowanetz M, Niimi H et al (2005) TGF-β and the Smad signaling pathway support transcriptomic reprogramming during epithelial-mesenchymal cell transition. Mol Biol Cell 16:1987–2002

van Dijke P, Yamashita H, Sampath TK, Reddi AH, Estevex M, Riddle DL, Ichijo H, Heldin CH, Miyazono K (1994) Identification of type I receptors for osteogenic protein-1 and bone morphogenetic protein-4. J Biol Chem 269:16985–16988

Vargas SJ, Gillespie MT, Powell GJ et al (1992) Localization of parathyroid hormone-related protein mRNA expression and metastatic lesions by in situ hybridization. J Bone Miner Res 7(8):971–980

Wai PY, Kuo PC (2004) The role of osteopontin in tumor metastasis. J Surg Res 121:228–241

Wiesner C, Nabha SM, Dos Santos EB et al (2008) C-kit and its ligand stem cell factor: potential contribution to prostate cancer bone metastasis. Neoplasia 10:996–1003

Wu JY, Scadden DT, Kronenberg M (2009) Role of the osteoblast lineage in the bone marrow hematopoietic niches. J Bone Min Res 24:759–763

Wyckoff JB (2007) Direct visualization of macrophageassisted tumor cell intravasation in mammary tumors. Cancer Res 67:2649–2656

Xie Y, Yin T, Wiegraebe W et al (2009) Detection of functional haematopoietic stem cell niche using real-time imaging. Nature 457:97–101

Xu J, Lamouille S, Derynck R (2009) TGF-beta-induced epithelial to mesenchymal transition. Cell Res 19(2):156–172

Yates AJ, Gutierrez GE, Smolens P et al (1988) Effects of a synthetic peptide of a parathyroid hormone-related protein on calcium homeostasis, renal tubular calcium reabsorption, and bone metabolism in vivo and in vitro in rodents. J Clin Invest 81:932–938

Yin T, Li L et al (2006) The stem cell niche in bone. J Clin Invest 116:1195–1201

Yin L, Raum E, Haug U et al (2009) Meta-analysis of longitudinal studies: serum vitamin D and prostate cancer risk. Cancer Epidem 33:435–445

Yin L, Grandi N, Raum E et al (2010) Meta-analysis: serum vitamin D and breast cancer risk. Eu J Cancer 46:2196–2205

Yu XF, Collin-Osdoby P, Osdoby P (2003a) SDF-1 increases recruitment of osteoclast precursors by upregulation of matrix metalloproteinase 9 activity. Connect Tissue Res 44:79–84

Yu XF, Huang YF, Collin-Osdoby P et al (2003b) Stromal cell derived factor 1 (SDF-1) recruits osteoclast precursors by inducing chemotaxis, matrix metalloproteinase 9 (MMP9) activity, and collagen transmigration. J Bone Miner Res 18(8):1404–1418

Yucha C, Guthrie D (2003) Renal homeostasis of calcium. Nephrol Nurs J 30:755–764

Zakalik D, Diep D, Hooks MA et al (1992) Transforming growth factor β increases stability of parathyroid hormone-related protein messenger RNA. J Bone Miner Res 7(Suppl 1): 104A, S118

Zavadil J, Cermak L, Soto-Nieveset N et al (2004) Integration of TGF-beta/Smad and Jagged1/Notch signalling in epithelial-to-mesenchymal transition. EMBO J 23(5):1155–1165

Zeisberg M, Hanai J, Sugimoto H, Mammoto T, Charytan D, Strutz F, Kalluri R (2003) BMP-7 counteracts TGF-b1-induced epithelial-to-mesenchymal transition and reverses chronic renal injury. Nat Med 9:964–968

Zhang J, Dai J, Qi Y, Lin DL et al (2001) Osteoprotegerin inhibits prostate cancer-induced osteoclastogenesis and prevents prostate tumor growth in the bone. J Clin Invest 107(10):1235–1244

Zhang J, Grindley JC, Yin T et al (2006) PTEN maintains haematopoietic stem cells and acts in lineage choice and leukaemia prevention. Nature 441:518–522

Zhang XH, Wang Q, Gerald W et al (2009) Latent bone metastasis in breast cancer tied to Src-dependent survival signals. Cancer Cell 16:67–78

Zheng H, Fu G, Dai T, Huang H (2007) Migration of endothelial progenitor cells mediated by stromal cell-derived factor-1alpha/CXCR4 via PI3 K/Akt/eNOS signal transduction pathway. J Cardiovasc Pharmacol 50(3):274–280

Zhou J, Wulfkuhle J, Zhang H et al (2007) Activation of the PTEN/mTOR/STAT3 pathway in breast cancer stem-like cells is required for viability and maintenance. Proc Natl Acad Sci USA 104(41):16158–16163

Zhu AJ, Watt FM (1999) β-catenin signalling modulates proliferative potential of human epidermal keratinocytes independently of intercellular adhesion. Development 126:2285–2298

Zunich SM, Douglas T, Valdovinos M, Chang T, Bushman W, Walterhouse D, Iannaccone P, Lamm ML (2009) Paracrine sonic hedgehog signalling by prostate cancer cells induces osteoblast differentiation. Mol Cancer 8:12

Bisphosphonates: Prevention of Bone Metastases in Breast Cancer

Michael Gnant, Peter Dubsky and Peyman Hadji

Abstract

Disease recurrence and distant metastases remain challenging for patients with breast cancer despite advances in early diagnosis, surgical expertise, and adjuvant therapy. Bone is the most common site for breast cancer metastasis, and the bone microenvironment plays a crucial role in harboring disseminated tumor cells (DTCs), a putative source of late relapse in and outside bone. Therefore, agents that affect bone metabolism might not only prevent the development of bone lesions but also provide meaningful reductions in the risk of relapse both in bone and beyond. Bisphosphonates bind to mineralized bone surfaces and are ingested by osteoclasts, wherein they inhibit osteolysis, thereby preventing the release of growth factors from the bone matrix. Therefore, the bone microenvironment becomes less conducive to survival and growth of DTCs and bone lesion formation. Recent trials of zoledronic acid in the adjuvant setting in breast cancer have demonstrated reduced disease recurrence in bone and other sites in premenopausal and postmenopausal women with early breast cancer. Based on the proven effect of bone protection during adjuvant endocrine therapy, new treatment guidelines recommend the routine use of bisphosphonates to prevent bone loss during adjuvant therapy, which may likely become the standard practice.

M. Gnant (✉) · P. Dubsky
Department of Surgery, Comprehensive Cancer Center Vienna,
Medical University of Vienna, Waehringer Guertel 18-20,
A-1090 Wien, Austria
e-mail: michael.gnant@meduniwien.ac.at

P. Hadji
Department of Gynecology, Gynecological Endocrinology and Oncology,
Philipps-University of Marburg, Marburg, Germany

Keywords

Adjuvant therapy · Anticancer · Bisphosphonate · Bone metastases · Breast cancer · Cancer prevention · Clodronate · Zoledronic acid

Abbreviations

ABCSG	Austrian Breast and Colorectal Cancer Study Group
AE	Adverse event
AI	Aromatase inhibitor
ANA	Anastrozole
BCINIS	Breast Cancer in Northern Israel Study
β-CTX	Beta C-terminal telopeptide of type I collagen
BM	Bone metastases
BMD	Bone mineral density
BP	Bisphosphonate
CI	Confidence interval
CLO	Clodronate
CTCs	Circulating tumor cells
CTIBL	Cancer treatment-induced bone loss
DFS	Disease-free survival
DTCs	Disseminated tumor cells
ER	Estrogen receptor
ESMO	European Society for Medical Oncology
HCM	Hypercalcemia of malignancy
HER2	Human epidermal growth factor receptor 2
HR	Hazard ratio
IBA	Ibandronate
LET	Letrozole
LN	Lymph node
NCIC CTG	National Cancer Institute of Canada Clinical Trials Group
NNT	Number needed to treat
NR	None reported
NS	Not significant
ONJ	Osteonecrosis of the jaw
OS	Overall survival
SRE	Skeletal-related events
TAM	Tamoxifen
VEGF	Vascular endothelial growth factor
WHI-OS	Women's Health Initiative Observational Study
Z-/ZO-/E-ZO-FAST	Zometa-Femara Adjuvant Synergy Trials
ZOL	Zoledronic acid

Contents

1	Introduction	67
2	Bone-Targeted Therapies for Breast Cancer	69
3	Anticancer Effects of Oral Bisphosphonates in Early Breast Cancer	70
	3.1 Oral Clodronate	70
	3.2 Oral Pamidronate	71
	3.3 Anticancer Benefits of Zoledronic Acid	72
	3.4 ABCSG-12	73
	3.5 ZO-FAST	74
	3.6 AZURE	74
	3.7 Is There a Subset of Patients More Likely to Benefit from ZOL Anticancer Effects?	76
	3.8 Neoadjuvant Therapy	78
	3.9 Further Data From Translational Studies in Early Breast Cancer	78
4	Can Bisphosphonates Prevent Cancer?	79
5	Tolerability and Safety of Bisphosphonates as Adjuvant Therapy	82
6	Other Uses of Antiresorptives in Women with Early Breast Cancer	84
7	Conclusions	84
References		85

1 Introduction

Despite progress in locoregional treatments resulting in a high rate of amelioration of all detectable traces of early breast cancer in patients, as well as progress in potent adjuvant therapy regimens, disease recurrence remains a challenge (Gerber et al. 2010). For example, early relapse has been reported in approximately 4.3% of women with successfully resected breast cancer during adjuvant tamoxifen therapy (rate peaks at 2 years postoperatively), and distant metastases (stage IV disease) account for approximately 75% of these early relapses (Baum et al. 2002; Mansell et al. 2009; Thurlimann et al. 2005). Distant recurrence is especially concerning given that, despite improvements in palliative treatment, cure is not possible after distant metastasis occurs (Lin et al. 2008; Rugo 2008). In general, survival rates for patients with breast cancer are directly correlated with disease stage, with 5-year survival rates decreasing from 98% for patients with localized disease (stage I and II) to 84% for stage III and to only 28% for patients with distant metastases from breast cancer (Garcia et al. 2007; Jemal et al. 2006). Therefore, identifying the source of the residual breast cancer and developing therapeutic strategies to target it and prevent its seeding of recurrent disease would provide important survival benefits. Bisphosphonates (BPs) are a class of bone-targeted agents that reduce rates of bone resorption (osteolysis) and have demonstrated promising anticancer potential. There is a growing body of clinical evidence supporting an expanded role for BPs not only as adjuvant therapy (Coleman 2011; Costa et al. 2011), but also—potentially—for preventing breast cancer. However, the relative contribution of the anticancer activities demonstrated by BPs in preclinical models (as described in Chaps. 1 and 7) in each of the cancer settings is unknown.

Even if the effects of BP therapy on the bone microenvironment were limited to effects on bone metastases (as described by Mundy et al. (2002) and discussed in Chap. 2), these effects could potentially lead to meaningful decreases in tumor burden and increases in survival (Diel et al. 2008). Bone is the most common site of distant metastasis in patients with breast cancer (Coleman 2001), and bone has many features that make it a fertile "soil" for the cancer "seed" (Paget 1889). Rates of osteoclast-mediated bone resorption can be substantially increased in patients with bone lesions from solid tumors (Clezardin 2005; Winter et al. 2008), and osteoclast-mediated osteolysis releases growth factors from within the bone matrix, thereby making the microenvironment more conducive to cancer cell proliferation (Guise and Mundy 1998).

Bisphosphonates, through blocking malignant osteolysis, prevent bone destruction and would be expected to render the "soil" less hospitable for growth of the cancer "seed" within bone. However, there is now a large body of clinical evidence demonstrating that the adjuvant therapy benefits of BPs extend beyond bone (Coleman et al. 2010a). There are multiple possible mechanisms that could contribute to these effects. In some patients with early breast cancer, >5 circulating tumor cells (CTCs) can be detected in samples (7.5 mL) of peripheral blood, and bone marrow biopsy reveals the presence of disseminated tumor cells (DTCs) within the bone marrow (Naume et al. 2007). In these patients, there are increased risks of distant disease recurrence and poorer outcomes compared with patients who are DTC-negative or who have CTC counts $\leq$5/7.5 mL (Bidard et al. 2009; Bidard et al. 2008; Janni et al. 2011; Schindlbeck et al. 2005; Schindlbeck et al. 2009), suggesting that these cells might be the source of breast cancer recurrence (Ross and Slodkowska 2009). Interestingly, there is also an increased risk of local recurrence in these patients (Bidard et al. 2009). Preclinical studies suggest that DTCs and CTCs can colonize their tissue of origin in a self-seeding process (Kim et al. 2009; Norton 2008). The self-seeding of breast cancer tumors is preferentially mediated by "aggressive" CTCs, including those with bone-, lung-, or brain-metastatic tropism, suggesting that DTCs in bone marrow and CTCs in blood may seed not only bone metastases but also local recurrence and visceral metastases (Kim et al. 2009). Clinical studies have shown that the potent nitrogen-containing BP zoledronic acid (ZOL) can reduce DTC levels in breast cancer adjuvant therapy settings (Aft et al. 2010; Greenberg et al. 2010; Solomayer et al. 2009), although further studies are needed to determine effects on disease outcomes. Additionally, bone-derived cells have been shown to migrate to tumor sites to generate tumor-supportive tissues in a "premetastatic niche", which fosters early transitions in the multistep process of tumor metastasis (Gnant 2009). By inhibiting growth-factor release from the bone matrix, BPs could also potentially block the mobilization of the cellular components of this premetastatic niche. Therefore, bone-targeted agents have the potential to affect the metastatic process throughout the body.

This chapter discusses the clinical evidence for anticancer benefits from BPs and provides insight into the possible underlying mechanisms. The potential benefits are also placed in the context of the safety profile of antiresorptive therapy in patients with early breast cancer.

2   Bone-Targeted Therapies for Breast Cancer

Breast cancer cells have an innate predilection for bone, with bone metastases developing in approximately 70% of patients with stage IV disease (Coleman 2004). Indeed, advanced breast cancer is associated with a heavy burden of skeletal disease, with annual rates of 1–4 potentially debilitating or life-limiting skeletal-related events (SREs) (Kohno et al. 2005; Theriault et al. 1999) such as spinal cord compression, pathologic fracture, hypercalcemia of malignancy, or the need for palliative radiotherapy or surgery to bone (Coleman 2001; Saad et al. 2007).

The bone microenvironment is a rich source of growth factors and matrix-derived growth factors that are released during osteolysis and can further support cancer cell growth in the bone (as described further in Chap. 1). Increased bone turnover has been associated with a higher risk of metastatic bone lesion formation in preclinical (Padalecki and Guise 2002) and clinical (Lipton et al. 2009) studies. Indeed, studies monitoring biochemical markers of bone resorption have shown significant correlations between elevated rates of osteolysis and risk of bone metastases in patients with early breast cancer. For example, in a substudy of the National Cancer Institute of Canada Clinical Trials Group (NCIC CTG) MA.14 trial comparing tamoxifen with octreotide to tamoxifen alone for adjuvant treatment of stage I or II breast cancer in postmenopausal patients, increased levels of the osteolysis marker beta C-terminal telopeptide of type I collagen (β-CTX) correlated with reduced bone metastasis-free survival (Lipton et al. 2009). Osteolysis rates have been shown to be elevated during adjuvant endocrine therapy for breast cancer (Santen 2011). In addition to directly supporting cancer cell growth and bone lesion formation, growth factors and other molecules released during osteolysis may also activate DTCs from a dormant to a proliferative state, seeding posttreatment relapses.

Bone marrow is a sanctuary for normal hematopoietic stem cells (Ehninger and Trumpp 2011), and this supportive niche can be usurped by DTCs. Although the underlying mechanisms are poorly understood, these cancer seeds, which lodge in the fertile soil of the bone marrow, can survive in a dormant state for extended periods of time before reactivating and metastasizing to other sites (Meads et al. 2008). Additionally, the hematopoietic niche within the bone marrow may provide a safe haven for tumor cells from immunosurveillance and cytotoxicity from chemotherapeutic agents (Meads et al. 2008) because of cell–cell interactions and signaling pathways that may contribute to reduced drug activity and the emergence of drug resistance (Meads et al. 2008).

Modification of the microenvironment surrounding cancer cells is emerging as an important anticancer strategy (Gnant 2009). Because DTCs can reside in the bone marrow, agents that modify the bone microenvironment (such as BPs) may potentially alter the ability of DTCs to survive and/or reactivate. Bisphosphonate-mediated inhibition of osteoclast-mediated bone resorption also blocks the release of cancer-supporting bone matrix-associated growth factors (Mundy 2002). In addition, BPs may directly inhibit cancer cell proliferation and induce apoptosis, as well as synergize with anticancer therapies (as described further in Chaps. 1 and 7) (Almubarak et al. 2011; Winter and Coleman 2009; Winter et al. 2008). Finally, BPs may also activate immune surveillance against cancer cells (Abe et al. 2009; Benzaid and Clezardin 2010). Therefore, there is a wealth of theoretical data supporting the potential of BPs to exert anticancer effects.

3 Anticancer Effects of Oral Bisphosphonates in Early Breast Cancer

Knowledge of the underlying pathophysiology of malignant bone lesions and the "seed and soil" hypothesis of tumor metastasis (as described in Chaps. 1 and 2) led pioneering oncologists to question whether, by reducing the release of growth factors from bone, antiresorptive agents could impede the formation of bone metastases. The earliest clinical studies of the bone-metastasis-preventing potential of BPs in early breast cancer used oral clodronate, which has received regulatory approval outside the United States for preventing SREs in patients with advanced breast cancer metastatic to bone (Bayer Plc 2010). Although clodronate is relatively weak compared with the intravenous BPs that were developed after these initial trials were initiated (Green 2004), its effects were sufficient to suggest that not only was there potential to prevent bone metastases, but that other effects on the disease course might be possible (Powles et al. 2002), thereby laying the groundwork for further clinical investigations.

3.1 Oral Clodronate

In the first large trial for the prevention of bone metastases, Powles et al. (2006, 2002) randomized 1,069 patients with stages I–III breast cancer to oral clodronate (1,600 mg/day) for 2 years in addition to standard therapy or to standard therapy alone (Table 1) (Diel et al. 2008; Powles et al. 2002, 2006; Saarto et al. 2004). Clodronate significantly reduced the risk of bone metastases both during the 2-year treatment period and at the 5-year time point, 3 years after clodronate had been discontinued (Powles et al. 2002, 2006). Moreover, at both time points, survival was significantly longer with clodronate versus standard therapy alone. A similar but smaller study that enrolled breast cancer patients with bone marrow micrometastases (e.g, positive histology results from bone marrow biopsies) reported similar results, although the decreased risk of metastases was not durable after the clodronate treatment period had concluded (Diel et al. 2008). The overall

Table 1 Summary of adjuvant clodronate trials in patients with breast cancer

	(Powles et al. 2002, 2006)	(Saarto et al. 2004)	(Diel et al. 2008)
Patients, N	1,069	299	290
Extent of disease[a]	Stage I–III	LN$^+$	Bone$^+$
Treatment duration, years	2	3	2
Follow-up time, years	2/5	10	8.5
Skeletal effect	+	NS	±[b]
Extraskeletal effect	NS	–	±[c]
Disease-free survival	NS	–(ER$^-$)	±[d]
Overall survival	+	NS	+

Abbreviations: *BM* bone metastases, *LN* lymph nodes, *NS* not significant, *ER* estrogen receptor, +, better than standard therapy alone, –, worse than standard therapy alone
[a] Bone$^+$ refers to primary breast cancer patients with positive bone marrow biopsies
[b] Effects were significant at 36 ($P = 0.003$) and 55 months ($P = 0.044$), but not at 103 months
[c] Effects were significant at 36 ($P = 0.003$) but not at 55 or 103 months
[d] Effects were significant at 36 and 55 months ($P < 0.001$ for each) but not at 103 months

survival (OS) benefit was maintained in long-term (20.4% mortality with clodronate vs. 40.7% mortality in the control group after 8.5 years; $P = 0.04$) followup in this smaller study (Diel et al. 2008). In contrast, a third trial produced results that were inconsistent with the other studies, with no difference in the rates of bone metastases ($P = 0.35$), but increased rates of visceral metastases in clodronate-treated patients (50% vs. 36% in the control group; $P = 0.005$) (Saarto et al. 2004). However, subsequent analyses of this trial population revealed baseline imbalances in poor-prognosis disease characteristics (e.g. hormone-receptor—negative tumors) between treatment groups, favoring the control arm of the study (Saarto et al. 2004). The effects of this imbalance could have been amplified by the trial-mandated endocrine therapy regimen, which would have been expected to have lower potential benefit in patients with hormone-receptor—negative tumors (Saarto et al. 2004). Therefore, the role of clodronate in adjuvant therapy for breast cancer will likely remain controversial until the maturation of ongoing clinical trials (Table 2).

3.2 Oral Pamidronate

The introduction of nitrogen-containing BPs, with antiresorptive activity orders of magnitude higher than the earlier-generation agents (Green 2004), provided additional tools to the therapeutic repertoire for testing in early breast cancer. Oral formulations of nitrogen-containing BPs were developed, such as oral ibandronate, which is now approved alongside its intravenous formulation for preventing SREs in patients with breast cancer in Europe (Roche 2006), and oral pamidronate,

Table 2 Ongoing trials evaluating the anticancer activity of bisphosphonates in breast cancer

Study	Agent(s)	Region	Accrual status	N (targeted or actual)
SWOG 0307	CLO vs IBA vs ZOL	US	Complete	6,097
SUCCESS	ZOL	Germany	Complete	3,754
NSABP B34	CLO	Canada/US	Complete	3,400
AZURE	ZOL	UK/Australia	Complete	3,360
GAIN	IBA	Germany	Complete	3,024
NATAN	Postoperative ZOL	Germany, Austria	Complete	693
ABCSG-18	Denosumab	Austria	Open	3,400
D-CARE	Denosumab	International	Open	4,500

Abbreviations: *CLO* clodronate, *IBA* ibandronate, *ZOL* zoledronic acid

which was subsequently abandoned in favor of intravenous regimens, which allow improved gastrointestinal tolerability and higher bioavailability (Major et al. 2000). Adjuvant oral pamidronate (150 mg twice daily for 4 years) was tested in 953 patients with lymph node-negative primary breast cancer, but neither improved OS nor prevented the occurrence of bone metastases (Kristensen et al. 2008). However, after this study was initiated, pamidronate was developed as an intravenous agent and received broad regulatory approval in the multiple myeloma and advanced breast cancer settings for preventing SREs. The effects of intravenous pamidronate on the disease course during adjuvant therapy for breast cancer have not been investigated.

3.3 Anticancer Benefits of Zoledronic Acid

Decades of innovation resulted in the development of multiple generations of BPs with increasing levels of potency and clinical utility (Green and Guenther 2011). Zoledronic acid was introduced into the oncology community when it demonstrated superiority over pamidronate, the former standard of care, for combating potentially life-threatening hypercalcemia of malignancy (HCM) in patients with advanced cancers (Major et al. 2001). Since then, it has developed the broadest oncology indication of any BP, receiving approval for the prevention of SREs in patients with bone lesions from multiple myeloma or bone metastases secondary to any solid tumor (Novartis Pharmaceuticals Corporation 2008). Therefore, several large clinical trials investigated the potential of adjuvant ZOL to prevent breast cancer recurrence. The majority of these studies used twice-yearly dosing, a schedule that was designed to protect against bone loss during adjuvant endocrine therapy. However, the AZURE study used a more intense upfront dosing regimen, which gradually tapered to the twice-yearly dosing schedule during the first

3 years of the study (every 3–4 weeks for 6 doses, every 3 months for 8 doses, then every 6 months for 5 doses) (Coleman et al. 2011b).

3.4 ABCSG-12

The Austrian Breast and Colorectal Cancer Study Group (ABCSG)-12 trial randomized 1,803 premenopausal women with early stage, endocrine-responsive breast cancer to four separate treatment regimens and evaluated disease-free survival (DFS) as the primary endpoint. Patients received goserelin and tamoxifen or anastrozole with or without ZOL (4 mg every 6 months) for 3 years. In the event-driven primary analysis at a median follow-up of 48 months, addition of ZOL to adjuvant endocrine therapy led to a relative reduction of 36% (log-rank $P = 0.01$) in the risk of DFS events versus endocrine therapy alone (Fig. 1a) (Gnant et al. 2009). Adding ZOL to adjuvant endocrine therapy was associated with an absolute DFS improvement of 3.2% compared with endocrine therapy alone (48-month absolute DFS rates were 94.0% in the ZOL group vs. 90.8% in the no-ZOL group; $P = 0.01$) (Gnant et al. 2009), resulting in a number-needed-to-treat (NNT) of 31 patients to prevent 1 DFS event with ZOL at a median follow-up of 48 months, which compares favorably with the NNT for prevention of 1 DFS event of 28 for paclitaxel (60–69 months' follow-up) and 31 for docetaxel (43–60 months' follow-up), two taxanes that are widely used for chemotherapy of breast cancer. Notably, anticancer effects with ZOL were seen both in bone and beyond—patients who received ZOL had fewer recurrences at all sites (locoregional recurrence [10 vs. 20], distant recurrence [29 vs. 41] including bone metastases [16 vs. 23], and contralateral breast cancer [6 vs. 10]) versus patients who did not receive ZOL (Gnant et al. 2009). Moreover, the longer-term follow-up results from ABCSG-12 at a median follow-up of 62 months demonstrated a continued 32% improvement in DFS ($P = 0.008$) in the ZOL-treated group. Because the adjuvant therapy regimen had been completed after 36 months, these effects, more than 2 years after completion of therapy, suggest a sustained, long-term "carryover" benefit from adding ZOL to endocrine therapy (Gnant et al. 2010). In addition, ZOL also produced a strong trend toward improved OS (hazard ratio [HR] = 0.67; $P = 0.094$). There were no cases of clinically significant renal impairment or osteonecrosis of the jaw (ONJ) reported at the 62-month follow-up of the study.

Further analyses were performed on the mature data set from ABCSG-12 to determine whether there are subsets more likely to receive DFS benefits from the addition of ZOL to adjuvant endocrine therapy. Exploratory subgroup analyses revealed a significant difference in ZOL treatment effects based on patient age at enrolment (Gnant et al. 2011). In the subgroup of women who were 40 years old or younger ($n = 413$), ZOL did not produce a significant decrease in the risk of DFS events (HR = 0.94; $P = 0.821$). In contrast, among patients who were older than 40 years of age at study entry ($n = 1,390$), ZOL produced a striking 42% reduction in the risk of DFS events (HR = 0.58; $P = 0.003$) versus no ZOL. Moreover, although the survival endpoint was underpowered because of the favorable survival profile in this study, ZOL produced a strong trend toward a 43% reduction in the risk of death versus no ZOL in this older subset of patients (HR = 0.57; P = 0.057).

3.5 ZO-FAST

The Zometa–Femara Adjuvant Synergy Trials (Z-FAST, ZO-FAST, and E-ZO-FAST) were initiated primarily to investigate the bone-preserving activity of ZOL during adjuvant therapy with aromatase inhibitors, and these studies have provided important additional insight into the anticancer potential of ZOL. Each of these studies enrolled postmenopausal women after surgical resection of their stage I–IIIa breast cancer and randomized them to 5 years of adjuvant letrozole (2.5 mg/day for 5 years) alone or with ZOL ("upfront ZOL"; 4 mg every 6 months; the same dose as that used in premenopausal women in ABCSG-12) (Eidtmann et al. 2010). Patients randomized to letrozole alone were to initiate ZOL if they developed clinically significant decreases in bone health that would place them at elevated risk for fractures (e.g, osteoporosis/severe osteopenia or a fragility fracture). Therefore, the control arms of these studies are referred to as the "delayed-ZOL" groups. In each of these trials, upfront ZOL significantly increased bone mineral density (BMD) relative to delayed ZOL in the overall trial population within the first year (Brufsky et al. 2008; Eidtmann et al. 2010; Schenk et al. 2007).

In ZO-FAST, the largest of these studies (N = 1,065), patients were stratified based on their menopausal status (recent or established postmenopausal), and patient follow-ups for disease recurrence and survival were continued even after patients had discontinued their study medication, allowing robust assessment of treatment benefits. After 3 years' median follow-up, in addition to the BMD benefits with ZOL (the trial's primary endpoint), the upfront-ZOL group had a significant 41% reduction in the risk of DFS events versus the delayed-ZOL group (HR = 0.588; log-rank P = 0.0314; Fig. 1b) (Eidtmann et al. 2010). Similar to the case in ABCSG-12, ZOL initiation at the start of adjuvant endocrine therapy was associated with a reduction in breast cancer recurrence in and outside bone, with distant recurrence in 20 upfront-ZOL versus 30 delayed-ZOL patients (of which bone metastases were in 9 upfront-ZOL versus 17 delayed-ZOL patients), and first recurrence locally in 2 upfront-ZOL versus 10 delayed-ZOL patients (Eidtmann et al. 2010). These DFS benefits with ZOL were maintained at 48 months (Coleman et al. 2009) and in the final 60-month analysis (HR = 0.66; log-rank P = 0.0375) (de Boer et al. 2010).

3.6 AZURE

The ongoing AZURE trial is evaluating the anticancer activity of a tapered schedule of ZOL (4 mg monthly for 6 months, then quarterly for 2 years, followed by twice yearly for 2.5 years, for a total of 5 years of treatment) in 3,360 patients

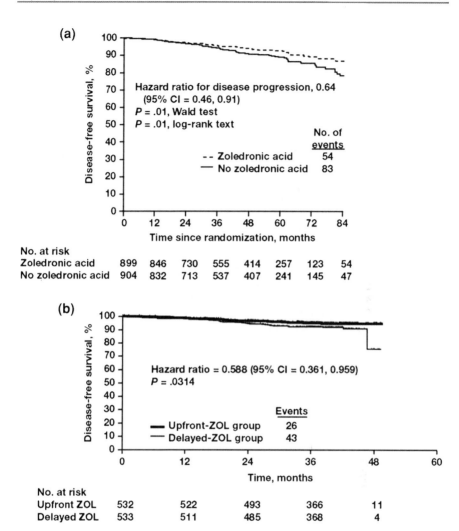

Fig. 1 *Addition of twice-yearly ZOL to adjuvant endocrine therapy improved disease-free survival compared with endocrine therapy alone in the (**a**) ABCSG-12 and (**b**) ZO-FAST trials. Abbreviations*: CI confidence interval, ZOL zoledronic acid. Panel (**a**) reprinted from Gnant et al. (2009) N Engl J Med 360: 679–691. © 2009 Massachusetts Medical Society (Gnant et al. 2009). Panel (**b**) reprinted from Eidtmann et al. Efficacy of zoledronic acid in postmenopausal women with early breast cancer receiving adjuvant letrozole: 36 month results of the ZO-FAST study. Ann Oncol (2010) 21(11): 2188–2194, by permission of the European Society for Medical Oncology (Eidtmann et al. 2010)

with high-risk, stage II/III BC receiving adjuvant chemotherapy and/or hormonal therapy (Coleman et al. 2011b). In the overall population of the AZURE trial, ZOL did not significantly increase DFS compared with standard therapy alone. The second interim analysis for this ongoing trial revealed no difference in DFS between ZOL and no ZOL in the overall trial population (HR = 0.98; $P = 0.79$) (Coleman et al. 2010b). However, there was an intriguing trend toward improved OS with ZOL (HR = 0.85; $P = 0.07$) (Coleman et al. 2010b). Prospective analyses evaluating treatment benefits in subgroups of patients revealed that there was a significant difference in ZOL benefits based on the menopausal status of the patients at study entry ($P = 0.02$), and preplanned analyses based on menopausal status were reported. Among pre- or perimenopausal patients, there was no appreciable difference in DFS or OS with ZOL treatment versus standard therapy alone. In contrast, among patients who were postmenopausal for at least 5 years before study entry ($n = 1,041$), ZOL significantly reduced the risk of DFS events by 24% (HR = 0.76; $P < 0.05$) and the risk of death by 29% (HR = 0.71; $P = 0.017$) (Coleman et al. 2010b). Although this subset constitutes only a relatively small proportion ($\sim 30\%$; $n = 1,041$) of the AZURE population, in the general population of patients with breast cancer the majority of patients ($\sim 70\%$) are in this older demographic subset and may echo the findings observed in the postmenopausal population of the AZURE trial (Voelker 2011).

3.7 Is There a Subset of Patients More Likely to Benefit From ZOL Anticancer Effects?

The treatment regimens used in each patient subgroup in the AZURE trial have yet to be reported. Because "standard therapy" was not defined in the protocol, patients received the standard of care at the treating institution. Based on usual treatment practices in the United Kingdom during the study period, it is likely that premenopausal women in the AZURE trial received chemotherapy (with or without targeted agents) without concomitant endocrine therapy (ovarian suppression and/or tamoxifen). Therefore, the premenopausal patient subset in AZURE was unlikely to be estrogen depleted and rendered amenorrheic or menopausal (unlike in ABCSG-12, wherein all patients underwent ovarian suppression with goserelin (Gnant et al. 2009)). In contrast, hormonal therapy with tamoxifen and/or aromatase inhibitors (AIs) was typically administered to older, established postmenopausal women in the institutions participating in the AZURE trial. Therefore, the established postmenopausal patient subset of AZURE in which the DFS and OS benefits were reported could be considered comparable with the patient populations in ABCSG-12 (Gnant et al. 2009) and potentially also ZO-FAST (Eidtmann et al. 2010) with respect to estrogen status (Fig. 2) (Coleman et al. 2010b; Eidtmann et al. 2010; Gnant et al. 2009). With this perspective, it is consistent that adding ZOL to anticancer therapy demonstrated a clear benefit in this estrogen-depleted patient subset, although the underlying mechanisms for this benefit have yet to be entirely elucidated. Indeed, benefits in a low-estrogen environment are consistent with the profound DFS benefits detected in the exploratory analyses of the older-patient subset of ABCSG-12 (Gnant et al. 2011), based on the prior observations that ovarian suppression with goserelin may not be sufficient to fully oblate estrogen production in younger premenopausal

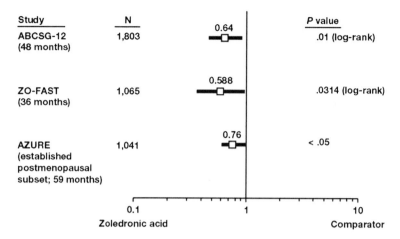

Fig. 2 *Hazard ratios for disease-free survival for zoledronic acid versus control in patients with early stage breast cancer.* Studies including populations with >1,000 patients who were postmenopausal or receiving ovarian suppression are summarized. Patients were randomized to zoledronic acid (ZOL) versus no ZOL in ABCSG-12 and AZURE, and to upfront versus delayed ZOL in ZO-FAST (Coleman et al. 2010b; Eidtmann et al. 2010; Gnant et al. 2009)

patients. For example, there have been case reports of very young premenopausal patients with breast cancer who became pregnant or resumed menses while receiving regimens of luteinizing hormone-releasing hormone–analogue therapy that would be expected to block ovarian function (Del Mastro et al. 1997, Uncu et al. 1996), suggesting that estrogen levels may not be completely suppressed. Similarly, there is a lower incidence of chemotherapy-induced amenorrhea in women less than 40 years of age (22–61%) versus women older than 40 (61–97%), suggesting that the effects of cancer therapies on ovarian function are heavily influenced by the proximity of patients' age to the anticipated date of menopause (Del Mastro et al. 1997). Further evaluations of the ZO-FAST database are underway to determine whether there is a difference in ZOL's effects on DFS in the stratum of patients who are postmenopausal versus patients in the earlier stages of menopause.

Thus, the outcomes from AZURE and exploratory analyses of the other trial databases underscore the importance of patient selection—identifying the subsets of patients most likely to benefit from each of the different therapeutic strategies is key to effective cancer control. An additional conclusion from the AZURE results is that the benefits of using a tapered ZOL dosing regimen versus the twice-yearly dosing used in ABCSG-12 and ZO-FAST are unclear, and further studies are necessary to determine whether there is additional benefit from the increased dose intensity used in the early years of AZURE.

The question of patient selection for ZOL therapy may persist throughout the breast cancer disease continuum. Retrospective analyses of the phase III trial database evaluating ZOL versus placebo in patients with bone metastases from solid tumors revealed that ZOL improved OS in patients with elevated bone turnover markers compared with placebo (Coleman et al. 2011a). Moreover, small studies of vascular endothelial growth factor (VEGF), a factor essential for angiogenesis, reported elevated levels in patients with bone metastases from solid tumors (Santini et al. 2007). In these patients, pamidronate and ZOL were shown to produce sustained and long-lasting decreases in circulating VEGF levels compared with baseline (Di Salvatore et al. 2011, Ferretti et al. 2005; Santini et al. 2002, 2003, 2007, 2006; Vincenzi et al. 2005).

3.8 Neoadjuvant Therapy

An exploratory subset analysis was performed among patients who received neoadjuvant chemotherapy in the AZURE trial. In this subset ($n = 205$), adding monthly ZOL significantly reduced the residual invasive tumor size at surgery ($P = 0.002$ vs. chemotherapy alone) (Coleman et al. 2010c). In addition, treatment with chemotherapy plus ZOL was associated with increased rates of pathologic complete response and reduced need for mastectomies compared with chemotherapy alone (Coleman et al. 2010c). Therefore, ZOL may have a role in the preoperative therapy of some patients with breast cancer to reduce tumor volume and possibly increase the rate of breast-conserving surgery (Coleman et al. 2010c). Notably, these effects were observed during the portion of the study in which ZOL was administered on a monthly basis. These results are hypothesis generating and consistent with the observations of anticancer synergy between ZOL and chemotherapy agents that have been demonstrated in preclinical models of human breast cancer (as discussed in Chap. 7). Further studies are needed to identify whether there are patient subgroups or tumor types that are more likely to benefit from neoadjuvant ZOL treatment.

3.9 Further Data From Translational Studies in Early Breast Cancer

Pilot and phase II studies in women with early stage, high-risk breast cancer (total $N = 435$) have reported that monthly ZOL, in combination with standard anticancer therapy, can effectively increase DTC clearance and reduce DTC number and persistence in bone marrow compared with standard therapy alone (Aft et al. 2010; Greenberg et al. 2010; Lin et al. 2008; Rack et al. 2010; Solomayer et al. 2009). One of these trials evaluated monthly ZOL combined with neoadjuvant epirubicin/docetaxel in 120 women with newly diagnosed stage II–III breast cancer (Aft et al. 2010). After 3 months, 17 of 56 patients receiving ZOL vs. 25 of 53 patients who did not receive ZOL had detectable DTCs ($P = 0.054$; Fig. 3a), and ZOL significantly improved the proportion of patients who maintained DTC-negative status from baseline to the 3-month assessment (Fig. 3b) (Aft et al. 2010). These ZOL-mediated decreases in DTC persistence might be one of the mechanisms underlying the observed clinical benefits in studies such as ABCSG-12 and ZO-FAST. However, bone marrow biopsies were not performed in these large clinical studies. Further studies are needed to determine whether the observed DFS benefits with ZOL correlate with decreases in DTC levels.

4 Can Bisphosphonates Prevent Cancer?

Exploratory analyses of clinical databases have provided intriguing insight into additional potential benefits of BPs as a class. Three such studies have suggested that, in addition to preserving BMD in postmenopausal women, BPs may actually impede the development of breast cancer. Each reported a reduction in breast cancer risk of approximately 30% for the BP-treated cohort versus women not treated with BPs, and benefits were maintained in multivariate analyses and after controlling for known confounding risk factors. Although prospective confirmation of these observations in randomized controlled trials is needed, the strength and consistency of the correlations are intriguing. The expanding theoretical framework for BP anticancer effects both inside and outside of bone includes mechanisms that could potentially apply to early stages of carcinogenesis and primary tumor development.

In the largest of these analyses ($N = 154{,}768$), Chlebowski et al. (2010) performed multivariate analyses of breast cancer rates using longitudinal data from the Women's Health Initiative Observational Study (WHI-OS). Women who received BPs for osteoporosis had a 32% relative reduction in the overall risk of breast cancer versus women who did not receive BPs (HR $= 0.68$; 95% confidence interval [CI] $= 0.52$, 0.88). Furthermore, BP-treated patients who did develop breast cancers had a higher proportion of in situ versus invasive disease compared with the disease pattern observed in the non–BP-treated women. Interestingly, both estrogen receptor (ER)-positive and ER-negative breast cancers occurred at lower rates among the BP-treated women, and the effects appeared more profound for ER-negative tumors. Concurrently, Rennert et al. (2010) performed a similar analysis using the Breast Cancer in Northern Israel Study (BCINIS) database ($N = 4{,}039$). Among postmenopausal women receiving BPs for more than 1 year, the risk of breast cancer was reduced by 28% (odds ratio $= 0.72$; 95% CI $= 0.57$, 0.90; $P < 0.01$). Moreover, the breast cancers that developed in BP-treated women generally had better prognostic features, including a lower proportion of human epidermal growth factor receptor 2 (HER2)-positive tumors, compared with those in women who did not receive BPs. In a population-based case–control study, Newcomb et al. (2010) compared 2,936 incident invasive breast cancer cases with 2,975 population controls who were younger than 70 years of age; breast cancer risk factors were assessed using multivariable logistic regression. The risk of breast cancer was 33% lower for current BP recipients compared with nonrecipients (odds ratio $= 0.67$; 95% CI $= 0.51, 0.89$). Moreover, longer duration of BP administration correlated with a significantly greater reduction in breast cancer risk (trend toward $P = 0.01$).

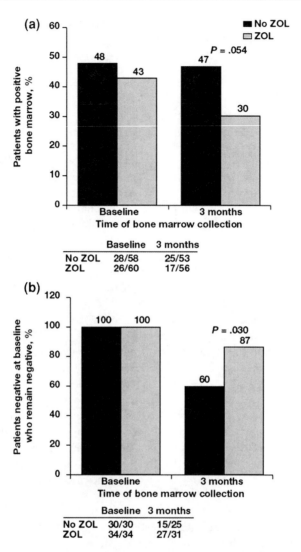

Fig. 3 *Effects of zoledronic acid on the presence of disseminated tumor cells (DTCs) in the bone marrow of patients with early breast cancer.* **a** Percentage of patients in each group with detectable DTCs in their bone marrow at baseline and 3 months. Compared with baseline, fewer patients in zoledronic acid than in the control group had positive DTCs at 3 months ($P = 0.054$ by Fisher's exact test). **b** Percentage of patients in each group with no DTCs detectable in their bone marrow at baseline who remained negative at 3 months ($P = 0.030$ by Fisher's exact test). Absolute numbers of patients at each time point are presented in the tables below each figure. Reprinted from Lancet Oncol (2010) vol 11, Aft et al., Effect of zoledronic acid on disseminated tumor cells in women with locally advanced breast cancer: an open label, randomised, phase 2 trial, pages 421–428, copyright 2010, with permission from Elsevier (Aft et al. 2010)

Each of these studies was based on clinical practice databases, and the types of BPs administered therefore varied based on local and regional practices. Thus, they contain an inherent assumption that the BP effect was consistent across the different agents, and it is possible that some BPs may have had stronger correlations with reduced breast cancer risk than others. Indeed, in preclinical assay systems, ZOL has consistently demonstrated higher anticancer activities compared with the earlier-generation BPs (Green and Lipton 2010; Green and Guenther 2011), which are widely used for the treatment of postmenopausal osteoporosis, and denosumab is yet to demonstrate any anticancer potential in the breast cancer setting (Brufsky 2010; Neville-Webbe et al. 2010; Terpos and Dimopoulos 2011). Indeed in the trial of denosumab to prevent cancer treatment-induced bone loss (CTIBL) in patients receiving adjuvant therapy for breast cancer, recurrence rates were slightly higher in the denosumab group versus the control treatment group (US Food and Drug Administration 2009). In each of these analyses, the authors attempted to control for confounders including age, ethnicity, tobacco use, alcohol use, physical activity, baseline BMD, body mass index, prior hormone therapy, calcium and vitamin D supplementation, number of pregnancies, duration of breastfeeding, and other unknown factors that may potentially interact with breast cancer risk. However, a major limitation of retrospective analyses such as these is that the relative and interrelated risk factors for breast cancer are not yet completely understood, and, therefore, it is impossible to ensure that all important factors have been considered. Nonetheless, these studies raise important questions and provide intriguing possibilities for future research. Among these are the assessment of which underlying activities of BPs may contribute to these observations and evaluation of whether there are subpopulations that would be most likely to benefit from preventive therapy.

As with the outcomes in the adjuvant therapy setting, the estrogen environment may affect the breast cancer outcomes in these studies. Lifetime exposure to estrogen influences not only breast cancer risk but also BMD, and there are clear correlations between high BMD and increased risk of breast cancer (Cauley et al. 1996; Chen et al. 2008; Lucas et al. 1998; Zmuda et al. 2001), presumably because estrogen can stimulate the growth of ER-positive breast cancer cells (Douchi et al. 2007). Indeed, in the WHI-OS database analysis, the breast cancer risk reduction with BPs was significant for ER-positive invasive breast cancers. However, there was also a similar (albeit not statistically significant) trend for reductions in ER-negative tumors (Chlebowski et al. 2010), although the role of estrogen in the development of ER-negative breast cancers is poorly understood. Moreover, Rennert et al. (2011) reported that, in a database similar to the one used for the BCINIS study, the rate of colorectal cancers was also lower among BP-treated women versus women who did not receive BPs, suggesting that the potential cancer-preventing benefits of BPs are not limited to breast cancers. Therefore, there are multiple aspects of this complex story that will need to be answered before breast cancer prevention with BPs can be effectively implemented in clinical practice.

Ongoing trials of the anticancer potential of ZOL in early breast cancer settings include SWOG 0307 (ZOL vs. CLO vs. ibandronate), NATAN (ZOL versus control), and SUCCESS (ZOL vs. no ZOL). As these trials mature, they are expected to provide additional insights into the anticancer activities of ZOL and other BPs, and the role of BP therapy will likely expand.

5 Tolerability and Safety of Bisphosphonates as Adjuvant Therapy

In general, BPs are well tolerated and have well-established safety profiles. The safety profiles of ZOL in the adjuvant therapy setting have been very consistent across the reported clinical trials (Table 3) (Coleman et al. 2009; Gnant et al. 2009).

Common adverse events of BPs vary by the administration route, dose, treatment duration, and drug characteristics (Body 2001). For example, all oral BPs are associated with gastrointestinal toxicities, whereas intravenous BPs are associated with dose- and infusion rate-dependent effects on renal function, and adherence to renal safety protocols for patient monitoring as well as dose adjustment, infusion volume, and infusion duration is crucial for maintaining patient safety and comfort (Berenson 2005). Each of the nitrogen-containing BPs is associated with an acute-phase reaction (characterized by flu-like symptoms) after the first infusion. This reaction is generally mild, preventable, or manageable with adequate hydration and over-the-counter analgesics (Hamdy 2010), and uncommon with subsequent treatment (Tanvetyanon and Stiff 2006).

Although the acute-phase reaction is a cluster of adverse events (e.g, flu-like symptoms, muscle ache), it may reflect a potentially beneficial anticancer effect of BPs. The acute-phase symptoms might be associated with activation of the immune system through phosphoantigen production (a consequence of inhibition of the mevalonate pathway by ZOL) and activation of gamma-delta T cells (Hewitt et al. 2005), a subset of T cells involved in immunologic surveillance against cancer cells. Indeed, phosphoantigen-mediated activation of gamma-delta T cells was found to contribute to the anticancer activities of ZOL in preclinical models of human breast cancer (Benzaid and Clezardin 2010; Vantourout et al. 2009). However, no correlative analyses between acute-phase reactions and cancer outcomes have yet been reported. Therefore, the relationship between acute-phase reactions and anticancer immune responses is purely speculative.

Osteonecrosis of the jaw, characterized by exposed bone within the oral cavity that does not heal despite at least 6 weeks of appropriate dental care, has been reported as an uncommon adverse event in patients with advanced cancer receiving complex therapeutic regimens including intravenous BPs for malignant bone disease (Hoff et al. 2008). Recent studies have demonstrated that the incidence of ONJ can be reduced by up to 70% by implementing preventive dental measures and regular dental care (Dimopoulos et al. 2009; Ripamonti et al. 2009). In the large clinical trials of adjuvant ZOL twice yearly, the overall ONJ incidence

Table 3 Adverse events of interest in clinical trials of zoledronic acid during adjuvant endocrine therapy

	ZO-FAST 48 months		Z-FAST 60 months		E-ZO-FAST 36 months		ABCSG-12 48 months				
Therapy	LET						ANA[a]			TAM[a]	
Patients, n (%)	Upfront (n = 525)	Delayed (n = 535)	Upfront (n = 300)	Delayed (n = 300)	Upfront (n = 254)	Delayed (n = 269)	ZOL (n = 453)	No ZOL (n = 450)	ZOL (n = 449)	No ZOL (n = 451)
Arthralgia	247 (47)	360 (67)	141 (47)	136 (45)	115 (45)	129 (48)	150 (33)	112 (25)	65 (15)	52 (12)
Myalgia	66 (13)	70 (13)	61 (20)	47 (16)	30 (12)	29 (11)	NR	NR	NR	NR
Pyrexia	81 (15)	18 (3)	29 (10)	14 (5)	19 (7)	2 (0.7)	46 (10)	11 (2)	34 (8)	9 (2)
Bone pain	90 (17)	61 (11)	48 (16)	24 (8)	24 (9)	19 (7)	185 (41)	128 (28)	132 (29)	94 (21)
Hot flashes	147 (28)	162 (30)	122 (41)	118 (39)	63 (25)	92 (34)	25 (6)	25 (6)	27 (6)	28 (6)
Renal AEs (≥grade 3)	2 (0.4)	3 (0.6)	1 (0.3)	0	1 (0.4)	0	0	0	0	0
Atrial fibrillation	2 (0.4)	5 (0.9)	0	0	0	1 (0.4)	NR	NR	NR	NR
ONJ[a]	3	0	0	0	2	0	0	0	0	0

Abbreviations: ANA anastrozole, AE adverse event, LET letrozole, NR none reported, ONJ osteonecrosis of the jaw, TAM tamoxifen, ZOL zoledronic acid
[a] All patients in ABCSG-12 were premenopausal and received ovarian suppression with goserelin

was 0.2% (5 confirmed cases in approximately 4,000 patients at a median follow-up of 62 months for ABCSG-12 (Gnant et al. 2010), 60 months for Z-FAST, 48 months for ZO-FAST, and 36 months for E-ZO-FAST) (Coleman et al. 2009). Furthermore, a meta-analysis of 15 randomized clinical trials of adjuvant BPs reporting cases of ONJ ($N = 10,694$) revealed that ONJ was uncommon for BPs as a class. Only 13 ($\sim 0.24\%$) of the 5,312 patients receiving BPs were reported to develop ONJ, versus 1 ($\sim 0.019\%$) of the 5,382 patients whose adjuvant therapy regimens did not include BPs (Mauri et al. 2009).

6 Other Uses of Antiresorptives in Women with Early Breast Cancer

Advances in adjuvant therapies for breast cancer have, on the one hand, led to favorable long-term survival, and on the other, necessitated the management of CTIBL to prevent long-term increases in fracture risks (Gnant et al. 2008; Sverrisdottir et al. 2004; Vehmanen et al. 2006). This is especially true among premenopausal patients receiving adjuvant endocrine therapy and postmenopausal patients receiving AIs (Forbes et al. 2008; Rabaglio et al. 2009; Santen 2011).

Several clinical trials have examined the use of antiresorptives to prevent bone loss associated with endocrine therapy in both pre-and postmenopausal women with breast cancer (Lipton 2010). The strongest clinical evidence to date for protecting bone health during adjuvant endocrine therapy for breast cancer is with ZOL at the same dose and schedule (twice-yearly ZOL concomitant with AI regimen) that produced reduced disease recurrence in ABCSG-12/ZO-FAST (Eidtmann et al. 2010; Gnant et al. 2010). Current guidelines for bone health in early breast cancer recommend the use of BPs in patients at high risk for fracture (Aebi et al. 2010; Gralow et al. 2009; Hadji et al. 2008, 2011; Hillner et al. 2003; Reid et al. 2008). For example, treatment guidelines from the European Society for Medical Oncology (ESMO) now support the potential use of adjuvant ZOL to prevent bone loss and disease recurrence in women who meet the criteria for ABCSG-12 or ZO-FAST (Aebi et al. 2010). However, the exact criteria for initiating therapy for BMD effects vary between the different society, local, and regional treatment guidelines (as discussed by Hadji et al. (2011)). Administering ZOL may therefore provide both BMD and anticancer benefits in this setting.

7 Conclusions

Bone plays a key role in harboring DTCs and supporting metastases in breast cancer, and elevated levels of bone turnover release growth factors that can support cancer cell growth in the bone. Bisphosphonates, alone or in combination with anticancer agents, have been shown to block multiple steps in the process of tumor metastasis. Modification of the bone marrow microenvironment (soil) with BPs may complement the effects of adjuvant therapy on the breast cancer cells (seeds), thereby further improving clinical outcomes. Results from recent clinical trials in patients with hormone-responsive breast cancer support the concomitant use of ZOL with adjuvant endocrine therapy to improve DFS, and ongoing trials are further evaluating the effects of antiresorptive agents in combination with endocrine therapy and/or chemotherapy in the adjuvant breast cancer setting.

Additionally, BPs and other antiresorptive agents can help prevent bone loss and fractures associated with adjuvant therapy for breast cancer patients, suggesting that patients may experience both anticancer and bone-health benefits from BPs during adjuvant therapy. Recent population-based and case–control studies suggest that long-term BP administration to treat postmenopausal osteoporosis may also reduce the risk of developing invasive breast cancer. However, prospective clinical trials are needed to confirm these correlations and to identify population subgroups most likely to derive such benefits.

The past decade has seen major developments in the treatment of patients with early breast cancer. In addition to advances in hormonal and cytotoxic adjuvant therapy regimens, ZOL has been shown to significantly improve DFS in patients receiving adjuvant hormonal therapy. Ongoing clinical studies are further evaluating the anticancer potential of ZOL; determining whether the anticancer effects demonstrated inconsistently with clodronate in early trials will be confirmed in studies of more modern design, and whether such anticancer effects extend to all BPs and other classes of antiresorptive agents. The role of these agents in the treatment of patients with breast cancer is likely to evolve as these studies mature.

Acknowledgments Financial support for medical editorial assistance was provided by Novartis Pharmaceuticals. We thank Catherine Browning, PhD, ProEd Communications, Inc.®, for her medical editorial assistance with this manuscript.

Conflict of Interest Dr. Gnant has served on advisory boards for and received consulting and lecture fees from AstraZeneca and Novartis, as well as lecture fees and research support from Roche, Schering, Pfizer, Novartis, AstraZeneca, sanofi-aventis, and Amgen. Dr. Dubsky has received honoraria for lectures and advisory boards from Novartis, Pfizer, AstraZeneca, and Roche, and other remuneration (travel) from Novartis, Roche, AstraZeneca, and Pfizer. Dr. Hadji has received honoraria, unrestricted educational grants, and research funding from Amgen, AstraZeneca, Eli Lilly, GlaxoSmithKline, Novartis, Pfizer, Roche, and sanofi-aventis.

References

Abe Y, Muto M, Nieda M et al (2009) Clinical and immunological evaluation of zoledronate-activated Vgamma9gammadelta T-cell-based immunotherapy for patients with multiple myeloma. Exp Hematol 37:956–968

Aebi S, Davidson T, Gruber G et al (2010) Primary breast cancer: ESMO clinical practice guidelines for diagnosis, treatment and follow-up. Ann Oncol 21(suppl 5):v9–v14

Aft R, Naughton M, Trinkaus K et al (2010) Effect of zoledronic acid on disseminated tumour cells in women with locally advanced breast cancer: an open label, randomised, phase 2 trial. Lancet Oncol 11:421–428

Almubarak H, Jones A, Chaisuparat R et al (2011) Zoledronic acid directly suppresses cell proliferation and induces apoptosis in highly tumorigenic prostate and breast cancers. J Carcinog 10:2

Baum M, Budzar AU, Cuzick J et al (2002) Anastrozole alone or in combination with tamoxifen versus tamoxifen alone for adjuvant treatment of postmenopausal women with early breast cancer: first results of the ATAC randomised trial. Lancet 359:2131–2139

Bayer Plc (2010) Bonefos [summary of product characteristics]. Bayer Plc, Newbury

Benzaid I, Clezardin P (2010) Nitrogen-containing bisphosphonates and human $\gamma\delta$ T cells. IBMS BoneKEy 7:208–217

Berenson JR (2005) Recommendations for zoledronic acid treatment of patients with bone metastases. Oncologist 10:52–62

Bidard FC, Kirova YM, Vincent-Salomon A et al (2009) Disseminated tumor cells and the risk of locoregional recurrence in nonmetastatic breast cancer. Ann Oncol 20:1836–1841

Bidard FC, Vincent-Salomon A, Sigal-Zafrani B et al (2008) Prognosis of women with stage IV breast cancer depends on detection of circulating tumor cells rather than disseminated tumor cells. Ann Oncol 19:496–500

Body JJ (2001) Dosing regimens and main adverse events of bisphosphonates. Semin Oncol 28:49–53

Brufsky A, Bundred N, Coleman R et al (2008) Integrated analysis of zoledronic acid for prevention of aromatase inhibitor-associated bone loss in postmenopausal women with early breast cancer receiving adjuvant letrozole. Oncologist 13:503–514

Brufsky AM (2010) The evolving role of bone-conserving therapy in patients with breast cancer. Semin Oncol 37(suppl 1):S12–S19

Cauley JA, Lucas FL, Kuller LH et al (1996) Bone mineral density and risk of breast cancer in older women: the study of osteoporotic fractures. Study of Osteoporotic Fractures Research Group. JAMA 276:1404–1408

Chen Z, Arendell L, Aickin M et al (2008) Hip bone density predicts breast cancer risk independently of Gail score: results from the Women's Health Initiative. Cancer 113:907–915

Chlebowski RT, Chen Z, Cauley JA et al (2010) Oral bisphosphonate use and breast cancer incidence in postmenopausal women. J Clin Oncol 28:3582–3590

Clezardin P (2005) Anti-tumour activity of zoledronic acid. Cancer Treat Rev 31(suppl 3):1–8

Coleman R (2011) The use of bisphosphonates in cancer treatment. Ann N Y Acad Sci 1218:3–14

Coleman RE (2001) Metastatic bone disease: clinical features, pathophysiology and treatment strategies. Cancer Treat Rev 27:165–176

Coleman RE (2004) Bisphosphonates: clinical experience. Oncologist 9(suppl 4):14–27

Coleman R, Bundred N, de Boer R et al (2009) Impact of zoledronic acid in postmenopausal women with early breast cancer receiving adjuvant letrozole: Z-FAST, ZO-FAST, and E-ZO-FAST [poster]. Presented at: 32nd Annual San Antonio Breast Cancer Symposium, San Antonio, 9–13 Dec 2009 Abstract 4082

Coleman RE, Lipton A, Roodman GD et al (2010a) Metastasis and bone loss: advancing treatment and prevention. Cancer Treat Rev 36:615–620

Coleman RE, Thorpe HC, Cameron D et al (2010b) Adjuvant treatment with zoledronic acid in stage II/III breast cancer. The AZURE trial (BIG 01/04) [oral presentation]. Presented at: 33rd Annual San Antonio Breast Cancer Symposium, San Antonio, 8–12 Dec 2010 Abstract S4-5

Coleman RE, Winter MC, Cameron D et al (2010c) The effects of adding zoledronic acid to neoadjuvant chemotherapy on tumour response: exploratory evidence for direct anti-tumour activity in breast cancer. Br J Cancer 102:1099–1105

Coleman R, Costa L, Saad F et al (2011a) Consensus on the utility of bone markers in the malignant bone disease setting. Crit Rev Oncol Hematol [Epub ahead of print]

Coleman R, Woodward E, Brown J et al (2011b) Safety of zoledronic acid and incidence of osteonecrosis of the jaw (ONJ) during adjuvant therapy in a randomised phase III trial (AZURE: BIG 01-04) for women with stage II/III breast cancer. Breast Cancer Res Treat 127:429–438

Costa L, Harper P, Coleman RE et al (2011) Anticancer evidence for zoledronic acid across the cancer continuum. Crit Rev Oncol Hematol 77(suppl 1):S31–S37

de Boer R, Bundred N, Eidtmann H et al (2010) The effect of zoledronic acid on aromatase inhibitor associated bone loss in postmenopausal women with early breast cancer receiving adjuvant letrozole: the ZO-FAST study 5-year final follow-up [poster]. Presented at: 33rd Annual San Antonio Breast Cancer Symposium, San Antonio, 8–12 Dec 2010 Abstract P5-11-01

Del Mastro L, Venturini M, Sertoli MR et al (1997) Amenorrhea induced by adjuvant chemotherapy in early breast cancer patients: prognostic role and clinical implications. Breast Cancer Res Treat 43:183–190

Di Salvatore M, Orlandi A, Bagala C et al (2011) Anti-tumour and anti-angiogenetic effects of zoledronic acid on human non-small-cell lung cancer cell line. Cell Prolif 44:139–146

Diel IJ, Jaschke A, Solomayer EF et al (2008) Adjuvant oral clodronate improves the overall survival of primary breast cancer patients with micrometastases to the bone marrow: a long-term follow-up. Ann Oncol 19:2007–2011

Dimopoulos MA, Kastritis E, Bamia C et al (2009) Reduction of osteonecrosis of the jaw (ONJ) after implementation of preventive measures in patients with multiple myeloma treated with zoledronic acid. Ann Oncol 20:117–120

Douchi T, Yonehara Y, Kosha S et al (2007) Bone mineral density in breast cancer patients with positive estrogen receptor tumor status. Maturitas 57:221–225

Ehninger A, Trumpp A (2011) The bone marrow stem cell niche grows up: mesenchymal stem cells and macrophages move in. J Exp Med 208:421–428

Eidtmann H, de Boer R, Bundred N et al (2010) Efficacy of zoledronic acid in postmenopausal women with early breast cancer receiving adjuvant letrozole: 36-month results of the ZO-FAST study. Ann Oncol 21:2188–2194

Ferretti G, Fabi A, Carlini P et al (2005) Zoledronic-acid-induced circulating level modifications of angiogenic factors, metalloproteinases and proinflammatory cytokines in metastatic breast cancer patients. Oncology 69:35–43

Forbes JF, Cuzick J, Buzdar A et al (2008) Effect of anastrozole and tamoxifen as adjuvant treatment for early-stage breast cancer: 100-month analysis of the ATAC trial. Lancet Oncol 9:45–53

Garcia M, Jemal A, Ward EM et al. (2007) Global Cancer Facts & Figures 2007. American Cancer Society, Atlanta

Gerber B, Freund M, Reimer T (2010) Recurrent breast cancer: treatment strategies for maintaining and prolonging good quality of life. Dtsch Arztebl Int 107:85–91

Gnant M (2009) Bisphosphonates in the prevention of disease recurrence: current results and ongoing trials. Curr Cancer Drug Targets 9:824–833

Gnant M, Mlineritsch B, Luschin-Ebengreuth G et al (2008) Adjuvant endocrine therapy plus zoledronic acid in premenopausal women with early-stage breast cancer: 5-year follow-up of the ABCSG-12 bone-mineral density substudy. Lancet Oncol 9:840–849

Gnant M, Mlineritsch B, Schippinger W et al (2009) Endocrine therapy plus zoledronic acid in premenopausal breast cancer. N Engl J Med 360:679–691

Gnant M, Mlineritsch B, Stoeger H et al (2010) Mature results from ABCSG-12: adjuvant ovarian suppression combined with tamoxifen or anastrozole, alone or in combination with zoledronic acid, in premenopausal women with endocrine-responsive early breast cancer [poster]. Presented at: 46th Annual Meeting of the American Society of Clinical Oncology, Chicago, 4–8 June 2010 Abstract 533

Gnant M, Mlineritsch B, Stoeger H et al (2011) Preplanned subgroup analysis of ABCSG-12 suggests that benefits of adjuvant zoledronic acid (ZOL) are most pronounced in lowest estrogen environment [poster]. Presented at: 12th St. Gallen International Breast Cancer Conference, St Gallen, Switzerland, 16–19 March 2011 Abstract P286

Gralow JR, Biermann JS, Farooki A et al (2009) NCCN Task Force report: bone health in cancer care. J Natl Compr Canc Netw 7(suppl 3):S1–S32 quiz S33-S35

Green J, Lipton A (2010) Anticancer properties of zoledronic acid. Cancer Invest 28:944–957
Green JR (2004) Bisphosphonates: preclinical review. Oncologist 9(suppl 4):3–13
Green JR, Guenther A (2011) The backbone of progress—preclinical studies and innovations with zoledronic acid. Crit Rev Oncol Hematol 77(suppl 1):S3–S12
Greenberg S, Park JW, Melisko ME et al (2010) Effect of adjuvant zoledronic acid (ZOL) on disseminated tumor cells (DTC) in the bone marrow (BM) of women with early-stage breast cancer (ESBC): updated results [abstract]. J Clin Oncol 28(15 suppl):114s Abstract 1002
Guise TA, Mundy GR (1998) Cancer and bone. Endocr Rev 19:18–54
Hadji P, Body JJ, Aapro MS et al (2008) Practical guidance for the management of aromatase inhibitor-associated bone loss. Ann Oncol 19:1407–1416
Hadji P, Aapro MS, Body JJ et al (2011) Management of aromatase inhibitor-associated bone loss in postmenopausal women with breast cancer: practical guidance for prevention and treatment. Ann Oncol (Epub ahead of print)
Hamdy RC (2010) Zoledronic acid: clinical utility and patient considerations in osteoporosis and low bone mass. Drug Des Devel Ther 4:321–335
Hewitt RE, Lissina A, Green AE et al (2005) The bisphosphonate acute phase response: rapid and copious production of proinflammatory cytokines by peripheral blood gd T cells in response to aminobisphosphonates is inhibited by statins. Clin Exp Immunol 139:101–111
Hillner BE, Ingle JN, Chlebowski RT et al (2003) American Society of Clinical Oncology 2003 update on the role of bisphosphonates and bone health issues in women with breast cancer. J Clin Oncol 21:4042–4057
Hoff AO, Toth BB, Altundag K et al (2008) Frequency and risk factors associated with osteonecrosis of the jaw in cancer patients treated with intravenous bisphosphonates. J Bone Miner Res 23:826–836
Janni WJ, Vogl FD, Wiedswang G et al (2011) Persistence of disseminated tumor cells in the bone marrow of breast cancer patients predicts increased risk for relapse—a European pooled analysis. Clin Cancer Res 17:2967–2976
Jemal A, Siegel R, Ward E et al (2006) Cancer statistics, 2006. CA Cancer J Clin 56:106–130
Kim MY, Oskarsson T, Acharyya S et al (2009) Tumor self-seeding by circulating cancer cells. Cell 139:1315–1326
Kohno N, Aogi K, Minami H et al (2005) Zoledronic acid significantly reduces skeletal complications compared with placebo in Japanese women with bone metastases from breast cancer: a randomized, placebo-controlled trial. J Clin Oncol 23:3314–3321
Kristensen B, Ejlertsen B, Mouridsen HT et al (2008) Bisphosphonate treatment in primary breast cancer: results from a randomised comparison of oral pamidronate versus no pamidronate in patients with primary breast cancer. Acta Oncol 47:740–746
Lin AY, Park JW, Scott J et al (2008) Zoledronic acid as adjuvant therapy for women with early stage breast cancer and disseminated tumor cells in bone marrow [abstract]. J Clin Oncol 26(15 suppl): 20s Abstract 559
Lipton A (2010) Should bisphosphonates be utilized in the adjuvant setting for breast cancer? Breast Cancer Res Treat 122:627–636
Lipton A, Chapman JW, Demers L et al (2009) Elevated bone resorption predicts shorter recurrence-free survival for bone metastasis in breast cancer [poster]. Presented at: Primary Therapy of Early Breast Cancer 11th International Conference, St. Gallen, Switzerland, 11–14 March 2009 Abstract 244
Lucas FL, Cauley JA, Stone RA et al (1998) Bone mineral density and risk of breast cancer: differences by family history of breast cancer. Study of Osteoporotic Fractures Research Group. Am J Epidemiol 148:22–29
Major P, Lortholary A, Hon J et al (2001) Zoledronic acid is superior to pamidronate in the treatment of hypercalcemia of malignancy: a pooled analysis of two randomized, controlled clinical trials. J Clin Oncol 19:558–567
Major PP, Lipton A, Berenson J et al (2000) Oral bisphosphonates: a review of clinical use in patients with bone metastases. Cancer 88:6–14

Mansell J, Monypenny IJ, Skene AI et al (2009) Patterns and predictors of early recurrence in postmenopausal women with estrogen receptor-positive early breast cancer. Breast Cancer Res Treat 117:91–98

Mauri D, Valachis A, Polyzos IP et al (2009) Osteonecrosis of the jaw and use of bisphosphonates in adjuvant breast cancer treatment: a meta-analysis. Breast Cancer Res Treat 116:433–439

Meads MB, Hazlehurst LA, Dalton WS (2008) The bone marrow microenvironment as a tumor sanctuary and contributor to drug resistance. Clin Cancer Res 14:2519–2526

Mundy GR (2002) Metastasis to bone: causes, consequences and therapeutic opportunities. Nat Rev Cancer 2:584–593

Naume B, Zhao X, Synnestvedt M et al (2007) Presence of bone marrow micrometastasis is associated with different recurrence risk within molecular subtypes of breast cancer. Mol Oncol 1:160–171

Neville-Webbe HL, Gnant M, Coleman RE (2010) Potential anticancer properties of bisphosphonates. Semin Oncol 37(suppl 1):S53–S65

Newcomb PA, Trentham-Dietz A, Hampton JM (2010) Bisphosphonates for osteoporosis treatment are associated with reduced breast cancer risk. Br J Cancer 102:799–802

Norton L (2008) Cancer stem cells, self-seeding, and decremented exponential growth: theoretical and clinical implications. Breast Dis 29:27–36

Novartis Pharmaceuticals Corporation (2008) Zometa (zoledronic acid) injection (package insert). Novartis Pharmaceuticals Corporation, East Hanover

Padalecki SS, Guise TA (2002) Actions of bisphosphonates in animal models of breast cancer. Breast Cancer Res 4:35–41

Paget S (1889) Secondary growths in cancer of breast. Lancet 133:571–573

Powles T, Paterson S, Kanis JA et al (2002) Randomized, placebo-controlled trial of clodronate in patients with primary operable breast cancer. J Clin Oncol 20:3219–3224

Powles T, Paterson A, McCloskey E et al (2006) Reduction in bone relapse and improved survival with oral clodronate for adjuvant treatment of operable breast cancer (ISRCTN83688026). Breast Cancer Res 8:R13

Rabaglio M, Sun Z, Price KN et al (2009) Bone fractures among postmenopausal patients with endocrine-responsive early breast cancer treated with 5 years of letrozole or tamoxifen in the BIG 1–98 trial. Ann Oncol 20:1489–1498

Rack B, Juckstock J, Genss EM et al (2010) Effect of zoledronate on persisting isolated tumour cells in patients with early breast cancer. Anticancer Res 30:1807–1813

Reid DM, Doughty J, Eastell R et al (2008) Guidance for the management of breast cancer treatment-induced bone loss: a consensus position statement from a UK expert group. Cancer Treat Rev 34(suppl 1):S3–S18

Rennert G, Pinchev M, Rennert HS (2010) Use of bisphosphonates and risk of postmenopausal breast cancer. J Clin Oncol 28:3577–3581

Rennert G, Pinchev M, Rennert HS et al (2011) Use of bisphosphonates and reduced risk of colorectal cancer. J Clin Oncol 29:1146–1150

Ripamonti CI, Maniezzo M, Campa T et al (2009) Decreased occurrence of osteonecrosis of the jaw after implementation of dental preventive measures in solid tumour patients with bone metastases treated with bisphosphonates. The experience of the National Cancer Institute of Milan. Ann Oncol 20:137–145

Roche (2006) Bondronat (package insert). Roche, Welwyn Garden City

Ross JS, Slodkowska EA (2009) Circulating and disseminated tumor cells in the management of breast cancer. Am J Clin Pathol 132:237–245

Rugo HS (2008) The importance of distant metastases in hormone-sensitive breast cancer. Breast 17(suppl 1):S3–S8

Saad F, Lipton A, Cook R et al (2007) Pathologic fractures correlate with reduced survival in patients with malignant bone disease. Cancer 110:1860–1867

Saarto T, Vehmanen L, Virkkunen P et al (2004) Ten-year follow-up of a randomized controlled trial of adjuvant clodronate treatment in node-positive breast cancer patients. Acta Oncol 43:650–656

Santen RJ (2011) Clinical review: effect of endocrine therapies on bone in breast cancer patients. J Clin Endocrinol Metab 96:308–319

Santini D, Vincenzi B, Avvisati G et al (2002) Pamidronate induces modifications of circulating angiogenetic factors in cancer patients. Clin Cancer Res 8:1080–1084

Santini D, Vincenzi B, Dicuonzo G et al (2003) Zoledronic acid induces significant and long-lasting modifications of circulating angiogenic factors in cancer patients. Clin Cancer Res 9:2893–2897

Santini D, Vincenzi B, Hannon RA et al (2006) Changes in bone resorption and vascular endothelial growth factor after a single zoledronic acid infusion in cancer patients with bone metastases from solid tumours. Oncol Rep 15:1351–1357

Santini D, Vincenzi B, Galluzzo S et al (2007) Repeated intermittent low-dose therapy with zoledronic acid induces an early, sustained, and long-lasting decrease of peripheral vascular endothelial growth factor levels in cancer patients. Clin Cancer Res 13:4482–4486

Schenk N, Lombart A, Frassoladti A et al (2007) The E-ZO-FAST trial: zoledronic acid (ZA) effectively inhibits aromatase inhibitor associated bone loss (AIBL) in postmenopausal women (PMW) with early breast cancer (EBC) receiving adjuvant letrozole (Let) [abstract]. Eur J Cancer 5:186–187 Abstract 2008

Schindlbeck C, Kampik T, Janni W et al (2005) Prognostic relevance of disseminated tumor cells in the bone marrow and biological factors of 265 primary breast carcinomas. Breast Cancer Res 7:R1174–R1185

Schindlbeck C, Rack B, Jueckstock J et al (2009) Prognostic relevance of circulating tumor cells (CTCs) in peripheral blood of breast cancer patients before and after adjuvant chemotherapy—translational research program of the German SUCCESS-trial [abstract]. Cancer Res 69(suppl 1):88s Abstract 303

Solomayer EF, Gebauer G, Hirnle P et al (2009) Influence of zoledronic acid on disseminated tumor cells (DTC) in primary breast cancer patients [abstract]. Cancer Res 69(suppl 2): 170s–171s Abstract 2048

Sverrisdottir A, Fornander T, Jacobsson H et al (2004) Bone mineral density among premenopausal women with early breast cancer in a randomized trial of adjuvant endocrine therapy. J Clin Oncol 22:3694–3699

Tanvetyanon T, Stiff PJ (2006) Management of the adverse effects associated with intravenous bisphosphonates. Ann Oncol 17:897–907

Terpos E, Dimopoulos MA (2011) Interaction between the skeletal and immune systems in cancer: mechanisms and clinical implications. Cancer Immunol Immunother 60:305–317

Theriault RL, Lipton A, Hortobagyi GN et al (1999) Pamidronate reduces skeletal morbidity in women with advanced breast cancer and lytic bone lesions: a randomized, placebo-controlled trial. Protocol 18 Aredia Breast Cancer Study Group. J Clin Oncol 17:846–854

Thurlimann B, Keshaviah A, Coates AS et al (2005) A comparison of letrozole and tamoxifen in postmenopausal women with early breast cancer. N Engl J Med 353:2747–2757

Uncu G, Benderli S, Esmer A (1996) Pregnancy during gonadotrophin-releasing hormone agonist therapy. Aust N Z J Obstet Gynaecol 36:484–485

US Food and Drug Administration (2009) Background document for meeting of Advisory Committee for Reproductive Health Drugs (August 13, 2009). Denosumab. Available at: http://www.fda.gov/downloads/AdvisoryCommittees/CommitteesMeetingMaterials/Drugs/ReproductiveHealthDrugsAdvisoryCommittee/UCM176595.pdf. Accessed 11 April 2011

Vantourout P, Mookerjee-Basu J, Rolland C et al (2009) Specific requirements for Vgamma9V-delta2 T cell stimulation by a natural adenylated phosphoantigen. J Immunol 183:3848–3857

Vehmanen L, Elomaa I, Blomqvist C et al (2006) Tamoxifen treatment after adjuvant chemotherapy has opposite effects on bone mineral density in premenopausal patients depending on menstrual status. J Clin Oncol 24:675–680

Vincenzi B, Santini D, Dicuonzo G et al (2005) Zoledronic acid-related angiogenesis modifications and survival in advanced breast cancer patients. J Interferon Cytokine Res 25:144–151

Voelker R (2011) "Disappointing" trial results offer hope for older women with breast cancer. JAMA 305:765–766

Winter MC, Coleman RE (2009) Bisphosphonates in breast cancer: teaching an old dog new tricks. Curr Opin Oncol 21:499–506

Winter MC, Holen I, Coleman RE (2008) Exploring the anti-tumour activity of bisphosphonates in early breast cancer. Cancer Treat Rev 34:453–475

Zmuda JM, Cauley JA, Ljung BM et al (2001) Bone mass and breast cancer risk in older women: differences by stage at diagnosis. J Natl Cancer Inst 93:930–936

Bisphosphonates: Prevention of Bone Metastases in Lung Cancer

Lynn Decoster, Filippo de Marinis, Kostas Syrigos, Vera Hirsh and Kristiaan Nackaerts

Abstract

In patients with lung cancer, bone is one of the most frequent sites of distant spread, with approximately 30% of patients developing skeletal metastases. About half of these patients will experience a skeletal-related event, the occurrence of which not only affects quality of life, but is also associated with poor prognosis. Bisphosphonates are currently the mainstay for treating bone metastases in patients with lung cancer, with proven beneficial effects on prevention and delay of skeletal complications. Their role in preventing the development of skeletal metastases, their anti-tumoral properties and their effect on survival remain to be elucidated. Other bone-targeted therapies are being investigated in phase II and III clinical trials and might expand the therapeutic arsenal in the near future.

L. Decoster · K. Nackaerts (✉)
Department of Pulmonology, Respiratory Oncology,
University Hospital Gasthuisberg, Herestraat 49,
B-3000, Leuven, Belgium
e-mail: kristiaan.nackaerts@uzleuven.be

F. de Marinis
Department of Lung Diseases, San Camillo High Specialization Hospital,
Rome, Italy

K. Syrigos
Oncology Unit, Sotiria General Hospital, Athens, Greece

V. Hirsh
Department of Medicine and Oncology, McGill University Health Centre,
Royal Victoria Hospital, Montreal, Canada

Abbreviations

AUC	Area under the curve
BALP	Bone-specific alkaline phosphatase
CT	Computed tomography (scan)
FDG-PET	Fluorine-18 deoxyglucose positron emission tomography
Gy	Gray
HR	Hazard ratio
IV	Intravenous
MRI	Magnetic resonance imaging
PD	Progressive disease
QOL	Quality of life
NSCLC	Non-small cell lung cancer
NTX	N-telopeptide of type I collagen
ONJ	Osteonecrosis of the jaw
RANKL	Receptor activator of nuclear factor kappa B ligand
RR	Relative risk
SCLC	Small cell lung cancer
SRE	Skeletal-related event

Contents

1	Introduction	95
2	Incidence of Bone Metastasis in Lung Cancer	95
3	Impact of Bone Metastases: The Rationale for Adequate Treatment	96
4	Diagnosis of Bone Metastases in Lung Cancer	97
5	Treatment of Bone Metastases in Lung Cancer: A Multidisciplinary Affair	99
6	Bisphosphonates in the Treatment of Bone Metastases: The Current Standard of Care	99
	6.1 Therapeutic Efficacy of Zoledronic Acid in Lung Cancer: Results From Clinical Trials	100
	6.2 Safety Issues and Recommendations for Use	101
	6.3 Biochemical Markers of Bone Turnover: Predictors of Clinical Outcome?	101
	6.4 Pharmaco-Economic Considerations	102
	6.5 Prevention of Bone Metastases: Under Investigation	103
	6.6 Evidence for Anti-Tumoral Activity in Lung Cancer?	104
7	Bone Metastasis Therapy in Lung Cancer: What the Future Might Bring	104
	7.1 Denosumab	104
	7.2 Other Small Molecules	105
8	Conclusion	105
References		106

1 Introduction

Lung cancer is still the leading cause of cancer-related death worldwide, with about 1.3 million patients dying from this disease each year. The majority of patients will present with advanced (i.e. inoperable stage IIIB or stage IV) disease at diagnosis, making them unsuitable for treatment with curative intent. But even when diagnosed at an early stage, a large number of patients will eventually experience disease relapse with metastases. As a consequence, the prognosis of lung cancer patients is dismal, with a five year survival rate of only 15%. Furthermore, during the course of their illness, patients with advanced lung cancer may experience debilitating symptoms, seriously affecting their quality of life. Skeletal metastases, a frequent site of distant spread in lung cancer, particularly cause significant morbidity and quality of life (QOL) impairment as well as a decline of performance status preventing further lines of treatments. Therefore, adequate assessment and treatment of bone disease is essential in the management of lung cancer patients.

2 Incidence of Bone Metastasis in Lung Cancer

Based on the results of autopsy reports, the incidence of bone metastases in lung cancer has been estimated at 30–40% (Coleman 2001). On the one hand, these data probably do not reflect the true incidence of bone metastases at diagnosis. On the other hand, treatment advances in the past decade have resulted in improved survival, leading to possibly even more patients being diagnosed with bone metastases throughout their disease course.

Detection rates of bone metastases also vary depending on the diagnostic modality used. Different studies using whole-body bone scans to evaluate the presence of bone metastases in non-small-cell lung cancer (NSCLC) yielded varying results with incidence rates between 8 and 34% (Kosteva and Langer 2008). In recent years, fluorine-18 deoxyglucose positron emission tomography (FDG-PET) has become a valuable tool for the detection of skeletal metastases. In a single-center retrospective review, 110 patients diagnosed with NSCLC underwent baseline FDG-PET and a bone metastases incidence rate of 19% was found (Bury et al. 1998).

Still, underestimation remains a problem, as current staging guidelines do not routinely recommend screening for bone metastases in all patients with newly diagnosed lung cancer.

Bone scans are mainly advised in symptomatic patients or in case of abnormal clinical or laboratory findings (e.g. high alkaline phosphatase levels or hypercalcemia). In a small retrospective study addressing this issue, whole-body bone scanning was performed in 49 patients who were believed to have potentially operable NSCLC after initial evaluation. Although these patients had no clinical or biochemical evidence of bone involvement, skeletal metastases were present in

8 of 49 patients or 16.3% (Iordanidou et al. 2006). Similar results were found in a prospective study of 100 patients with NSCLC: using whole-body bone scans, bone metastases were detected in 7 of the 26 patients (27%) who did not report bone pain, whereas the prevalence was 32% among the 74 patients who were symptomatic (Schirrmeister et al. 2004).

3   Impact of Bone Metastases: The Rationale for Adequate Treatment

Patients with skeletal metastases are at increased risk for so-called skeletal-related events (SREs). This term groups all complications from bone metastases as well as any therapeutic intervention required for palliation. SREs include pathologic fractures, spinal cord and nerve root compression, hypercalcemia of malignancy and the requirement for surgery or radiotherapy. In a large prospective study assessing the efficacy of zoledronic acid in the treatment of skeletal metastases in patients with NSCLC and other solid tumors (except carcinoma of breast and prostate), 48% of patients in the placebo group experienced at least one SRE (Rosen et al. 2004). Many patients have multiple SREs during the course of their disease, with a mean of 2.71 SREs per year for lung cancer patients (Langer and Hirsh 2010). The median time to first SRE is approximately 5 months (Rosen et al. 2004). Bone pain, although usually not considered a SRE, is the most common presentation of skeletal metastases, with 80% of NSCLC patients complaining of pain at the affected site. The most common 'true' SREs are need for radiation therapy (34%) and occurrence of pathologic fractures (22%). Need for surgery (5%), spinal cord compression (4%) and hypercalcemia of malignancy (4%) seem to be less common complications (Kosteva and Langer 2004). All SREs have considerable impact on quality of life (QOL), survival and healthcare costs.

QOL-issues of SREs have not yet been investigated in NSCLC patients specifically, but data may be well extrapolated from the experience in prostate cancer patients, in whom a significant decline in physical, emotional and functional well-being was demonstrated in patients who developed a SRE compared to patients who did not (Weinfurt et al. 2006).

The occurrence of a SRE is a poor prognostic factor. Although in NSCLC patients with metastatic (stage IV) disease, overall survival was comparable between patients with or without bone involvement (237 days versus 268 days, $p = 0.733$), SREs were associated with a 50% decrease in survival (366 days versus 187 days), albeit not statistically significant (Tsuya et al. 2007).

The presence of skeletal metastases greatly increases the total *costs* of care for patients. In a retrospective analysis using a large United States health insurance claims database, the costs of SREs in patients with bone metastases from lung cancer were examined. The estimated life-time cost per patient for the management of SREs was approximately $12000 (based on 2004 cost estimations). Radiotherapy accounted for 60% of total costs, bone surgery for 21% and treatment of fracture for 4% (Delea et al. 2004). Since this study focused on expenses directly attributable to SREs, indirect costs, such as increased use of other medical care services due to loss of functionality were not included. When total costs of care were calculated, including those not directly related to the acute treatment of SREs, medical costs were almost $28000 higher in patients with SREs compared to patients without SREs (Delea et al. 2006).

4 Diagnosis of Bone Metastases in Lung Cancer

Current American Society of Clinical Oncology (ASCO) guidelines for staging of lung cancer recommend the use of FDG-PET when there is no evidence of distant metastatic disease on CT scan of the chest and abdomen. A bone scan is optional when FGD-PET is used, but remains necessary in patients with suspicious symptoms in regions not imaged by FDG-PET (Pfister et al. 2004). The European Society for Medical Oncology (ESMO) still advocates the use of bone scans, but only in patients with bone pain or clinical or biochemical suspicion of bone metastases (D'Addario and Felip 2008). Symptom-based screening practices, however, might well be inaccurate as demonstrated by Schirrmeister et al. (2004). In a prospective study in 100 patients with NSCLC, 74 patients either reported complaints related to the skeletal system or had abnormal findings at physical examination. Only in 38 patients (22%) did 2 separate specialists consider the symptoms suspicious for metastatic bone disease (Schirrmeister et al. 2004). Therefore, a European Expert Panel recently recommended to screen for the presence of bone metastases in every newly diagnosed lung cancer patient (de Marinis et al. 2009). Furthermore, the same panel suggested that screening should preferentially be based on FDG-PET as different studies have demonstrated the superior accuracy of FGD-PET. In a retrospective review by Bury et al. (1998) FDG-PET was compared with bone scintigraphy for the detection of bone metastases in patients with NSCLC. FDG-PET was found to have a sensitivity of 90%, which compared to the sensitivity of bone scintigraphy. However, FDG-PET was more specific (specificity 98% for FDG-PET versus 61% for bone scintigraphy) and had a higher positive predictive value (90% versus 35%). In a prospective study by Hetzel et al. (2003) 103 newly diagnosed NSCLC patients were evaluated by bone scan and FDG-PET. Bone scan proved false negative in 13 of 33 patients compared to 2 false negative results with FDG-PET. Furthermore, FDG-PET detected 11 of 13 bone metastases missed by bone scan.

Another diagnostic modality that has recently been introduced for the assessment of distant metastases is whole-body magnetic resonance imaging (MRI) (Fig. 1). This technique, especially with diffusion-weighted imaging, compared favorably to whole-body FDG-PET/CT when sensitivity is considered and might have higher specificity (Takenaka et al. 2008), although specificity for FGD-PET/CT was rather low in this trial. The main advantage of MRI is that it does not require the use of ionizing radiation whereas availability is currently a major disadvantage.

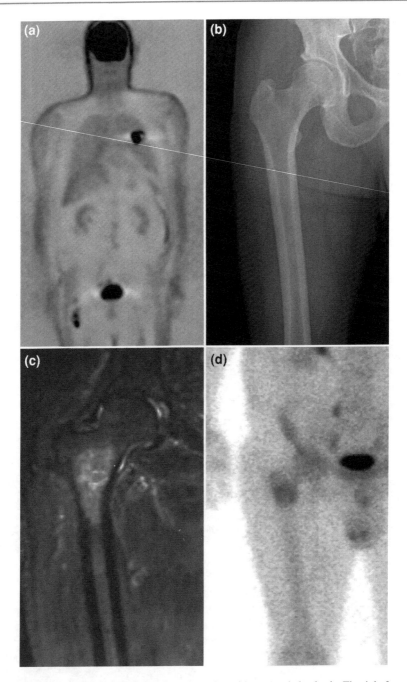

Fig. 1 Bone metastasis in a NSCLC patient presenting without any skeletal pain. The right femoral bone metastasis was first described on PET scan (**a**) and later confirmed by MRI (**c**), but not visuable by standard radiography of the femur (**b**). A whole-body bone scan was also positive (**d**)

5 Treatment of Bone Metastases in Lung Cancer: A Multidisciplinary Affair

The ultimate goal in bone care would be the prevention of developing skeletal metastases. Until this becomes possible, management of bone metastases involves palliation of pain and prevention or treatment of SREs. For this purpose, different treatment modalities are often employed.

Medical treatment consists mainly of analgesics (non-steroidal anti-inflammatory drugs in combination with narcotic analgesics) and intravenous bisphosphonates. Bisphosphonates have become the mainstay of treatment of skeletal metastases and will be discussed more extensively in the next section. In patients with refractory pain, impending pathologic fractures or spinal cord compression, radiation therapy is often required. A meta-analysis by the Cochrane Collaboration, found that radiotherapy produced complete pain relief in 25% of patients at 1 month and at least 50% relief in 41% (McQuay et al. 2000). Different dose-fractionation schemes are currently being used, varying from single fractions (usually 8 Gy) over short fractionation schedules (20 to 30 Gy in 5–10 fractions) to more radical treatment schemes of up to 50 Gy over 5 weeks (Bezjak 2003). A meta-analysis of radiotherapy dose-fractionation trials found no difference in terms of pain control between patients receiving single or multiple fractions (Chow et al. 2007). However, it remains unclear if this is also true for other indications of radiotherapy such as the prevention of pathologic fractures or neurologic decompression.

A major limitation of external radiotherapy is its inability to safely cover multiple affected sites with optimal irradiation doses. Radiopharmaceuticals such as strontium-89 chloride (^{89}SrCl) accumulate in metastatic bone lesions and have been shown to have analgesic effects mainly in patients with skeletal metastases from prostate cancer. In a small trial by Kasalicky and Krasjka (1998) 31 lung cancer patients were treated with strontium-89 chloride. Mild improvement occurred in 38.7% of patients, substantial improvement in 51.7%, with 2 patients (6.4%) reporting dramatic improvement (i.e. complete resolution of symptoms). The mean duration of the beneficial effects was 3.3 months, with myelosuppression being the most common adverse event.

When weight-bearing bones are involved or pathologic fractures occur, palliative surgery is the preferred treatment. Surgery may also be considered when conservative measures fail to prevent neurologic complications of spinal cord compression.

6 Bisphosphonates in the Treatment of Bone Metastases: The Current Standard of Care

In the past decades, the use of bisphosphonates has become common practice for the treatment of hypercalcemia of malignancy and prevention of skeletal complications in patients with proven bone metastases. For lung cancer in particular, zoledronic acid is the only bisphosphonate that has been extensively studied and that has gained regulatory approval based on the results of a large pivotal trial by Rosen et al. Little evidence in lung cancer exists for other bisphosphonates, although a retrospective trial in 104 patients with NSCLC found a survival benefit (15.4 months versus 2.1 months; $p < 0.001$) in patients receiving pamidronate (Spizzo et al. 2009).

6.1 Therapeutic Efficacy of Zoledronic Acid in Lung Cancer: Results From Clinical Trials

The efficacy of zoledronic acid for the treatment of bone metastases in patients with lung cancer was demonstrated in a large, randomized, placebo-controlled trial, in which 773 patients with bone metastases from solid tumors other than breast and prostate were randomized to receive either zoledronic acid (4 or 8 mg IV) or placebo every 3 weeks for up to 21 months. Approximately 50% of enrolled patients had NSCLC and 8% had small-cell lung cancer (SCLC). Due to safety issues concerning renal toxicity in the high dose group, patients receiving 8 mg were subsequently switched to a dose of 4 mg. Efficacy analyses were finally based on the comparison of the 4 mg-dose group versus placebo. The primary endpoint of the study was the reduction in patients developing one or more SRE at 21 months. In the overall population, 48% of patients in the placebo group had experienced a SRE compared to 39% in the zoledronic acid group ($p = 0.039$). Moreover, a 31% risk reduction for the development of skeletal complications was observed. Treatment with zoledronic acid significantly reduced all types of SREs as well as the annual incidence of SREs (1.74 SREs per year for the zoledronic acid-treated patients versus 2.71 SREs per year for placebo, $p = 0.012$). Furthermore, the median time to both first SRE (236 days versus 155 days, $p = 0.009$) and first pathologic fracture (294 days versus 161 days, $p = 0.020$) was significantly delayed in the zoledronic acid group. Patients receiving zoledronic acid also reported bone pain less frequently than patients treated with placebo. This trial could not demonstrate any benefit regarding time to disease progression nor an effect on overall survival (Rosen et al. 2004).

Time to disease progression and overall survival were the primary endpoints in a prospective trial by Zarogoulidis et al. (2009). In this study, 144 patients with stage IV disease and positive bone scan were consecutively recruited. Patients were treated with combination chemotherapy carboplatin (AUC = 6) and docetaxel (100 mg/m^2) every 4 weeks for up to 8 cycles, with symptomatic bone pain patients also receiving zoledronic acid 4 mg IV every 4 weeks during chemotherapy, and every 3 weeks as maintenance thereafter. Median time to disease progression was significantly delayed in the treatment group (265 days versus 150 days, $p < 0.001$) and a survival benefit of almost 3 months (578 days versus 384 days, $p < 0.001$) was seen in the patients receiving zoledronic acid. Moreover, a positive correlation was found between the number of zoledronic acid infusions received and survival and time to progression ($p < 0.01$ Pearson correlation).

6.2 Safety Issues and Recommendations for Use

Bisphosphonates are generally safe and well-tolerated. The most frequently reported adverse events in the Rosen trial were nausea, anemia, emesis, obstipation and dyspnea. These symptoms were mostly mild to moderate in severity.

Reports of renal dysfunction in patients treated with bisphosphonates raised concerns about renal safety. However, when an infusion time of 15 min was respected, the rate of grade 3/4 serum creatinine increases was identical in the zoledronic acid 4 mg group (1.8%) compared to the placebo group (1.8%) (Rosen et al. 2004). Assessment of renal function before the start of treatment and monthly before each dose is recommended. Furthermore, dose adjustments should be made in patients with mild to moderate renal dysfunction whereas zoledronic acid should not be used in patients with severe renal impairment (creatinine clearance <30 ml/min).

Osteonecrosis of the jaw (ONJ) may occur in up to 5% of patients treated with bisphosphonates, with dental trauma and suboptimal dental hygiene increasing the risk of developing ONJ. Preventive measures have shown to result in a significant reduction of the occurrence of ONJ: when comparing pre- and post-implementation of a preventive measures program, incidence rates for ONJ were 3.2% and 1.3%, respectively, (Ripamonti et al. 2009). Therefore, a dental examination prior to initiation of treatment should be performed whenever bisphosphonate treatment is considered.

6.3 Biochemical Markers of Bone Turnover: Predictors of Clinical Outcome?

Biochemical markers of bone turnover may provide prognostic information in patients with bone metastases. The value of N-telopeptide of type I collagen (NTX), a bone resorption marker and bone-specific alkaline phosphatase (BALP), a bone formation marker, as predictors of clinical outcome, has been investigated in NSCLC patients. Data were obtained from the placebo arm of two phase III trials of zoledronic acid for the treatment of bone metastases from prostate cancer, NSCLC and other solid tumors. When the NSCLC patient stratum was analyzed separately, patients with high baseline urinary levels of NTX (≥ 100 nmol/mmol creatinine) had a non-statistically significant increased risk of a SRE (RR = 1.66, $p = 0.183$) and time to first SRE (RR = 1.99, $p = 0.140$), a statistically significant increased risk of bone disease progression (RR 3.49, $p = 0.007$) and a significant 4.7-fold increase in risk of death (RR = 4.67, $p < 0.001$) compared to those with low NTX levels. Comparable results were found for increased levels (≥ 146 IU/l) of BALP. When the total patient population was considered (prostate cancer, NSCLC and other solid tumors), both baseline and on-study marker values were predictive for the risk of a negative clinical outcome, with on-study values probably being even more significant. Furthermore, NTX levels seemed to be stronger prognostic indicators for negative clinical outcomes than BALP levels (Brown et al. 2005).

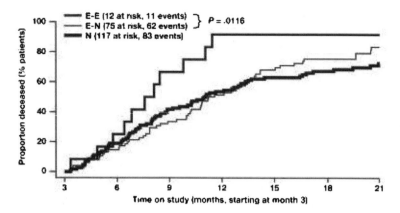

Fig. 2 Patients with NSCLC whose elevated baseline levels of N-telopeptide of type I collagen (*NTX*) normalize under treatment with zoledronic acid (*E–N*) have improved survival compared to patients with persistently elevated NTX levels (*E–E*). E–E indicates patients with elevated baseline and 3-month NTX; E–N, patients with elevated baseline and normalized 3-month NTX; N, patients with normal baseline NTX (From Lipton et al. Cancer 2008; 113(1):193–201, with permission)

Lipton et al. (2008) demonstrated that in NSCLC patients with elevated NTX levels (≥ 64 nmol/mmol creatinine), zoledronic acid normalized NTX levels within 3 months in 81% of patients (compared to 17% in the placebo group). Normalization of NTX levels was associated with a significantly reduced risk of death in patients treated with zoledronic acid (RR = 0.43, p = 0.0116) (Fig. 2). Similar associations were found for SRE-free survival (45% relative increase) and bone lesion progression-free survival (61% relative increase). In another retrospective analysis of the Rosen-trial, the effect of baseline NTX levels on treatment effect was assessed. In patients with high baseline NTX (≥ 64 nmol/mmol creatinine), treatment with zoledronic acid significantly reduced the risk of death by 35% (RR = 0.652, p = 0.025) compared to placebo, an effect that could not be demonstrated in patients with low baseline NTX (Hirsh et al. 2008). Different explanations have been proposed for these findings: patients with high NTX levels might have bone disease more responsive to the effect of bisphosphonates or might be more likely to benefit from treatment because of their higher risk for life-limiting SREs. Furthermore, reduced osteolysis could result in decreased release of growth factors from the bone matrix.

6.4 Pharmaco-Economic Considerations

Several recent studies have addressed the economic impact of treatment with zoledronic acid. In a retrospective analysis in lung cancer patients in France, Germany and the United Kingdom, drug-related costs were € 1,610, € 1.510 and € 1.597 per patient, respectively. However, the use of zoledronic acid resulted in a

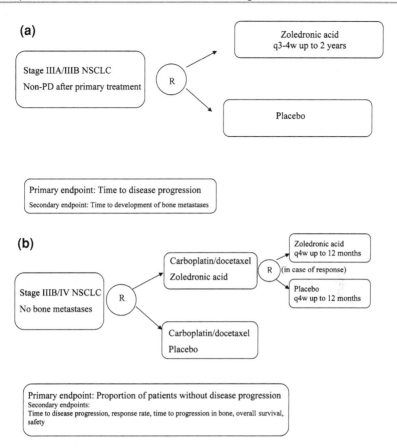

Fig. 3 Outline of two clinical trials evaluating the ability of zoledronic acid to prevent or delay the development of bone metastases in NSCLC patients. **a** NCT00172042 **b** NCT00086268. (US National Institutes of Health 2011a)

net reduction of SRE-related costs of € 2,221, € 2,031 and € 2,014 per patient, leading to average overall cost savings of € 598 per patient in France, € 521 in Germany and € 417 in the United Kingdom. The use of zoledronic acid can therefore be considered highly cost-effective (Stephens et al. 2009).

6.5 Prevention of Bone Metastases: Under Investigation

Currently, the results of two clinical trials evaluating the ability of zoledronic acid to prevent or delay the development of bone metastases are eagerly awaited (Fig. 3) (US National Institutes of Health 2011b). In a European trial (NCT00172042), patients with newly diagnosed stage IIIA and IIIB NSCLC, once successfully treated with surgical or non-surgical combined modality treatment, were then randomly assigned to zoledronic acid 4 mg IV every 3–4 weeks or placebo for up to 2 years. Patients in the placebo arm who developed bone metastases were crossed over to receive zoledronic acid monthly. The primary endpoint of this study is to evaluate the efficacy of zoledronic acid in delaying disease progression, disease recurrence or death, with one of the secondary endpoints being the time to bone metastases development. The US-ZPACT trial (NCT0086268) has also completed enrollment and recruited patients with stage IIIB or IV NSCLC (not metastatic to the bone), who were treated with chemotherapy (carboplatin/docetaxel). Patients were randomized to either zoledronic acid or placebo for up to six cycles. Patients in the zoledronic acid arm who responded to treatment were further randomized to zoledronic acid or placebo monthly for up to 12 months. The primary endpoint is the proportion of patients without disease progression (Fig. 3).

6.6 Evidence for Anti-Tumoral Activity in Lung Cancer?

There is a growing amount of preclinical evidence that zoledronic acid has intrinsic anti-tumoral properties. In vitro, zoledronic acid was able to induce apoptosis and inhibit cell growth in 16 different NSCLC cell lines (Berger et al. 2005) and in 8 out of 12 small cell lung cancer (SCLC) cell lines. Zoledronic acid also inhibited SCLC cell lines growth in vivo in animal models.

Furthermore, there was in vitro evidence of an augmentation of the effects of different chemotherapeutic agents frequently used in the treatment of lung cancer such as paclitaxel, etoposide, cisplatinum (Matsumoto et al. 2005) and gemcitabine (Budman and Calabro 2006).

In addition to preclinical data, post hoc analysis from clinical trials also pointed toward a possible direct anti-cancer activity of bisphosphonates. We already discussed the potential effect on disease progression and survival (see Sect. 6.1). Moreover, Karamanos et al. (2010) found higher partial response rates in the primary tumor (32% versus 16%) after completion of first-line chemotherapy in patients who additionally received zoledronic acid.

7 Bone Metastasis Therapy in Lung Cancer: What the Future Might Bring

7.1 Denosumab

Denosumab is a fully human monoclonal antibody that inhibits osteoclast function and bone resorption by targeting receptor activator of nuclear factor kappa B ligand (RANKL) (Fizazi et al. 2009; Lipton et al. 2007). The efficacy and safety of denosumab in patients with solid tumors (other than breast and prostate) or multiple myeloma was assessed in a phase III trial by Henry et al. 2009. In total, 1776 bisphosphonate naïve patients were randomized to receive subcutaneous denosumab 120 mg or intravenous zoledronic acid 4 mg (dose adjusted for creatinine clearance) every 4 weeks. Denosumab proved to be noninferior to zoledronic acid (HR: 0.84; 95% CI 0.71–0.98, $p = 0.0007$) in delaying the time to first on-study SRE. Although statistically non-significant, a trend towards prolonged time to first on-study SRE (20.6 months for denosumab versus 16.3 months for zoledronic acid) was seen in favor of denosumab. The incidence of osteonecrosis of the jaw was similar between both groups (1.1% for denosumab, 1.3% for zoledronic acid).

7.2 Other Small Molecules

Different other pathways and agents for the treatment of neoplastic bone disease are currently being investigated. Potential new molecular targets are c-Src, cathepsin K and $\alpha_v\beta_3$ integrins (Kawatani and Osada 2009).

c-Src is a non-receptor tyrosine kinase that plays a key role not only in osteoclast activation but also in various oncogenic cellular activities such as proliferation, invasion and survival. Therefore, targeting this pathway is believed to result in both anti-resorptive as well as anti-neoplastic effects. In preclinical trials, dasatinib, an oral broadspectrum tyrosine kinase inhibitor, has demonstrated both anti-osteoclast activity as well as anti-proliferative effects in a wide variety of cell lines, including NSCLC. A phase II trial is ongoing in NSCLC with progression-free survival being the primary endpoint. Preliminary data reported 1 patient with partial response and 6 patients with stable disease among 25 patients with metastasized NSCLC treated with dasatinib (Johnson et al. 2009).

Cathepsin K is a proteinase that is crucial in the collagen breakdown during bone resorption. A phase II trial with a cathepsin K inhibitor in patients with breast cancer was withdrawn before enrollment because of administrative reasons.

$\alpha_v\beta_3$ Integrins belong to a family of cell-surface adhesion receptors that mediate cell–cell and cell–matrix interactions. Preclinical data in breast cancer suggest that these agents may be useful in the treatment and prevention of breast cancer skeletal metastases.

8 Conclusion

Bone metastases are common in patients with lung cancer. They cause significant morbidity and their skeletal complications may negatively influence life expectancy. Early detection, preferably with FDG-PET in all newly diagnosed lung cancer patients, will allow for prompt initiation of bone-targeted treatment. The beneficial effects of zoledronic acid on prevention and delay of skeletal complications have sufficiently been proven in large clinical trials. There is also some, though so far limited, clinical evidence for a survival benefit in zoledronic acid-treated NSCLC patients, supported by preclinical evidence for direct anti-cancer properties of bisphosphonates. Based on the currently available data, the routine use of zoledronic acid is recommended in all lung cancer patients with proven bone metastases. Preventive use of zoledronic acid in non-skeletal metastasized lung cancer patients is not yet to be recommended. With the advent of newer targeted agents for the treatment of bone metastases, such as RANKL antibodies, the optimal treatment regimens for stage IV lung cancer with bone metastases may become more complex in the near future.

References

Berger W, Kubista B, Elbling L et al (2005) The N-containing bisphosphonate zoledronic acid exerts potent anticancer activity against non-small cell lung cancer cells by inhibition of protein geranylgeranylation. Proc Am Assoc Cancer Res 46: Abstr 4981

Bezjak A (2003) Palliative therapy for lung cancer. Semin Surg Oncol 21:138–147

Brown JE, Cook RJ, Major P (2005) Bone turnover markers as predictors of skeletal complications in prostate cancer, lung cancer and other solid tumors. J Natl Cancer Inst 97:59–69

Budman DR, Calabro A (2006) Zoledronic acid (Zometa®) enhances the cytotoxic effect of gemcitabine and fluvastatin: in vitro isobologram studies with conventional and nonconventional cytotoxic agents. Oncology 70:147–153

Bury T, Barreto A, Daenen F et al (1998) Fluorine-18 deoxyglucose positron emission tomography for the detection of bone metastases in patients with non-small cell lung cancer. Eur J Nucl Med 25:1244–1247

Chow E, Harris K, Fan G et al (2007) Meta-analysis of palliative radiotherapy trials for bone metastases. Clin Oncol 19:S26

Coleman RE (2001) Metastatic bone disease: clinical features, pathophysiology and treatment strategies. Cancer Treat Rev 27:165–176

D'Addario G, Felip E (2008) Non-small-cell lung cancer: ESMO clinical recommendations for diagnosis, treatment and follow-up. Ann Oncol 19 (Suppl 1):ii39–ii40

Delea T, Langer C, McKiernan J et al (2004) The cost of treatment of skeletal-related events in patients with bone metastases from lung cancer. Oncology 67:390–396

Delea TE, McKiernan J, Brandman J et al (2006) Impact of skeletal complications on total medical care costs among patients with bone metastases of lung cancer. J Thorac Oncol 1:571–576

de Marinis F, Eberhardt W, Harper PG et al (2009) Bisphosphonate use in patients with lung cancer and bone metastases. Recommendations of a European expert panel. J Thorac Oncol 4(10):1280–1288

Fizazi K, Lipton A, Mariete X et al (2009) Randomized phase II trial of denosumab in patients with bone metastases from prostate cancer, breast cancer or other neoplasms after intravenous bisphosphonates. J Clin Oncol 27:1534–1546

Henry D, von Moos R, Vadhan-Ray S et al (2009) A double-blind, randomized study of denosumab versus zoledronic acid for the treatment of bone metastases in patients with advanced cancer (excluding breast and prostate cancer) or multiple myeloma. Eur J Cancer 7(suppl):11

Hetzel M, Arslandemir C, König HH et al (2003) F-18NaF PET for detection of bone metastases in lung cancer: accuracy, cost-effectiveness, and impact on patient management. J Bone Miner Res 18(12):2206–2214

Hirsh V, Major PP, Lipton A et al (2008) Zoledronic acid and survival in patients with metastatic bone disease from lung cancer and elevated markers of osteoclast activity. J Thorac Oncol 3:228–236

Iordanidou L, Trivizaki E, Saranti S et al (2006) Is there a role of whole body bone scan in early stages of non small cell lung cancer patients. J BUON 11:491–497

Johnson FM, Tang X, Tran H et al (2009) Phase II study of dasatinib in non-small cell lung cancer (NSCLC). J Clin Oncol 27(Suppl 15):e19015

Karamanos N, Zarogoulidis K, Boutsikou E et al (2010) Prolonged survival and time to disease progression with zoledronic acid in patients with bone metastases from non-small cell lung cancer. J Clin Oncol 28(15):e18077

Kasalicky J, Krajska V (1998) The effect of repeated strontium-89 chloride therapy on bone palliation in patients with skeletal cancer metastases. Eur J Nuc Med 25:1362–1367

Kawatani M, Osada H (2009) Osteoclast-targeting small molecules for the treatment of neoplastic bone metastases. Cancer Sci 100:1999–2005

Kosteva J, Langer CJ (2004) Incidence and distribution of skeletal metastases in NSCLC in the era of PET. Lung Cancer 46(1):S45

Kosteva J, Langer C (2008) The changing landscape of the medical management of skeletal metastases in non small cell lung cancer. Curr Opin Oncol 20:155–161

Langer C, Hirsh V (2010) Skeletal morbidity in lung cancer patients with bone metastases: demonstrating the need for early diagnosis and treatment with bisphosphonates. Lung Cancer 67:4–11

Lipton A, Steger GG, Figueroa J et al (2007) Randomized active-controlled phase II study of denosumab efficacy and safety in patients with breast cancer-related bone metastases. J Clin Oncol 25:4431–4437

Lipton A, Cook R, Saad F et al (2008) Normalization of bone markers is associated with improved survival in patients with bone metastases from solid tumors and elevated bone resorption receiving zoledronic acid. Cancer 113(1):193–201

Matsumoto S, Kimura S, Segawa H et al (2005) Efficacy of the third-generation bisphosphonate, zoledronic acid alone and combined with anti-cancer agents against small cell lung cancer cell lines. Lung Cancer 47:31–37

McQuay HJ, Collins SL, Carroll D et al (2000) Radiotherapy for the palliation of painful bone metastases. Cochrane Database Syst Rev CD001793

Pfister DG, Johnson DH, Azzoli CG et al (2004) American Society of Clinical Oncology treatment of unresectable non-small-cell lung cancer guideline: update 2003. J Clin Oncol 22(2):330–353

Ripamonti CI, Maniezzo M, Campa T et al (2009) Decreased occurrence of osteonecrosis of the jaw after implementation of preventive measures in solid tumour patients with bone metastases treated with bisphosphonates. The experience of the National Cancer Institute of Milan. Ann Oncol 20:137–145

Rosen LS, Gordon D, Tchekmedyian NS et al (2004) Long-term efficacy and safety of zoledronic acid in the treatment of skeletal metastases in patients with nonsmall cell lung carcinoma and other solid tumors. Cancer 100(12):2613–2621

Schirrmeister H, Arslandemir C, Glatting G et al (2004) Omission of bone scanning according to staging guidelines leads to futile therapy in non-small cell lung cancer. Eur J Nucl Med Mol Imaging 31:964–968

Spizzo G, Seeber A, Mitterer M (2009) Routine use of pamidronate in NSCLC with bone metastasis: results from a retrospective analysis. Anticancer Res 29(12):5245–5249

Stephens J, Kaura S, Botteman MF (2009) Cost-effectiveness of zoledronic acid versus placebo in the management of skeletal metastases in lung cancer patients (LC pts): Comparison across three European countries. J Clin Oncol 27(15S):8081

Takenaka D, Ohno Y, Matsumoto K et al (2008) Detection of bone metastases in non-small cell lung cancer patients: comparison of whole-body diffusion-weighted imaging (DWI), whole-body MRI imaging without and with DWI, whole-body FDG-PET/CT, and bone scintigraphy. J Magn Reson Imaging 30:298–308

Tsuya A, Kurata T, Tamura K (2007) Skeletal metastases in non-small cell lung cancer: a retrospective study. Lung Cancer 57:229–232

US National Institutes of Health (2011a). A study to evaluate the safety and efficacy of zoledronic acid in the prevention or delaying of bone metastasis in patients with stage IIIA and IIIB non-small cell lung cancer. Available at: http://clinicaltrials.gov/ct2/show/NCT00172042?term=zoledronic+acid+AND+lung+cancer&rank=1

US National Institutes of Health (2011b). Non-small cell lung cancer study US75(Z-PACT). Available at: http://clinicaltrials.gov/ct2/show/NCT00086268?term=zoledronic+acid+AND+lung+cancer&rank=9

Weinfurt KP, Anstrom KJ, Castel LD et al (2006) Effect of zoledronic acid on pain associated with bone metastasis in patients with prostate cancer. Ann Oncol 17:986–989

Zarogoulidis K, Boutsikou E, Zarogoulidis P et al (2009) The impact of zoledronic acid therapy on survival of lung cancer patients with bone metastasis. Int J Cancer 125:1705–1709

Bisphosphonates: Prevention of Bone Metastases in Prostate Cancer

Fred Saad and Jean-Baptiste Lattouf

Abstract

Bone metastases and their associated morbidities are common in patients with advanced prostate cancer and other genitourinary (GU) malignancies. Zoledronic acid (a bisphosphonate) has long been the mainstay of treatment for reducing the risk of skeletal-related events in patients with bone metastases from GU cancers, and denosumab (a monoclonal antibody directed against the receptor activator of nuclear factor kappa B ligand [RANKL]) has recently received approval for this indication in the United States. Preclinical data indicate that modifying the bone microenvironment may render it less conducive to metastasis, and emerging clinical findings suggest that the potential benefits from bone-directed therapies are not limited to reducing skeletal morbidity—these agents might help to improve survival and delay bone disease progression or even development of bone metastases (if used earlier in the disease course). This chapter reviews the rationale and recent clinical data supporting an antimetastatic role for bone-directed therapies in patients with GU malignancies.

Keywords

Anticancer · Bisphosphonate · Bone metastases · Genitourinary cancer · Prostate cancer · Zoledronic acid

---

F. Saad (✉) · J.-B. Lattouf
Centre Hospitalier de l'Université de Montréal, Hôpital Notre-Dame,
1560 Rue Sherbrooke East, Montréal, QC, Canada H2L 4M,
e-mail: fred.saad@umontreal.ca

Abbreviations

ADT	Androgen-deprivation therapy
BALP	Bone-specific alkaline phosphatase
BMD	Bone mineral density
BP	Bisphosphonate
CRPC	Castration-resistant prostate cancer
CTC	Circulating tumor cell
DM	Distant metastasis
DTC	Disseminated tumor cell
E-E	Patients with elevated baseline and 3-month NTX
E-N	Patients with elevated baseline and normalized 3-month NTX
$\gamma\delta$	Gamma-delta (T cells)
GU	Genitourinary
HR	Hazard ratio
MM	Multiple myeloma
N-BP	Nitrogen-containing bisphosphonate
NTX	N-telopeptide of type I collagen
OS	Overall survival
PC	Prostate cancer
PO	Oral(ly)
PSA	Prostate-specific antigen
RANKL	Receptor activator of nuclear factor kappa B ligand
RCC	Renal cell carcinoma
RP	Radical prostatectomy
SC	Subcutaneous(ly)
SRE	Skeletal-related event
ZOL	Zoledronic acid

Contents

1 Introduction 111
   1.1 Genitourinary Malignancies: Burden of Disease and Challenges to Bone Health 111
   1.2 Hormonal Therapy for Prostate Cancer 113
2 Anticancer Activity of Antiresorptive Agents in Prostate Cancer 114
   2.1 Preclinical and Translational Data Suggesting Potential Anticancer Activity of Bone-Targeted Agents 114
   2.2 Insights From Early Bisphosphonate Trials 115
   2.3 Exploratory Analyses From Phase III, Placebo-Controlled Trials of Zoledronic Acid: Benefits in Patients with Elevated Levels of Bone Turnover Markers 115
   2.4 Ongoing Clinical Trials Evaluating the Anticancer Potential of Bone-Directed Therapies in the Prostate Cancer Setting 118

3 Anticancer Activity of Bisphosphonates in Other Genitourinary Cancers 119
   3.1 Proof-of-Principle Data From Clinical Studies 119
   3.2 Normalization of Bone Markers 120
4 Conclusions 121
References 121

1 Introduction

1.1 Genitourinary Malignancies: Burden of Disease and Challenges to Bone Health

Genitourinary (GU) malignancies represent a considerable health burden, with prostate cancer (PC) being the most commonly diagnosed malignancy among men (782,647 new cases diagnosed worldwide every year) (Garcia et al. 2007). These cancers have a marked predilection for metastasis to the skeleton—bone metastases have been reported to develop in 65–75% of patients with advanced PC and 20–40% of patients with other advanced GU cancers (Coleman 2001). Malignant bone lesions disrupt normal bone homeostasis, the balanced and spatially coupled interactions between osteoclasts (bone resorption) and osteoblasts (bone formation) responsible for normal bone maintenance and repair, resulting in weakening of the skeleton (Coleman 2001). In imaging studies, bone lesions from GU cancers, such as PC, renal cell carcinoma (RCC), or bladder cancer, may appear to be osteolytic, osteoblastic, or a combination thereof. Regardless of their appearance, all bone lesions are associated with localized elevations in bone turnover (Mundy 2002). Bone metastases can lead to skeletal-related events (SREs), including pathologic fractures, spinal cord compression, the need for surgery to bone or palliative radiotherapy, and hypercalcemia of malignancy (Coleman 2001). In the absence of bone-directed therapy, most patients with advanced PC will experience a SRE during the course of their disease (Saad et al. 2004). Bisphosphonates (BPs) are antiresorptive agents that block pathologic bone resorption by inhibiting osteoclast activation and function (Boyle et al. 2003; Rogers et al. 2000). These agents thereby interrupt the vicious cycle of increased osteolysis coupled with increased tumor growth (Mundy 2002). Bisphosphonates are the standard of care for maintaining bone health in patients with bone metastases from solid tumors and bone lesions from multiple myeloma (MM) (Aapro et al. 2008). Denosumab, a monoclonal antibody against the receptor activator of nuclear factor kappa-B ligand (RANKL) has received regulatory approval in the United States for preventing SREs in patients with bone metastases from solid tumors (Fizazi et al. 2011; Henry et al. 2011). Although the mechanism of action of denosumab is different from that of BPs, the end effect is inhibition of pathologic bone turnover, resulting in reduced skeletal morbidity.

Emerging evidence also suggests that, in addition to preserving skeletal integrity in patients with malignant bone lesions, antiresorptive agents may help delay the development of skeletal and other metastases, potentially by making the

Table 1 Correlations between CTC/DTC levels and clinical outcomes in prostate cancer

Setting	N	Result
Newly diagnosed nonmetastatic PC (Kollermann et al. 2008)	193	DTC status before neoadjuvant endocrine therapy predicted PSA relapse after RP
PC with no evidence of disease after RP (Morgan et al. 2009)	98	DTC status after RP predicted recurrence
Nonmetastatic PC (Berg et al. 2007)	131	DTC status at baseline correlated with Gleason score and with risk of DM after RP
Progressive CRPC (chemotherapy naive) (Anand et al. 2010)	65	CTC status at baseline correlated with radiographic progression-free survival
Metastatic CRPC (Danila et al. 2010)	54	CTC status during treatment correlated with time to PSA progression
Localized or metastatic PC (Lee et al. 2009)	42	CTC levels correlated with radiographic and biochemical disease parameters in patients with metastatic PC
CRPC (Olmos et al. 2009)	119	Baseline CTC levels and treatment-associated changes in CTC levels correlated with OS
Newly diagnosed PC (Weckermann et al. 2009)	384	DTC levels before RP (but not after RP) correlated with risk of PC recurrence within 48 months

Abbreviations CRPC castration-resistant prostate cancer, CTC circulating tumor cells, DTC disseminated tumor cells, DM distant metastasis, OS overall survival, PC prostate cancer, PSA prostate-specific antigen, RP radical prostatectomy

bone microenvironment less conducive to tumor growth. The preferential metastasis of cancer cells to bone is best explained theoretically in the "seed and soil" hypothesis (Paget 1889), first described more than a century ago, but still relevant as our understanding of the metastatic process grows. According to this theory, the skeleton provides a fertile "soil" for the germination and growth of cancer "seeds". It is now believed that circulating tumor cells (CTCs) may act as "seeds" for subsequent local and distant relapse in supportive "soil"; the sites of future tumor growth may be the primary tumor site (tumor "self seeding") or distant metastasis (such as in the bone or visceral organs such as the liver) (Mundy 2002; Norton and Massague 2006). Moreover, CTCs often take up residence in the bone marrow (referred to as disseminated tumor cells [DTCs]) because the bone microenvironment and specialized signaling mechanisms and cell–cell contacts therein provide a secure niche for DTCs to survive for prolonged periods of time, and even allow them to evade the cytotoxic or proapoptotic effects of systemic anticancer therapy (Clines and Guise 2008; Meads et al. 2008; Mundy 2002; Shiozawa et al. 2008). Furthermore, CTCs and DTCs have been associated with increased risk of recurrence and distant metastases in patients with PC (Table 1) (Anand et al. 2010; Berg et al. 2007; Danila et al. 2007; Danila et al. 2010; Kollermann et al. 2008; Lee et al. 2009; Morgan et al. 2009; Olmos et al. 2009; Weckermann et al. 2009), suggesting that manipulating the bone microenvironment to make it less supportive of DTC survival might provide a means to prevent or delay the development of overt bone disease.

1.2 Hormonal Therapy for Prostate Cancer

Bone metastases and their associated SREs are of substantial concern for patients with advanced PC. Several BPs have been evaluated in patients with bone metastases from PC (Donat et al. 2006; Ernst et al. 2003; Hatoum et al. 2011; Hering et al. 2003; Lipton et al. 2002; Rodrigues et al. 2004; Saad 2008; Saad et al. 2004); although both oral (PO) and intravenous (IV) BPs have shown palliative activity in this setting, zoledronic acid (ZOL) is the only BP to have demonstrated significant objective and durable benefits and to have received broad regulatory approval for preventing SREs in patients with bone metastases from castration-resistant PC (CRPC) (Saad et al. 2002, 2004). Current treatment options for patients with bone metastases from CRPC and other GU malignancies include ZOL (Novartis Pharmaceuticals Corporation 2009) (4 mg IV every 3–4 weeks) worldwide, and denosumab (120 mg subcutaneously [SC] every 4 weeks) in the United States and the European Union (Amgen Inc 2010a; Amgen Europe BV 2011).

Patients with PC may face additional challenges to skeletal health even before they develop bone metastases. Osteoporosis is prevalent among men diagnosed with PC (Diamond et al. 2004). Androgen-deprivation therapy (ADT) is frequently used to treat high-risk PC or for rising prostate-specific antigen after primary therapy (Heidenreich et al. 2009). However, ADT is associated with decreased bone mineral density (BMD), which is a cumulative effect during long-term treatment. A number of antiresorptive agents (PO alendronate and risedronate; IV ZOL; SC denosumab) are approved for treating osteoporosis in men and women (Merck & Co. Inc 2010; Novartis Pharmaceuticals Corporation 2008; Procter & Gamble Pharmaceuticals Inc 2009). Although several of these agents maintain BMD in patients with PC during ADT, studies show that alendronate, denosumab, and ZOL also improve BMD in patients with PC receiving ADT (Bhoopalam et al. 2009; Casey et al. 2010; Greenspan et al. 2007; Israeli et al. 2007; Izumi et al. 2009; Planas et al. 2009; Ryan et al. 2006; Smith et al. 2003; Smith et al. 2001; Smith et al. 2009; Taxel et al. 2010). Based on preclinical data, it is possible that increased bone turnover (as observed during ADT) may increase the risk of developing bone metastases (Padalecki et al. 2002), potentially by increasing the release of bone matrix-derived growth factors that may support tumor cell survival and proliferation (Mundy 2002). Such physiology may help render the bone microenvironment more conducive to cancer cell growth. Thus, using a BP or other antiresorptive agent to reduce the rate of bone turnover may help delay the development of bone metastases.

2 Anticancer Activity of Antiresorptive Agents in Prostate Cancer

The preclinical rationale and mechanisms supporting the anticancer potential of BPs and other antiresorptive agents were discussed in detail in Chap. 1, and are therefore only mentioned briefly here. The clinical data supporting these preclinical observations will be discussed in the following sections.

2.1 Preclinical and Translational Data Suggesting Potential Anticancer Activity of Bone-Targeted Agents

Using bone-targeted agents to alter the bone microenvironment may disrupt interactions between PC cells and bone that are central to metastatic tumor formation (Josson et al. 2010; Mundy 2002; Rucci and Teti 2010), thereby reducing the risk of disease progression. For example, in a preclinical model, orchiectomy was associated with elevated rates of bone loss and PC metastasis to bone (Padalecki et al. 2002). Treatment with ZOL was associated with reversal of the bone loss and a reduced rate of metastasis to bone (Padalecki et al. 2002). Bisphosphonates may also inhibit disease progression by stimulating innate antitumor immune mechanisms. One important component of anticancer immunosurveillance is the gamma-delta ($\gamma\delta$) T cell; the predominant subtype, $V\gamma9\ V\delta2$, is activated by phosphoantigens and by metabolic and signaling intermediates often overexpressed in cancer cells (Clezardin and Massaia 2010). Treatment with nitrogen-containing BPs (N-BPs) such as ZOL blocks the mevalonate biosynthesis pathway, leading to accumulation of phosphoantigens and potentially to clinically relevant effects on $\gamma\delta$ T-cell activity (Clezardin and Massaia 2010). For example, small studies in patients with PC showed that ZOL treatment prompts a significant long-term shift of peripheral $\gamma\delta$ T cells toward an activated effector memory-like state associated with improved immune surveillance against transformed or malignant cells (Dieli et al. 2007; Naoe et al. 2010). Preclinical studies suggest that, in addition to their potential to render the bone microenvironment less conducive to tumor growth, BPs may also have direct anticancer activity (e.g., induction of cancer cell apoptosis) and synergy with cytotoxic chemotherapy; these effects are especially profound for ZOL (Boissier et al. 2000; Clyburn et al. 2010; Coxon et al. 2004; Facchini et al. 2010; Morgan et al. 2007; Neville-Webbe et al. 2005). For example, ZOL reduced the proliferation and survival of both androgen-independent and androgen-dependent PC cell lines (Koul et al. 2010). In other preclinical studies in PC cell lines, clinically relevant doses of doxorubicin and ZOL had proapoptotic synergy (Clyburn et al. 2010; Neville-Webbe et al. 2005).

2.2 Insights From Early Bisphosphonate Trials

The first evidence for a potential clinical anticancer benefit from BP therapy in patients with PC came from early trials of clodronate, an oral BP. Two studies evaluated the effect of clodronate on skeletal health and overall survival (OS) in men receiving hormonal therapy for stage M0 (localized disease) or M1 (bone metastases) PC (Dearnaley et al. 2009a). In long-term follow-up, clodronate improved OS in men with M1 disease beginning hormonal therapy, but not in men with M0 disease (Fig. 1) (Dearnaley et al. 2009b). These observations further support a possible benefit from BP effects on the "soil" (the bone microenvironment) in patients with PC.

The phase III, placebo-controlled trial of ZOL for reducing the risk of SREs in men with bone metastases from CRPC also evaluated OS as a secondary endpoint. In this study, ZOL produced a trend toward improved OS (median survival, 546 vs. 469 days with placebo; $P = 0.103$) (Saad 2008). Although this improvement in survival might be partially attributable to the prevention of potentially life-limiting SREs (Saad et al. 2007), these data support further investigation of bone-targeted agents for delaying disease progression and/or death in patients with CRPC.

2.3 Exploratory Analyses From Phase III, Placebo-Controlled Trials of Zoledronic Acid: Benefits in Patients with Elevated Levels of Bone Turnover Markers

Biochemical markers of bone turnover provide a window into the ongoing dynamics of bone remodeling. These markers include peptides (e.g., N-telopeptide of type I collagen [NTX]) and enzymes (e.g., bone-specific alkaline phosphatase [BALP]) that are highly specific to bone and are released during bone remodeling into serum and secreted in urine. These markers can be assessed relatively non-invasively. Retrospective exploratory studies showed that bone marker levels are often elevated in patients with bone metastases from PC or in patients receiving ADT for locally advanced disease (Lipton et al. 2008; Michaelson et al. 2004). Furthermore, small studies suggest that the patterns of bone marker changes during ADT in patients with localized disease may be distinct from the changes in patients with bone metastases. For example, compared with hormone-naive men, levels of NTX and BALP were elevated in men undergoing ADT for PC; however, BALP levels were substantially higher in men with than without bone metastases, whereas NTX levels did not differ based on bone involvement (Michaelson et al. 2004).

In exploratory analyses of the databases from phase III trials comparing ZOL versus placebo in patients with bone metastases from CRPC or other solid tumors, elevated bone marker levels (at baseline or during BP treatment) were associated with increased risk of SREs and reduced survival (Brown et al. 2005; Coleman et al. 2005; Cook et al. 2006; Smith et al. 2007). In addition, pilot trials suggest that elevated bone markers may be associated with increased risks of disease

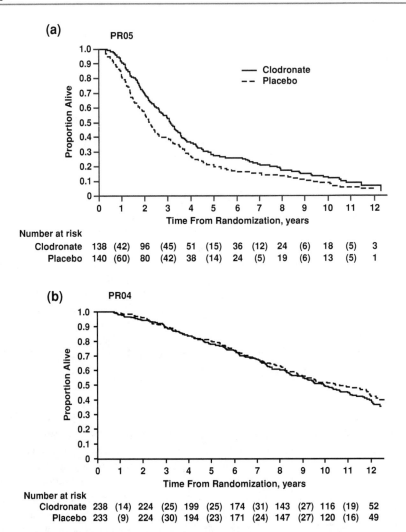

Fig. 1 *Clodronate treatment improved overall survival in men with metastatic (a; study PR05), but not localized (b; study PR04), hormone-sensitive prostate cancer.* Patients at risk (alive) are presented at 2-year intervals; the numbers of events (deaths) during the respective intervals are presented in parentheses. Reprinted from Lancet Oncol, vol. 10, Dearnaley et al. Adjuvant therapy with oral sodium clodronate in locally advanced and metastatic prostate cancer: long-term overall survival results from the MRC PR04 and PR05 randomised controlled trials, pp 872–876, copyright 2009, with permission from Elsevier (Dearnaley et al. 2009b)

recurrence or progression (Costa et al. 2009; Noguchi et al. 2003). For example, in a study in patients with bone metastases from PC receiving hormonal therapy, elevated bone marker levels correlated with biochemical recurrence and progression of bone metastases (Noguchi et al. 2003). These observations support the hypothesis that normalization of elevated bone turnover might correlate with better

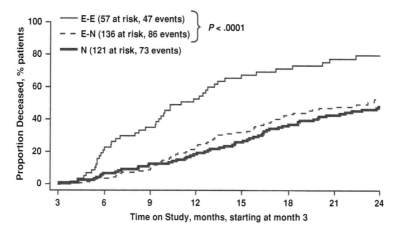

Fig. 2 *Kaplan-Meier survival estimates, stratified by baseline and 3-month N-telopeptide of type I collagen (NTX) levels in patients with bone metastases from castration-resistant prostate cancer.* Patients received zoledronic acid (4 mg via intravenous infusion every 3 weeks for up to 2 years). Abbreviations E–E, patients with elevated baseline and 3-month NTX E-N, patients with elevated baseline and normalized 3-month NTX N, patients with normal baseline NTX. Reprinted from Lipton et al. (2008) Cancer 113:193–201, with permission from John Wiley and Sons (Lipton et al. 2008)

disease outcomes. Indeed, in a recent study in patients with bone metastases receiving continuous ZOL treatment, OS was prolonged in patients whose bone marker levels decreased by the 3-month assessment (Izumi et al. 2010). Furthermore, in exploratory analyses of data from the phase III trial of ZOL versus placebo in patients with bone metastases from CRPC ($N = 314$), of ZOL-treated patients ($n = 193$) who had elevated baseline NTX (≥ 64 nmol/mmol creatinine) 70% normalized their NTX levels within 3 months, compared with only 8% in the placebo group. Normalization of NTX levels was associated with 59% decrease in the risk of death ($P < 0.0001$; Fig. 2) compared with persistently elevated NTX levels (Lipton et al. 2008), and any NTX decrease over the first 3 months was associated with a corresponding improvement in survival (Lipton et al. 2008). Interestingly, further retrospective analyses of the phase III trial database of ZOL showed that ZOL treatment was associated with improved survival in patients with aggressive bone disease as defined by markedly elevated NTX levels (≥ 100 nmol/mmol creatinine) at baseline (Body et al. 2009). Although such correlative data are not available for changes of BALP during ZOL therapy, baseline and on-study BALP levels showed strong prognostic potential in exploratory analyses of the same trial database (Coleman et al. 2005), suggesting that monitoring BALP level changes during treatment might also provide insights into the underlying biology of PC-associated bone disease and response to BPs.

Table 2 Ongoing Phase III trials of antiresorptive agents in the prostate cancer setting

Study (Agent)	N	Accrual status	Key endpoints
ZEUS (ZOL)	1,498	Complete	Time to bone metastasis in high-risk, nonmetastatic disease (± ADT)
RADAR (ZOL)	1,071	Complete	Relapse-free survival in patients receiving short- or long-term ADT
STAMPEDE (ZOL)	3,300	Enrolling; current n = 1,469	Failure-free survival in patients receiving ADT ± chemotherapy
AMG 147 (Denosumab)	1,435	Complete	Time to bone metastasis or death in high-risk, nonmetastatic CRPC

Abbreviations ADT androgen-deprivation therapy, CRPC castration-resistant prostate cancer, ZOL zoledronic acid

2.4 Ongoing Clinical Trials Evaluating the Anticancer Potential of Bone-Directed Therapies in the Prostate Cancer Setting

Several ongoing trials are evaluating the potential for BPs and other bone-targeted therapies to delay or prevent PC progression (Table 2). The STAMPEDE trial (ISRCTN78818544) is assessing the anticancer activity of ZOL in combination with various chemotherapy regimens (Dearnaley et al. 2009b), and the RADAR study is evaluating whether ZOL can prevent bone loss and bone metastases in patients with PC initiating ADT (US National Institutes of Health 2009). Furthermore, the ZEUS study is examining the ability of ZOL to prevent bone metastases in patients with asymptomatic recurrent PC (US National Institutes of Health 2008).

In addition to the ongoing studies with BPs, a large, placebo-controlled, phase III study (AMG 147) is investigating the role of denosumab in prolonging time to bone metastases in patients with CRPC (Harper and Dansey 2010). In a preliminary data release from this trial, denosumab (60 mg every 4 weeks per study design and in the initial portion of the trial; increased on-study to 120 mg every 4 weeks) was reported to improve bone-metastasis-free survival by 4.2 months (hazard ratio [HR] = 0.85; $P = .03$) versus placebo but had no effect on OS (Amgen Inc 2010b). Further details about this study (e.g., patient and baseline disease characteristics, detailed clinical outcomes) were presented at recent peer-reviewed scientific forums (Smith et al. 2011; Oudard et al. 2011). These initial "positive" results from AMG 147 support the "seed and soil" concept of bone metastasis and suggest that inhibiting bone resorption may inhibit the development or progression of metastases in bone. However, given the additional potential anticancer activities of N-BPs, the outcomes from ongoing trials such as STAMPEDE, ZEUS, and RADAR are eagerly awaited.

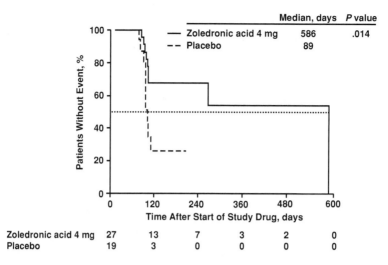

Fig. 3 *Zoledronic acid treatment delayed the progression of bone lesions in patients with bone metastases from renal cell carcinoma.* Reprinted from Saad and Lipton (2005) BJU Int 96:964–969, with permission from John Wiley and Sons (Saad and Lipton 2005)

3 Anticancer Activity of Bisphosphonates in Other Genitourinary Cancers

Preclinical studies using models of GU cancers showed that ZOL can inhibit overall tumor progression, proliferation, invasion, and adhesion; activate immune response against cancer cells; promote apoptosis; and produce synergistic anticancer effects with cytotoxic agents (Guise 2008; Ullen et al. 2009; Yuasa et al. 2009). Furthermore, in a mouse model of RCC, ZOL reduced blood vessel density compared with control mice, suggesting that ZOL may have antiangiogenic properties in the RCC setting (Soltau et al. 2008). This observation is especially intriguing given the extensive vascularization characteristic of RCC and the success of antiangiogenic therapies to treat metastatic RCC (Choueiri et al. 2010). In addition to these preclinical data, pilot studies and exploratory analyses from phase III trials in patients with bone metastases from GU cancers suggest potential anticancer effects with ZOL treatment.

3.1 Proof-of-Principle Data From Clinical Studies

Retrospective analyses of the RCC subset of patients enrolled in a phase III trial of ZOL in patients with lung cancer or other solid tumors showed that ZOL significantly extended time to disease progression (586 vs. 89 days; $P = .014$; Fig. 3) (Saad and Lipton 2005) and demonstrated a trend toward prolonged OS (347 vs. 216 days; $P = 0.104$) compared with placebo (Lipton et al. 2004; Saad 2008; Saad and Lipton 2005). Additionally, a prospective, placebo-controlled trial in patients with bone metastases from bladder cancer ($N = 40$) showed that ZOL (4 mg IV monthly for 6 months) significantly increased the 1-year survival rate ($P = 0.004$) compared with placebo (Zaghloul et al. 2010). These findings suggest that ZOL has anticancer activity in patients with advanced RCC or bladder cancer.

3.2 Normalization of Bone Markers

Exploratory studies suggest that elevated levels of bone turnover markers may reflect the presence and extent of bone metastases regardless of the primary cancer type (Saad and Lipton 2007). Indeed, in retrospective analyses from phase III clinical trials of ZOL, a majority of patients with solid tumors and confirmed bone metastases had urinary NTX levels at or above the normal threshold for young healthy adults (50 nmol/mmol creatinine) (Coleman et al. 2005). Furthermore, especially elevated levels of bone turnover markers may predict worse prognosis. In a retrospective subset analysis in patients with PC, lung cancer, or other solid tumors, a larger proportion of patients with markedly elevated (≥ 100 nmol/mmol creatinine) baseline NTX levels experienced SREs compared with patients with normal NTX levels (Brown et al. 2005). Moreover, exploratory analyses in patients with bone metastases from RCC showed that patients with elevated (≥ 64 nmol/mmol creatinine) NTX on study also had increased risks of death (HR = 13.370; $P = 0.0001$), bone disease progression (HR = 11.137; $P = 0.0087$), first pathologic fracture (HR = 7.650; $P = 0.0217$), and any pathologic fracture (HR = 5.085; $P = 0.0031$) compared with patients with normal baseline NTX levels (Brown et al. 2009). In addition to reducing the risk of SREs, ZOL treatment was associated with improved cancer-related outcomes in some patient populations. In exploratory analyses of the phase III, placebo-controlled trials in patients with bone metastases from solid tumors, ZOL treatment was associated with a reduced risk of disease progression and death in patients with baseline NTX ≥ 100 nmol/mmol creatinine (Body et al. 2009; Costa et al. 2009). Although SREs (especially pathologic fractures) are associated with increased mortality (Saad et al. 2007), the survival benefit with ZOL in patients with elevated baseline NTX levels was maintained in analyses adjusting for SRE incidence (Body et al. 2009), thereby suggesting an underlying anticancer effect.

Similar to the previously reported finding in patients with bone metastases from CRPC, exploratory analyses in patients with bone metastases from other solid tumors (including RCC and bladder cancer) also show that ZOL therapy is associated with normalization of elevated NTX levels in a majority of patients, and that normalization of NTX levels might be correlated with a potential survival benefit (Hirsh et al. 2008; Lipton et al. 2008; Lipton et al. 2007). Among patients with bone metastases from lung cancer or other solid tumors (excluding breast and prostate) and elevated baseline NTX levels, approximately 80% of ZOL-treated patients experienced normalization of NTX levels within 3 months of therapy compared with only 17% of patients who received placebo (Lipton et al. 2008).

Normalization of NTX levels at 3 months versus baseline was associated with a 57% reduced risk of death compared with persistently elevated NTX ($P = 0.0116$) (Lipton et al. 2008). Similarly, rapid normalization of NTX levels was associated with a 48% reduced risk of death compared with persistently elevated NTX ($P = 0.0017$) among patients with bone metastases from breast cancer. These data indicate that further studies are warranted to evaluate the potential of antiresorptive agents to alter the disease course in GU malignancies, as well as to better elucidate the clinical utility and prognostic value of bone turnover markers during bone-targeted therapy.

4 Conclusions

Traditionally, anticancer therapies have been targeted against the malignant cells. It is becoming evident, however, that the microenvironment is key to metastatic tumor growth and provides an additional target for anticancer therapy. Although hormonal therapy could be considered a means to alter the systemic environment supporting tumor growth and progression, this principle is currently best recognized for antiangiogenic therapies used to treat metastatic RCC. Nevertheless, it is becoming evident that using antiresorptive agents to alter the bone microenvironment may help prevent the development and/or progression of skeletal metastases from PC and other GU malignancies, and initial clinical data suggest a possible expanded role for bone-targeted agents in GU cancers. Ongoing clinical trials are further evaluating the anticancer potential of bone-targeted therapies, and results are eagerly awaited.

Acknowledgments Financial support for medical editorial assistance was provided by Novartis Pharmaceuticals. We thank Shalini Murthy, PhD, ProEd Communications, Inc., for her medical editorial assistance with this manuscript.

Conflict of Interest Dr. Saad has served as an advisor and conducted research for Novartis and Amgen and has received funding for medical editorial assistance from Novartis. Dr. Lattouf has served as a consultant for and received research funding from Novartis and Amgen.

References

Aapro M, Abrahamsson PA, Body JJ et al (2008) Guidance on the use of bisphosphonates in solid tumours: recommendations of an international expert panel. Ann Oncol 19:420–432

Amgen Inc (2010a) Xgeva (denosumab) injection [package insert]. http://www.accessdata.fda.gov/drugsatfda_docs/label/2010/125320s007lbl.pdf. Accessed 8 Feb 2011

Amgen Inc (2010b) Xgeva™ (denosumab) significantly improved bone metastasis-free survival in men with prostate cancer [press release]. http://wwwext.amgen.com/media/media_pr_detail.jsp?year=2010&releaseID=1507379. Accessed 8 Feb 2011

Amgen Europe BV (2011) XGEVA 120 mg solution for injection [summary of product characteristics]. http://www.ema.europa.eu/docs/en_GB/document.library/EPAR_-_Product_Information/human/002173/WC500110381.pdf. Accessed 21 Oct 2011

Anand A, Scher HI, Beer TM, et al (2010) Circulating tumor cells (CTC) and prostate specific antigen (PSA) as response indicator biomarkers in chemotherapy-naive patients with progressive castration-resistant prostate cancer (CRPC) treated with MDV3100. J Clin Oncol 28(suppl):353 s, Abstract 4546

Berg A, Berner A, Lilleby W et al (2007) Impact of disseminated tumor cells in bone marrow at diagnosis in patients with nonmetastatic prostate cancer treated by definitive radiotherapy. Int J Cancer 120:1603–1609

Bhoopalam N, Campbell SC, Moritz T et al (2009) Intravenous zoledronic acid to prevent osteoporosis in a veteran population with multiple risk factors for bone loss on androgen deprivation therapy. J Urol 182:2257–2264

Body J-J, Cook R, Costa L, et al (2009) Possible survival benefits from zoledronic acid treatment in patients with bone metastases from solid tumors and poor prognostic features [poster]. Presented at: the IX International Meeting on Cancer Induced Bone Disease,Arlington, 28–31 Oct 2009, Poster 71

Boissier S, Ferreras M, Peyruchaud O et al (2000) Bisphosphonates inhibit breast and prostate carcinoma cell invasion, an early event in the formation of bone metastases. Cancer Res 60:2949–2954

Boyle WJ, Simonet WS, Lacey DL (2003) Osteoclast differentiation and activation. Nature 423:337–342

Brown JE, Cook RJ, Major P et al (2005) Bone turnover markers as predictors of skeletal complications in prostate cancer, lung cancer, and other solid tumors. J Natl Cancer Inst 97:59–69

Brown JE, Lipton A, Cook RJ, et al (2009) N-telopeptide of type I collagen (NTX) correlates with survival and fractures in patients (pts) with bone metastases from renal cell carcinoma (RCC) [poster]. Presented at: American Society of Clinical Oncology 2009 Genitourinary Cancers Symposium,Orlando, 26–28 Feb 2009, Poster A66

Casey R, Gesztesi Z, Rochford J (2010) Long term zoledronic acid during androgen blockade for prostate cancer. Can J Urol 17:5170–5177

Choueiri TK, Duh MS, Clement J et al (2010) Angiogenesis inhibitor therapies for metastatic renal cell carcinoma: effectiveness, safety and treatment patterns in clinical practice-based on medical chart review. BJU Int 105:1247–1254

Clezardin P, Massaia M (2010) Nitrogen-containing bisphosphonates and cancer immunotherapy. Curr Pharm Des 16:3007–3014

Clines GA, Guise TA (2008) Molecular mechanisms and treatment of bone metastasis. Expert Rev Mol Med 10:e7

Clyburn RD, Reid P, Evans CA et al (2010) Increased anti-tumour effects of doxorubicin and zoledronic acid in prostate cancer cells in vitro: supporting the benefits of combination therapy. Cancer Chemother Pharmacol 65:969–978

Coleman RE (2001) Metastatic bone disease: clinical features, pathophysiology and treatment strategies. Cancer Treat Rev 27:165–176

Coleman RE, Major P, Lipton A et al (2005) Predictive value of bone resorption and formation markers in cancer patients with bone metastases receiving the bisphosphonate zoledronic acid. J Clin Oncol 23:4925–4935

Cook RJ, Coleman R, Brown J et al (2006) Markers of bone metabolism and survival in men with hormone-refractory metastatic prostate cancer. Clin Cancer Res 12:3361–3367

Costa L, Cook R, Body JJ, et al (2009) Zoledronic acid treatment delays disease progression and improves survival in patients with bone metastases from solid tumors and elevated levels of bone resorption [poster]. Presented at: the IX International Meeting on Cancer Induced Bone Disease, Arlington, 28–31 Oct 2009, Poster 50

Coxon JP, Oades GM, Kirby RS et al (2004) Zoledronic acid induces apoptosis and inhibits adhesion to mineralized matrix in prostate cancer cells via inhibition of protein prenylation. BJU Int 94:164–170

Danila DC, Heller G, Gignac GA et al (2007) Circulating tumor cell number and prognosis in progressive castration-resistant prostate cancer. Clin Cancer Res 13:7053–7058

Danila DC, Anand A, Sung CC, et al (2010) Molecular profiling of circulating tumor cells (CTC) in patients with castrate metastatic prostate cancer (CMPC) receiving abiraterone acetate (AA) after failure of docetaxel-based chemotherapy [abstract]. J Clin Oncol 28(suppl): 375 s, Abstract 4635

Dearnaley DP, Mason MD, Parmar MK, et al (2009a) Survival benefit with oral sodium clodronate in metastatic but not localised prostate cancer: long-term results of MRC PR04 & PR05 [poster]. Presented at: American Society of Clinical Oncology 2009 Genitourinary Cancers Symposium,Orlando, 26–28 Feb 2009, Abstract 6

Dearnaley DP, Mason MD, Parmar MKB et al (2009b) Adjuvant therapy with oral sodium clodronate in locally advanced and metastatic prostate cancer: long-term overall survival results from the MRC PR04 and PR05 randomised controlled trials. Lancet Oncol 10:872–876

Diamond TH, Higano CS, Smith MR et al (2004) Osteoporosis in men with prostate carcinoma receiving androgen-deprivation therapy: recommendations for diagnosis and therapies. Cancer 100:892–899

Dieli F, Vermijlen D, Fulfaro F et al (2007) Targeting human gd T cells with zoledronate and interleukin-2 for immunotherapy of hormone-refractory prostate cancer. Cancer Res 67: 7450–7457

Donat DA, Pesic JM, Tesanovic SM, et al (2006) Low-dose clodronate as adjunctive therapy in prostate cancer patients with painful bone metastases [abstract]. Ann Oncol 17(suppl 9):ix156 Abstract 484

Ernst DS, Tannock IF, Winquist EW et al (2003) Randomized, double-blind, controlled trial of mitoxantrone/prednisone and clodronate versus mitoxantrone/prednisone and placebo in patients with hormone-refractory prostate cancer and pain. J Clin Oncol 21:3335–3342

Facchini G, Caraglia M, Morabito A et al (2010) Metronomic administration of zoledronic acid and Taxotere combination in castration resistant prostate cancer patients: phase I ZANTE trial. Cancer Biol Ther 10:543–548

Fizazi K, Carducci M, Smith M, et al (2011) Denosumab versus zoledronic acid for treatment of bone metastases in men with castration-resistant prostate cancer: a randomised, double-blind study. Lancet 377:813–822

Garcia M, Jemal A, Ward EM, et al (2007) Global cancer facts and figures 2007. American Cancer Society. http://www.cancer.org/acs/groups/content/@nho/documents/document/globalfactsand figures2007rev2p.pdf. Accessed 8 Feb 2011

Greenspan SL, Bone HG, Ettinger MP et al (2007) Effect of recombinant human parathyroid hormone (1–84) on vertebral fracture and bone mineral density in postmenopausal women with osteoporosis: a randomized trial. Ann Intern Med 146:326–339

Guise TA (2008) Antitumor effects of bisphosphonates: promising preclinical evidence. Cancer Treat Rev 34:S19–S24

Harper S, Dansey R (2010) Amgen investor meeting: 2010 ASCO annual meeting. http://phx.corporate-ir.net/External.File?item=UGFyZW50SUQ9NDkyMTh8Q2hpbGRJRD0tMXxUeXBlPTM=&t=1. Accessed 8 Feb 2011

Hatoum HT, Lin SJ, Guo A et al (2011) Zoledronic acid therapy impacts risk and frequency of skeletal complications and follow-up duration in prostate cancer patients with bone metastasis. Curr Med Res Opin 27:55–62

Heidenreich A, Bolla M, Joniau S et al (2009) Guidelines on prostate cancer. European Association of Urology. http://www.uroweb.org/fileadmin/tx_eauguidelines/2009/Full/Prostate_Cancer.pdf. Accessed 8 Feb 2011

Henry DH, Costa L, Goldwasser F et al (2011) Randomized, double-blind study of denosumab versus zoledronic acid in the treatment of bone metastases in patients with advanced cancer (excluding breast and prostate cancer) or multiple myeloma. J Clin Oncol 29:1125–1132

Hering F, Rodrigues PRT, Lipay M (2003) Clodronate for treatment of bone metastases in hormone refractory prostate cancer. Int Braz J Urol 29:228–233

Hirsh V, Major PP, Lipton A et al (2008) Zoledronic acid and survival in patients with metastatic bone disease from lung cancer and elevated markers of osteoclast activity. J Thorac Oncol 3:228–236

Israeli RS, Rosenberg SJ, Saltzstein DR et al (2007) The effect of zoledronic acid on bone mineral density in patients undergoing androgen deprivation therapy. Clin Genitourin Cancer 5:271–277

Izumi K, Mizokami A, Sugimoto K et al (2009) Risedronate recovers bone loss in patients with prostate cancer undergoing androgen-deprivation therapy. Urology 73:1342–1346

Izumi K, Mizokami A, Narimoto K, et al (2010) The role of bone turnover markers in patients with bone metastatic prostate cancer receiving zoledronate infusion [poster]. Presented at: American Society of Clinical Oncology 2010 Genitourinary Cancers Symposium, San Francisco, 5–7 March 2010, Abstract 196

Josson S, Matsuoka Y, Chung LW et al (2010) Tumor-stroma co-evolution in prostate cancer progression and metastasis. Semin Cell Dev Biol 21:26–32

Kollermann J, Weikert S, Schostak M et al (2008) Prognostic significance of disseminated tumor cells in the bone marrow of prostate cancer patients treated with neoadjuvant hormone treatment. J Clin Oncol 26:4928–4933

Koul HK, Koul S, Kumar B, et al (2010) Direct effects of zoledronic acid on hormone-responsive and hormone-refractory prostate cancer cells [poster]. Presented at: American Society of Clinical Oncology 2010 Genitourinary Cancers Symposium, San Francisco, 5–7 March 2010, Abstract 184

Lee RJ, Stott SL, Nagrath S, et al (2009) Analyses of circulating tumor cell (CTC) dynamics and treatment response in prostate cancer using CTC-chip microfluidic device [abstract]. J Clin Oncol 27(suppl):271 s Abstract 5149

Lipton A, Small E, Saad F et al (2002) The new bisphosphonate, zometa (zoledronic acid), decreases skeletal complications in both osteolytic and osteoblastic lesions: a comparison to pamidronate. Cancer Invest 20(suppl 2):45–54

Lipton A, Seaman J, Zheng M (2004) Efficacy and safety of zoledronic acid in patients with bone metastases from renal cell carcinoma [poster]. Presented at: What is New in Bisphosphonates? Seventh Workshop on Bisphosphonates–From the Laboratory to the Patient, Davos, Switzerland, 24–26 Mar 2004 Abstract 28

Lipton A, Cook RJ, Major P et al (2007) Zoledronic acid and survival in breast cancer patients with bone metastases and elevated markers of osteoclast activity. Oncologist 12:1035–1043

Lipton A, Cook R, Saad F et al (2008) Normalization of bone markers is associated with improved survival in patients with bone metastases from solid tumors and elevated bone resorption receiving zoledronic acid. Cancer 113:193–201

Meads MB, Hazlehurst LA, Dalton WS (2008) The bone marrow microenvironment as a tumor sanctuary and contributor to drug resistance. Clin Cancer Res 14:2519–2526

Merck & Co. Inc (2010) Fosamax (alendronate sodium) tablets and oral solution [package insert]. http://www.accessdata.fda.gov/drugsatfda_docs/label/2010/020560s051s055s057,021575s012s016s018lbl.pdf. Accessed 8 Feb 2011

Michaelson MD, Marujo RM, Smith MR (2004) Contribution of androgen deprivation therapy to elevated osteoclast activity in men with metastatic prostate cancer. Clin Cancer Res 10:2705–2708

Morgan C, Lewis PD, Jones RM et al (2007) The in vitro anti-tumour activity of zoledronic acid and docetaxel at clinically achievable concentrations in prostate cancer. Acta Oncol 46:669–677

Morgan TM, Lange PH, Porter MP et al (2009) Disseminated tumor cells in prostate cancer patients after radical prostatectomy and without evidence of disease predicts biochemical recurrence. Clin Cancer Res 15:677–683

Mundy GR (2002) Metastasis to bone: causes, consequences and therapeutic opportunities. Nat Rev Cancer 2:584–593

Naoe M, Ogawa Y, Takeshita K et al (2010) Zoledronate stimulates gamma delta T cells in prostate cancer patients. Oncol Res 18:493–501

Neville-Webbe HL, Rostami-Hodjegan A, Evans CA et al (2005) Sequence- and schedule-dependent enhancement of zoledronic acid induced apoptosis by doxorubicin in breast and prostate cancer cells. Int J Cancer 113:364–371

Noguchi M, Yahara J, Noda S (2003) Serum levels of bone turnover markers parallel the results of bone scintigraphy in monitoring bone activity of prostate cancer. Urology 61:993–998

Norton L, Massague J (2006) Is cancer a disease of self-seeding? Nat Med 12:875–878

Novartis Pharmaceuticals Corporation (2008) Reclast (zoledronic acid) injection [package insert]. http://www.accessdata.fda.gov/drugsatfda_docs/label/2008/021817s001lbl.pdf. Accessed 8 Feb 2011

Novartis Pharmaceuticals Corporation (2009) Zometa (zoledronic acid) injection [package insert]. http://www.accessdata.fda.gov/drugsatfda_docs/label/2009/021223s018lbl.pdf. Accessed 8 Feb 2011

Olmos D, Arkenau HT, Ang JE et al (2009) Circulating tumour cell (CTC) counts as intermediate end points in castration-resistant prostate cancer (CRPC): a single-centre experience. Ann Oncol 20:27–33

Oudard S, Smith MR, Karsh L et al (2011) Denosumab and bone metastases-free survival in men with castration-resistant prostate cancer: Subgroup analyses from an international, double-blind, randomized phase 3 trial. Presented at: The European Multidisciplinary Cancer Congress. Stockholm, Sweden, 23–27 Sept 2011. Abstract 7003 [oral]

Padalecki SS, Carreon MR, Grubbs B, et al (2002) Androgen deprivation causes bone loss and increased prostate cancer metastases to bone: prevention by zoledronic acid [abstract]. Presented at: 24th annual meeting of the American Society for Bone and Mineral Research, San Antonio, 20–24 Sept 2002, Abstract SU072

Paget S (1889) The distribution of secondary growths in cancer of the breast. Lancet 1:571–573

Planas J, Trilla E, Raventos C et al (2009) Alendronate decreases the fracture risk in patients with prostate cancer on androgen-deprivation therapy and with severe osteopenia or osteoporosis. BJU Int 104:1637–1640

Procter & Gamble Pharmaceuticals Inc (2009) Actonel (risedronate sodium) tablets [package insert]. http://www.accessdata.fda.gov/drugsatfda_docs/label/2009/020835s036lbl.pdf. Accessed 8 Feb 2011

Rodrigues P, Hering F, Campagnari JC (2004) Use of bisphosphonates can dramatically improve pain in advanced hormone-refractory prostate cancer patients. Prostate Cancer Prostatic Dis 7:350–354

Rogers MJ, Gordon S, Benford HL et al (2000) Cellular and molecular mechanisms of action of bisphosphonates. Cancer 88:2961–2978

Rucci N, Teti A (2010) Osteomimicry: how tumor cells try to deceive the bone. Front Biosci (Schol Ed) 2:907–915

Ryan CW, Huo D, Demers LM, et al (2006) Zoledronic acid initiated during the first year of androgen deprivation therapy increases bone mineral density in patients with prostate cancer. J Urol 176:972–978, discussion follows

Saad F (2008) New research findings on zoledronic acid: survival, pain, and anti-tumour effects. Cancer Treat Rev 34:183–192

Saad F, Lipton A (2005) Zoledronic acid is effective in preventing and delaying skeletal events in patients with bone metastases secondary to genitourinary cancers. BJU Int 96:964–969

Saad F, Lipton A (2007) Clinical benefits and considerations of bisphosphonate treatment in metastatic bone disease. Semin Oncol 34(4):S17–S23

Saad F, Gleason DM, Murray R et al (2002) A randomized, placebo-controlled trial of zoledronic acid in patients with hormone-refractory metastatic prostate carcinoma. J Natl Cancer Inst 94:1458–1468

Saad F, Gleason DM, Murray R et al (2004) Long-term efficacy of zoledronic acid for the prevention of skeletal complications in patients with metastatic hormone-refractory prostate cancer. J Natl Cancer Inst 96:879–882

Saad F, Lipton A, Cook R et al (2007) Pathologic fractures correlate with reduced survival in patients with malignant bone disease. Cancer 110:1860–1867

Shiozawa Y, Havens AM, Pienta KJ et al (2008) The bone marrow niche: habitat to hematopoietic and mesenchymal stem cells, and unwitting host to molecular parasites. Leukemia 22:941–950

Smith MR, McGovern FJ, Zietman AL et al (2001) Pamidronate to prevent bone loss during androgen-deprivation therapy for prostate cancer. N Engl J Med 345:948–955

Smith MR, Eastham J, Gleason DM et al (2003) Randomized controlled trial of zoledronic acid to prevent bone loss in men receiving androgen deprivation therapy for nonmetastatic prostate cancer. J Urol 169:2008–2012

Smith MR, Cook RJ, Coleman R et al (2007) Predictors of skeletal complications in men with hormone-refractory metastatic prostate cancer. Urology 70:315–319

Smith MR, Egerdie B, Hernandez Toriz N et al (2009) Denosumab in men receiving androgen-deprivation therapy for prostate cancer. N Engl J Med 361:745–755

Smith MR, Saad F, Coleman R, et al (2009) Denosumab to prolong bone metastases-free survival in men with castrate-resistant prostate cancer: Results of a global phase 3, randomized, double-blind trial. Presented at: American Urological Association Annual Meeting. Washington, DC, 14–19 May 2011. Late Breaking News

Soltau J, Zirrgiebel U, Esser N et al (2008) Antitumoral and antiangiogenic efficacy of bisphosphonates in vitro and in a murine RENCA model. Anticancer Res 28:933–941

Taxel P, Dowsett R, Richter L et al (2010) Risedronate prevents early bone loss and increased bone turnover in the first 6 months of luteinizing hormone-releasing hormone-agonist therapy for prostate cancer. BJU Int 106:1473–1476

US National Institutes of Health (2008) Zoledronate plus standard therapy compared with placebo plus standard therapy to prevent bone metastases in patients with recurrent prostate cancer that has no symptoms. http://clinicaltrials.gov/ct2/show/NCT00005073. Accessed 8 Feb 2011

US National Institutes of Health (2009) RADAR trial—randomised androgen deprivation and radiotherapy. http://clinicaltrials.gov/ct2/show/NCT00193856. Accessed 8 Feb 2011

Ullen A, Schwarz S, Lennartsson L et al (2009) Zoledronic acid induces caspase-dependent apoptosis in renal cancer cell lines. Scand J Urol Nephrol 43:98–103

Weckermann D, Polzer B, Ragg T et al (2009) Perioperative activation of disseminated tumor cells in bone marrow of patients with prostate cancer. J Clin Oncol 27:1549–1556

Yuasa T, Sato K, Ashihara E et al (2009) Intravesical administration of gammadelta T cells successfully prevents the growth of bladder cancer in the murine model. Cancer Immunol Immunother 58:493–502

Zaghloul MS, Boutrus R, El-Hossieny H et al (2010) A prospective, randomized, placebo-controlled trial of zoledronic acid in bony metastatic bladder cancer. Int J Clin Oncol 15:382–389

Targeting Bone in Myeloma

G. J. Morgan and Ping Wu

Abstract
Myeloma bone disease (BD) not only impairs quality of life, but is also associated with impaired survival. Studies of the biology underlying BD support the notion that the increased osteoclastogenesis and suppressed osteoblastogenesis is both a consequence and a necessity for tumour growth and clonal expansion. Survival and expansion of the myeloma clone are dependent on its interactions with bone elements; thus, targeting these interactions should have anti-myeloma activities. Indeed, both experimental and clinical findings indicate that bone-targeted therapies, not only improve BD, but also create an inhospitable environment for myeloma cell growth and survival, favouring improved clinical outcome. This chapter summarizes recent progress in our understandings of the biology of myeloma BD, highlighting the role of osteoclasts and osteoblasts in this process and how they can be targeted therapeutically. Unravelling the mechanisms underlying myeloma–bone interactions will facilitate the development of novel therapeutic agents to treat BD, which as a consequence are likely to improve the clinical outcome of myeloma patients.

Contents

1	Bone Disease in Myeloma	128
2	Mechanism of Bone Disease in Myeloma	128
3	Pathogenesis and Targeting of Bone Disease in Myeloma	130
	3.1 What is the Impact of the "Novel Therapies" on Bone Disease	131
	3.2 The Anti-Myeloma Effects of Bisphosphonates	132

G. J. Morgan (✉) · P. Wu
Haemato-oncology Unit, The Royal Marsden NHS Foundation Trust,
Downs Road Sutton, Surrey SM2 5PT, United Kingdom
e-mail: gareth.morgan@icr.ac.uk

    3.3   Rank/RANKL System 133
    3.4   MIP1a.. 133
    3.5   Anti-BAFF-Neutralizing Antibody 133
    3.6   Bone Anabolic Agents 134
4   Conclusions.. 136
References.. 137

1 Bone Disease in Myeloma

Myeloma is unique among haematological malignancies, being characterized by osteolytic bone lesions and the development of skeletal-related events (SREs). At presentation, 70% of patients have bone disease and 60% patients report a pathologic fracture over the course of their disease (Melton et al. 2005). The presence of bone disease (BD) is a defining characteristic of myeloma requiring treatment; moreover, the extent of BD and bone resorption activity has been shown to be an important risk factor for overall survival (OS) (Durie and Salmon 1975; Jakob et al. 2008; Zhan et al. 2006). BD has been linked to poor prognosis in myeloma patients. Bone resorption activity has been shown to be an independent risk factor for OS in MM patients (Jakob et al. 2008). Results from the MRC myeloma IX trial show that patients with presenting BD have a significantly shorter OS compared to those without BD, with a shorter survival from relapse being the main contributor to this effect (median 12.2 vs. 23.4 months) (Wu et al. 2011).

The genetic lesions associated with subgroups of myeloma also seem to modulate rates of BD possibly by modifying the interaction of the myeloma cells with the BM milieu. For example, MM cells harbouring the t(14;16) translocation overexpress the transcription factor c-maf, which activates cyclin D2 expression and increases MM cell proliferation. In addition, c-maf up-regulates b7-integrin expression and potentiates MM cell adhesion to BM stromal cells (BMSCs) (Hurt et al. 2004). It has been shown that cases characterized by MAF deregulation have less BD as do cases with the t(4;14) (Robbiani et al. 2004; Wu et al. 2011). In contrast, MM cells characterized by the t(11;14) and hyperdiploid karyotypes have more BD and seem to depend on the BM microenvironment for the induction of cyclin D1 expression (Wu et al. 2010; Bergsagel et al. 2005). Furthermore, the hyperdiploid subgroup and cases with cyclin D1 overexpression are underrepresented in plasma cell leukaemia (Bergsagel and Kuehl 2003), where microenvironmental interactions are clearly less important.

2 Mechanism of Bone Disease in Myeloma

Studies of the biology underlying BD support the notion that the increased osteoclastogenesis and suppressed osteoblastogenesis is both a consequence and a necessity for tumour growth and clonal expansion. Thus, as BD is the major contributor to morbidity and mortality in MM, in addition to chemotherapy targeting the myeloma cells, bone-supportive treatment is also an essential component of the therapy, and accumulating evidence suggests that bone targeted therapies not only reduce skeletal complications but also improve survival.

On binding to their stromal environment, myeloma cells have been shown to induce changes in several cell types that are intimately involved in the induction of bone lesions, including BMSCs, BM endothelial cells, immune cells, osteoblasts and osteoclasts. The induced changes, in turn, offer the MM cells a supportive stromal environment, access to vascular networks, and locally produced growth factors and cytokines (Mitsiades et al. 2007), favouring their growth and survival. These examples support the notion that the genetics of MM cells and their interactions with the BM microenvironment are not completely independent of each other, but rather they functionally interact to influence the biology and clinical behaviour of the disease.

The mechanism underlying myeloma BD is an uncoupling of bone resorption from bone formation as a consequence of increased osteoclastic activity and inhibition of osteoblast function (Bataille et al. 1989). Several osteoclast activating factors have been found to be important in regulating bone resorption. The most significant system, in this respect, consists of the receptor activator of NF-κB (RANK), its ligand RANKL and a soluble decoy receptor, osteoprotegerin (OPG) (Roodman 2004). We are now beginning to understand that this dysregulation of the normal interactions within the bone marrow microenvironment is not only responsible for the bone destruction, but also for the initiation, maintenance and expansion of the myeloma clone. This pro-survival effect is thought to be mediated via direct cell–cell contact between myeloma and bone cells, as well as via positive cytokine feedback loops set up during the bone resorption process, creating a vicious cycle of bone resorption and tumour growth. The ability of BMSCs to support proliferation, survival and drug resistance of MM should be viewed as pathological recapitulation of their natural role in supporting haematopoiesis.

Myeloma cells either directly produce or induce other cells to produce "osteoclast activating factors", which drive the differentiation of haemopoietic stem/precursor cells to mature osteoclasts as well as increasing their bone resorbing activity. Osteoclast activation significantly increases the growth and survival of the myeloma clone, an effect that is mediated both by direct cell–cell contact and indirectly via the release of soluble factors. Soluble growth factors and cytokines in the MM microenvironment, such as interleukin 6 (IL-6), osteopontin, B cell activating factor of the TNF family (BAFF) and a proliferation-inducing ligand (APRIL), have been implicated in osteoclast-induced myeloma cell survival (Yaccoby 2010). Other important factors produced as a consequence of these interactions include vascular endothelial growth factor (VEGF), tumour necrosis factor- α (TNF-α), stromal cell-derived factor 1α (SDF-1a), fibroblast growth factor (FGF), Interleukin-1 (IL-1) and macrophage inflammatory protein 1 alpha (MIP-1α) (Mitsiades et al. 2007).

Cell adhesion-mediated drug resistance (CAMDR) is a feature of the myeloma cell interaction with osteoclasts in the BM. In this context, it has been observed that co-culturing osteoclasts with myeloma cells is able to protect them from drug-induced apoptosis (Yaccoby et al. 2004). Of interest in this respect is that after in vitro interaction with osteoclasts or stromal cells, myeloma cells acquire a more immature phenotype (Yaccoby 2005; Dezorella et al. 2009). Such observations are clinically relevant as high resolution imaging approaches have shown that plasma cells can persist in focal lesions in the BM of patients who have otherwise achieved a complete remission (Walker et al. 2007; Bartel et al. 2009). Such a process could also be responsible for maintaining myeloma stem cells within a stromal cell niche in the BM, mediating chemo-resistance and subsequent disease relapse (Zipori 2010).

Mature osteoblasts are suppressed in MM and differ from BMSCs and immature osteoblasts with a different pattern of cytokines and "osteoclast activating factors" being expressed which would inhibit the growth of the myeloma clone. Terminally differentiated osteoblasts produce high levels of OPG and reduced levels of RANKL, consequently reducing osteoclastogenesis, therefore, inhibiting bone resorption (Glass et al. 2005; Qiang et al. 2008; Spencer et al. 2006). The production of pro-survival growth factors, such as IL-6 and IGF1, are reduced as BMSCs differentiate into osteoblasts (Gunn et al. 2006), also favouring an anti-myeloma effect. This effect may also be enhanced by the fact that mature osteoblasts produce factors such as decorin, that directly inhibit the survival of myeloma cells as well as inhibit the pro-survival impact of osteoclasts (Yaccoby et al. 2006; Li et al. 2008). These observations suggest that the inhibition of osteoblast differentiation in MM not only contributes to the induction of osteolytic lesions, but also creates favourable conditions for myeloma cell survival and proliferation. Thus, therapeutic approaches to stimulate osteoblast differentiation may be able to reduce the levels of myeloma growth factors and osteoclastogenic factors in BM microenvironment, therefore, restraining myeloma clone growth and consequently improving clinical outcome.

Therefore, MM is currently viewed as a prototypical disease model for studying tumour–microenvironment interactions and the complex interactions present in the BM microenvironment bring with them the potential for their therapeutic targeting. We make the case for the potential for additional therapeutic benefit to be achieved by the combination of traditional antimyeloma agents targeting the interactions with the BM microenvironment and bone elements. This approach may not only be beneficial during induction treatment, by increasing the sensitivity of the myeloma cells to the cytotoxic agents used to kill the myeloma cells, but may also be important during the maintenance phase by targeting the plasma cell niche in the BM, such that the biology of residual clonal cells is modified.

3   Pathogenesis and Targeting of Bone Disease in Myeloma

BD in myeloma is characterized by purely osteolytic lesions with no new bone formation, an effect that is mediated via increased osteoclastic activity and inhibition of osteoblast function. Interestingly, in respect of the pattern of BD, myeloma cells lie in close proximity to the sites of active bone resorption and seem to play a key role in altering the balance of bone resorption and bone formation (Roodman 2004).

3.1 What is the Impact of the "Novel Therapies" on Bone Disease

The important contributions of the BM microenvironment to disease progression can explain, to a certain extent, why the "novel drugs" that target the bone microenvironment as well as myeloma cells, have been more effective than conventional approaches. Apart from their direct anti-tumour activities, the immunomodulatory agents (IMiDs) thalidomide and lenalidomide and the proteasome inhibitor bortezomib, seem to affect osteoclast and osteoblast activity in myelomatous bones (Zangari et al. 2005; Anderson et al. 2006; Terpos et al. 2007; Breitkreutz et al. 2008).

3.1.1 Immunomodulatory Drugs

Immunomodulatory drugs (IMiDs), such as Thalidomide, Actimid and Revlimid, are effective agents for treating MM. Apart from their well-known anti-tumour activity, these drugs may directly interfere with osteoclast differentiation via the reduction of PU.1 expression, a critical transcription factor during osteoclast development (Anderson et al. 2006; Breitkreutz et al. 2008). Moreover, the exposure of BMSCs derived from MM patients to Revlimid decreases their secretion of RANKL, consequently impairs osteoclastogenesis and favours myeloma cell suppression (Breitkreutz et al. 2008). These data were related to the clinical findings that in the serum of MM patients treated with Revlimid, RANK/RANKL levels were reduced, whereas OPG levels were increased. However, both Thalidomide and Revlimid have been shown to induce DKK1 expression of myeloma cells after 48 h of treatment in a GEP study, which could potentially impair osteoblast function (Shaugnessy et al. 2002).

3.1.2 Bortezomib

Possible informative data on the role of stimulating bone formation as a therapeutic strategy has come indirectly from the use of the proteosome inhibitor Bortezomib which was incidentally shown to have anabolic bone activities. Bortezomib is a proteasome and NF-κB signalling inhibitor with potent anti-MM activity. Since RANKL enhances osteoclast differentiation by activating NF-κB pathway, it is not surprising that bortezomib, by reducing NF-κB activity, can impair osteoclast survival and differentiation (Zavrski et al. 2005; von Metzler et al. 2007). In addition to decreasing osteoclast activity in MM, bortezomib also has "anabolic" bone effects by inducing osteoblast differentiation (Zangari et al. 2005; Mukherjee et al. 2008). Although the mechanism(s) by which proteasome inhibition leads to increased osteoblast activity has not been firmly established, previous work suggests that proteasome inhibition can upregulate Runx2 and osterix, two critical transcription factors in osteoblast differentiation (Mukherjee et al. 2008; Giuliani et al. 2007a; De Matteo et al. 2010). Bortezomib also appears to decrease the serum levels of DKK-1 and RANKL in patients with MM (Terpos et al. 2006). Taken together, these preclinical data provide an explanation for the increased bone formation markers and reduced bone resorption markers seen in MM patients treated with bortezomib (Shimazaki et al. 2005; Heider et al. 2006; Boissy et al. 2008; Uy et al. 2007). Although these findings suggest that bortezomib has the capacity to prevent myeloma BD, at present there is only one report showing the effectiveness of bortezomib on SREs in myeloma patients (Delforge et al. 2011), and interestingly radiological evidence of bone healing was observed in some of the bortezomib-treated patients.

3.2 The Anti-Myeloma Effects of Bisphosphonates

Bisphosphonates (BPs) are the current standard care for the prevention and treatment of malignant BD (Kyle et al. 2007; Morgan 2011), strong preclinical evidences from various models of MM suggest that nitrogen-containing BPs (N-BPs) such as zoledronic acid (ZOL) may have anticancer activity including inhibiting angiogenesis, enhancing antitumour immune responses, and directly or indirectly modulating the proliferation and survival of myeloma cells (Morgan 2011). This has been confirmed by a number of clinical trials showing bisphosphonates improve both OS and PFS in myeloma patients (Aviles et al. 2007; McCloskey et al. 2001; Berenson et al. 1998; Morgan et al. 2010; Berenson et al. 2006). These findings further support the notion that the interactions between myeloma cell and surrounding BM microenvironment constitute an important factor that needs to be taken into account in the development of novel therapeutic strategies.

BPs naturally bind to mineralized surfaces such as bone and inhibit osteoclast-mediated bone resorption. The second generation N-BPs (e.g. ZOL, pamidronate) have been proven more effective at reducing SREs compared to the first generation BPs (e.g. CLO) (Rosen et al. 2001). Moreover, strong preclinical evidence, from various models of MM, suggest that the N-BPs may have anticancer activity via the inhibition of angiogenesis, enhanced anti-tumour immune responses, inhibition of tumour cell migration and directly modulating the proliferation and survival of myeloma cells (Baulch-Brown et al. 2007; Shipman et al. 1997; Tassone et al. 2000; Ural et al. 2003; Corso et al. 2005; Zwolak et al. 2010). In vivo N-BPs may also affect MM progression by blocking the release of cytokines and growth factors from the bone matrix, thereby breaking the vicious cycle of bone destruction and cancer growth (Morgan 2011). In addition, the anticancer effects of BPs have been demonstrated to have synergy with agents that are used in the treatment of myeloma, including dexamethasone, thalidomide and bortezomib (Ural et al. 2003; Schmidmaier et al. 2006; Moschetta et al. 2010). Preclinical mouse models of MM indicate that the anti-myeloma effect of N-BPs may be mediated via the inhibition of protein prenylation and consequent inhibition of the RAS–RAF–MARK pathway (Guenther et al. 2010), a mechanism of action not shared by non-N-BPs. Based on the BP anticancer theory and promising early results, a large randomized trial (N = 1960) was conducted to evaluate the role of BPs in newly diagnosed MM patients receiving either intensive or non-intensive regimens (Morgan et al. 2010). Results show that ZOL significantly reduces skeletal morbidity and significantly improves both PFS and OS (HR 1.19, 95% CI 1.04–1.35) versus CLO. Notably, the survival benefit with ZOL remained significant after adjustment for SREs, consistent with clinically meaningful antimyeloma activity.

3.3 Rank/RANKL System

In the myeloma BM microenvironment, the interaction between BMSCs and MM cells results in increased RANKL expression and decreased OPG production, favouring bone resorption. A human neutralizing antibody against RANKL, denosumab, which mimics the endogenous effect of OPG, has been tested in myeloma patients (Raje and Roodman 2011). Denosumab has been investigated in two phase II studies of myeloma patients previously treated with BPs, and both studies confirmed its efficacy in reducing SREs (Fizazi et al. 2009; Vij et al. 2009). In one of the trials using denosumab as a single agent in patients with plateau phase or progressive MM, although denosumab did not significantly decrease tumour burden, some patients with progressive disease experienced disease stabilization (Vij et al. 2009). More recently Henry et al. (2011) reported the results of a phase III randomized trial that directly compared denosumab with ZOL on SRE development and survival in patients with myeloma. Consistent with the other studies denosumab was at least as effective as ZOL in reducing the time to first SREs; however, the ZOL treated group had a more favourable survival (HR 2.26; 95% CI 1.13 to 4.50). Therefore, current findings indicate that both BPs and denosumab can effectively reduce SREs, but denosumab treatment was not associated with a significant survival benefit in MM patients.

3.4 MIP1a

MIP1α, largely produced by myeloma cells and osteoclasts is a potent inducer of osteoclast formation independently of RANKL by promoting osteoclast precursor cell migration and fusion (Han et al. 2001). It also has multiple roles in myeloma cell, including promoting myeloma cell growth, survival and migration (Lentzsch et al. 2003). Targeting MIP1a could have important effects on improving patients' outcome. A clinical grade small molecule CCR1 antagonist, MLN3897, inhibits MIP1α-induced osteoclastogenesis and myeloma cell proliferation in vitro (Vallet et al. 2007). Recent report shows that MIP1α also inhibits osteoblast function by impairing matrix mineralization and suppressing osteocalcin production (Vallet et al. 2011), an effect mediated via downregulation of the osteogenic transcription factor osterix and downstream ERK signalling. MLN3897 blocks ERK phosphorylation and restores, at least partially, osteocalcin expression in vitro and in vivo.

3.5 Anti-BAFF-Neutralizing Antibody

Osteoclasts and myeloma cells interact by stimulating each others' growth and survival, and a critical mediator in this interplay is a TNF family member BAFF. BAFF is an MM growth factor derived from osteoclast and BMSC that mediates both myeloma cell survival and myeloma cell-BMSC adhesion (Abe et al. 2004; Tai et al. 2006). A neutralizing antibody against BAFF has been shown to significantly inhibit tumour burden in vivo and, importantly, reduce the number of lytic lesions and osteoclast differentiation (Neri et al. 2007). On the basis of these results, a phase I study of this BAFF-neutralizing antibody (LY2127399) combined to bortezomib is currently ongoing in drug resistant MM patients (NCT00689507) (www.clinicaltrials.gov).

3.6 Bone Anabolic Agents

While the N-BP ZOL is the current gold standard for the treatment of MM bone disease not all patients respond to the treatment. Despite being on ZOL up to 30% newly diagnosed MM patients still develop SREs within 2 years (Morgan et al. 2010). This observation has led researchers to focus activity on agents able to promote anabolic bone activity as a way of treating BD. In this respect, there are an abundance of growth factors either produced by myeloma cells or the other cells within the BM microenvironment, which can be targeted and have the potential to contribute to the suppression of osteoblast function and bone formation in myeloma (e.g. activin A, HGF, TNF-α, IL-7 and IL-3) (Raje and Roodman 2011).

3.6.1 The Pathogenesis of Impaired Bone Formation in Myeloma

Pathologically, myeloma BD seems to be related not only to the increased activity of osteoclast but also to a lack of an appropriate compensatory osteoblastic response. Bone formation is inhibited in myeloma via two distinct mechanisms, the first being the functional inhibition of already existing osteoblasts (Bataille et al. 1986, 1990a; Evans et al. 1989) and the second via the impaired differentiation of MSCs (mesenchymal stem cells) into new mature osteoblasts (Bataille et al. 1986, 1990b, 1991). In addition to reducing new bone formation, the excess of immature osteoblasts provides a rich source of the osteoclastogenic factor RANKL, favouring bone resorption and myeloma cell survival (Atkins et al. 2003). The differentiation to a mature osteoblast is inhibited by factors secreted by both myeloma cells (e.g. DKK1, sFRP2-3, sclerostin, IL-7 and HGF) and microenvironmental cells (e.g. IL-3, activin A), as well as by direct cell–cell contact between MM cells and osteoblast precursors. A full understanding of the mechanisms underlying this process should provide a rich source of therapeutic targets able to treat BD and also to improve the survival of myeloma patients.

The differentiation of MSCs to osteoblastic cells requires the transcriptional activity of Runx2/Cbfa1. Apart from Runx2 there is at least one more transcription factor, osterix, whose activity is absolutely required for osteoblast differentiation. Osterix acts downstream of Runx2 in the transcriptional cascade of osteoblast differentiation and osterix expression can be directly regulated by the binding of Runx2 to a response element in the promoter of the *osterix* gene (Karsenty 2008). A positive signal delivered by the Wnt signaling pathway is crucial in osteoblasts differentiation (Westendorf et al. 2004). Wnt signalling has been also demonstrated as the key mediator of parathyroid hormone (PTH)-induced bone formation, as the expression of DKK1, sclerostin, FRZB and several other components of the canonical Wnt signaling pathway have been shown to be negatively regulated by PTH (Bellido et al. 2005; Guo et al. 2010; Keller and Kneissel 2005; Kulkarni et al. 2005; Qin et al. 2003; Pennisi et al. 2010).

The sFRP family proteins are also soluble inhibitors of Wnt signalling, sFRP-2 and sFRP-3/FRZB have been investigated as possible mediators of osteoblast inhibition in myeloma. FRZB as well as DKK1 have been reported to be upregulated in MM samples compared to normal plasma cells and MGUS samples (Tian et al. 2003; Davies et al. 2003; De Vos et al. 2001). Sclerostin has, more recently, been identified as another major Wnt signalling pathway inhibitor (Li et al. 2009). While sclerostin was thought to be exclusively expressed in osteocytes; it has recently been shown to be expressed in myeloma cells. Sclerostin has been demonstrated to reduce bone formation marker in an in vitro co-culture system of BMSCs and myeloma cells and a neutralizing sclerostin antibody has been shown to improve bone formation markers (Colucci et al. 2010). These results suggest that anti-sclerostin represents a promising therapy for the anabolic treatment and warrant the assessment of this approach in myeloma BD.

3.6.2 Targeting the Wnt Pathway

The Canonical Wnt signalling has been identified as an important pathway in normal osteoblast differentiation; the two basic therapeutic strategies for enhancing bone regeneration through the Wnt signalling pathways are adding agonists or blocking naturally occurring antagonists.

A role for DKK1 in the inhibition of osteoblast activity in MM was first suggested based on GEP of myeloma patients (Tian et al. 2003). A correlation between increased DKK1 expression and the extent of BD seen in this study was confirmed by various other detection methods (ELISA, qRT-PCR, western blot and immunostaining) and in different data sets (Giuliani et al. 2007b; Haaber et al. 2008). More recently, in addition to its effects on osteoblast differentiation, DKK1 has also been shown to enhance osteoclast activity via an increase in RANKL/OPG ratio (Qiang et al. 2008; Spencer et al. 2006). Importantly in terms of targeting BD as a potential anti-myeloma therapy, it has been shown that administration of an anti-DKK-1 antibody in a mouse model of myeloma inhibits bone destruction, increases bone formation and also inhibits tumour growth (Yaccoby et al. 2007). DKK1 is a soluble inhibitor of the Wnt pathway produced by MM cells. Recently, a DKK1 neutralizing antibody (BHQ880) has been tested in myeloma in the context of the bone microenvironment (Fulciniti et al. 2009). This antibody was able to enhance osteoblast differentiation, inhibit osteoclast differentiation, as well as reduce IL-6 levels in a co-culturing system, which are potentially therapeutically relevant. While the antibody did not demonstrate direct cytotoxic effects on MM cells, it did inhibit MM cell growth when the MM cells were cocultured with BMSCs and this was associated with reduced IL-6 secretion by BMSCs, suggesting that it may have anti-myeloma effects in vivo. Indeed, a few studies using murine MM models show that DKK1-neutralizing antibody increases osteoblast numbers and bone formation, as well as inhibits MM cell growth (Yaccoby et al. 2007; Fulciniti et al. 2009). BHQ880 is being tested in an ongoing phase I/II clinical trial for patients with relapsed and refractory MM who are receiving ZOL and anti-MM therapy (NCT00741377) (www.clinicaltrials.gov).

The inhibition of GSK3β is necessary for effective canonical Wnt signalling and subsequent osteogenic differentiation, GSK3β inhibitors which enhance Wnt signalling are, therefore, good candidates for bone anabolic therapy in MM. GSK3β inhibition has also been shown to reduce myeloma-induced BD as well as inducing tumour cell death in a murine plasmacytoma model (Gunn et al. 2011). An orally active, small molecule GSK3β inhibitor, 603281-31-8, has been reported to increase bone mass and bone formation markers, lower adiposity and reduce fracture risk in ovariectimized mice (Kulkarni et al. 2006, 2007). These promising results from preclinical studies warrant the testing of GSK3β inhibitors in clinical settings.

3.6.3 Activin A

Activin A is a member of the transforming growth factor-β (TGF-β) superfamily and is released from BMSCs and osteoclasts. It signals through the activin type 2A receptor and has dual effects of stimulating osteoclast activity and inhibiting osteoblast differentiation. Activin A levels have been demonstrated to be elevated in the BM of MM patients and correlate with the extent of osteolytic lesions (Vallet et al. 2010). Effects of Activin A inhibition in MM were investigated using a soluble receptor RAP-011. RAP-011 treatment leads to increased OB differentiation and inhibits OC development in vitro. It has also been shown to increase bone volume and decrease MM tumour burden in a number of murine models of MM (Vallet et al. 2010; Chantry et al. 2007). Furthermore, RAP-011 also increased bone formation in macaques, demonstrating the capacity of this agent to enhance bone formation in vivo (Lotinun et al. 2010). As a result of these studies, a phase II trial of the humanized counterpart of RAP-011, ACE-011, in bisphosphonate naive MM patients with osteolytic lesions has been carried out, the results show that the bone formation markers are increased while the bone resorption markers are decreased in patients treated with the antagonist (Abdulkadyrov et al. 2009).

4 Conclusions

Tumour burden and BD are inextricably linked in MM, understanding the biology of MM BD and its roles in tumour growth and drug resistance is crucial for the development of novel anti-myeloma strategies. Some of the current therapies, such as N-BPs, IMiDs and bortezomib, have been shown being able to target both the tumour and bone cells (e.g. osteoblast and osteoclast), and consequently reduce the tumour burden and BD. Additionally, more novel bone-targeted agents, such as BHQ880 (anti-DKK1), denosumab (anti-RANKL), ACE-011 (anti-activin A) and LY2127399 (anti-BAFF) are under development, and will significantly improve the care of MM patients in the future.

Acknowledgments Thanks to these organizations who have provided funding support to this article: Myeloma UK, Cancer Research UK, the Bud Flanagan Leukaemia Fund and the Biological Research Centre of the National Institute for Health Research at the Royal Marsden Hospital.

References

Abdulkadyrov KM, Salogub GN, Khuazheva NK, Woolf R, Haltom E, Borgstein NG, Knight R, Renshaw G, Yang Y, Sherman ML (2009) ACE-011, a soluble activin receptor type IIa IgG-Fc fusion protein, increases hemoglobin (Hb) and improves bone lesions in multiple myeloma patients receiving myelosuppressive chemotherapy: preliminary analysis. Blood (ASH Meeting Abstracts) 114:1

Abe M, Hiura K, Wilde J, Shioyasono A, Moriyama K, Hashimoto T, Kido S, Oshima T, Shibata H, Ozaki S, Inoue D, Matsumoto T (2004) Osteoclasts enhance myeloma cell growth and survival via cell–cell contact: a vicious cycle between bone destruction and myeloma expansion. Blood 104(8):2484–2491. doi:10.1182/blood-2003-11-38392003-11-3839[pii]

Anderson G, Gries M, Kurihara N, Honjo T, Anderson J, Donnenberg V, Donnenberg A, Ghobrial I, Mapara MY, Stirling D, Roodman D, Lentzsch S (2006) Thalidomide derivative CC-4047 inhibits osteoclast formation by down-regulation of PU.1. Blood 107(8):3098–3105. doi:2005-08-3450[pii]10.1182/blood-2005-08-3450

Atkins GJ, Kostakis P, Pan B, Farrugia A, Gronthos S, Evdokiou A, Harrison K, Findlay DM, Zannettino AC (2003) RANKL expression is related to the differentiation state of human osteoblasts. J Bone Miner Res 18(6):1088–1098. doi:10.1359/jbmr.2003.18.6.1088

Aviles A, Nambo MJ, Neri N, Castaneda C, Cleto S, Huerta-Guzman J (2007) Antitumor effect of zoledronic acid in previously untreated patients with multiple myeloma. Med Oncol 24(2):227–230. doi:MO:24:2:227[pii]

Bartel TB, Haessler J, Brown TL, Shaughnessy JD Jr, van Rhee F, Anaissie E, Alpe T, Angtuaco E, Walker R, Epstein J, Crowley J, Barlogie B (2009) F18-fluorodeoxyglucose positron emission tomography in the context of other imaging techniques and prognostic factors in multiple myeloma. Blood 114(10):2068–2076. doi:blood-2009-03-213280[pii]10.1182/blood-2009-03-213280

Bataille R, Chappard D, Alexandre C, Dessauw P, Sany J (1986) Importance of quantitative histology of bone changes in monoclonal gammopathy. Br J Cancer 53(6):805–810

Bataille R, Chappard D, Marcelli C, Dessauw P, Sany J, Baldet P, Alexandre C (1989) Mechanisms of bone destruction in multiple myeloma: the importance of an unbalanced process in determining the severity of lytic bone disease. J Clin Oncol 7(12):1909–1914

Bataille R, Delmas PD, Chappard D, Sany J (1990a) Abnormal serum bone Gla protein levels in multiple myeloma. Crucial role of bone formation and prognostic implications. Cancer 66(1):167–172

Bataille R, Chappard D, Marcelli C, Rossi JF, Dessauw P, Baldet P, Sany J, Alexandre C (1990b) Osteoblast stimulation in multiple myeloma lacking lytic bone lesions. Br J Haematol 76(4):484–487

Bataille R, Chappard D, Marcelli C, Dessauw P, Baldet P, Sany J, Alexandre C (1991) Recruitment of new osteoblasts and osteoclasts is the earliest critical event in the pathogenesis of human multiple myeloma. J Clin Invest 88(1):62–66. doi:10.1172/JCI115305

Baulch-Brown C, Molloy TJ, Yeh SL, Ma D, Spencer A (2007) Inhibitors of the mevalonate pathway as potential therapeutic agents in multiple myeloma. Leuk Res 31(3):341–352. doi: S0145-2126(06)00268-2[pii]10.1016/j.leukres.2006.07.018

Bellido T, Ali AA, Gubrij I, Plotkin LI, Fu Q, O'Brien CA, Manolagas SC, Jilka RL (2005) Chronic elevation of parathyroid hormone in mice reduces expression of sclerostin by osteocytes: a novel mechanism for hormonal control of osteoblastogenesis. Endocrinology 146(11):4577–4583. doi:en.2005-0239[pii]10.1210/en.2005-0239

Berenson JR, Lichtenstein A, Porter L, Dimopoulos MA, Bordoni R, George S, Lipton A, Keller A, Ballester O, Kovacs M, Blacklock H, Bell R, Simeone JF, Reitsma DJ, Heffernan M, Seaman J, Knight RD (1998) Long-term pamidronate treatment of advanced multiple myeloma patients reduces skeletal events. Myeloma Aredia Study Group. J Clin Oncol 16(2):593–602

Berenson J, Dimopoulos M, Chen YM (2006) Improved survival in patients with multiple myeloma and high BALP levels treated with zoledronic acid compared with pamidronate: univariate and multivariate models of hazard ratios. Blood (ASH Meeting Abstracts) 1

Bergsagel PL, Kuehl WM (2003) Critical roles for immunoglobulin translocations and cyclin D dysregulation in multiple myeloma. Immunol Rev 194:96–104. doi:052[pii]

Bergsagel PL, Kuehl WM, Zhan F, Sawyer J, Barlogie B, Shaughnessy J Jr (2005) Cyclin D dysregulation: an early and unifying pathogenic event in multiple myeloma. Blood 106(1):296–303. doi:2005-01-0034[pii]10.1182/blood-2005-01-0034

Boissy P, Andersen TL, Lund T, Kupisiewicz K, Plesner T, Delaisse JM (2008) Pulse treatment with the proteasome inhibitor bortezomib inhibits osteoclast resorptive activity in clinically relevant conditions. Leuk Res 32(11):1661–1668. doi:S0145-2126(08)00093-3[pii]10.1016/j.leukres.2008.02.019

Breitkreutz I, Raab MS, Vallet S, Hideshima T, Raje N, Mitsiades C, Chauhan D, Okawa Y, Munshi NC, Richardson PG, Anderson KC (2008) Lenalidomide inhibits osteoclastogenesis, survival factors and bone-remodeling markers in multiple myeloma. Leukemia 22(10): 1925–1932. doi:leu2008174[pii]10.1038/leu.2008.174

Chantry A, Heath D, Coulton L, Gallagher O, Evans H, Seehra J, Vanderkerken KI CP (2007) A soluble activin type II receptor prevents myeloma bone disease. Haematologica (Abstract) 92 (suppl2):1

Colucci S, Brunetti G, Oranger A, Mori G, Sardone F, Liso V, Curci P, Miccolis RM, Rinaldi E, Specchia G, Passeri G, Zallone A, Rizzi R, Grano M (2010) Myeloma Cells Induce Osteoblast Suppression through Sclerostin Secretion. Blood (ASH Meeting Abstracts) 116:1

Corso A, Ferretti E, Lunghi M, Zappasodi P, Mangiacavalli S, De Amici M, Rusconi C, Varettoni M, Lazzarino M (2005) Zoledronic acid down-regulates adhesion molecules of bone marrow stromal cells in multiple myeloma: a possible mechanism for its antitumor effect. Cancer 104(1):118–125. doi:10.1002/cncr.21104

Davies FE, Dring AM, Li C, Rawstron AC, Shammas MA, O'Connor SM, Fenton JA, Hideshima T, Chauhan D, Tai IT, Robinson E, Auclair D, Rees K, Gonzalez D, Ashcroft AJ, Dasgupta R, Mitsiades C, Mitsiades N, Chen LB, Wong WH, Munshi NC, Morgan GJ, Anderson KC (2003) Insights into the multistep transformation of MGUS to myeloma using microarray expression analysis. Blood 102(13):4504–4511. doi:10.1182/blood-2003-01-00162003-01-0016[pii]

De Matteo M, Brunetti AE, Maiorano E, Cafforio P, Dammacco F, Silvestris F (2010) Constitutive down-regulation of Osterix in osteoblasts from myeloma patients: in vitro effect of Bortezomib and Lenalidomide. Leuk Res 34(2):243–249. doi:S0145-2126(09)00362-2 [pii]10.1016/j.leukres.2009.07.017

De Vos J, Couderc G, Tarte K, Jourdan M, Requirand G, Delteil MC, Rossi JF, Mechti N, Klein B (2001) Identifying intercellular signaling genes expressed in malignant plasma cells by using complementary DNA arrays. Blood 98(3):771–780

Delforge M, Terpos E, Richardson PG, Shpilberg O, Khuageva NK, Schlag R, Dimopoulos MA, Kropff M, Spicka I, Petrucci MT, Samoilova OS, Mateos MV, Magen-Nativ H, Goldschmidt H, Esseltine DL, Ricci DS, Liu K, Deraedt W, Cakana A, van de Velde H, San Miguel JF (2011) Fewer bone disease events, improvement in bone remodeling, and evidence of bone healing with bortezomib plus melphalan-prednisone vs. melphalan-prednisone in the phase III VISTA trial in multiple myeloma. Eur J Haematol. doi:10.1111/j.1600-0609.2011.01599.x

Dezorella N, Pevsner-Fischer M, Deutsch V, Kay S, Baron S, Stern R, Tavor S, Nagler A, Naparstek E, Zipori D, Katz BZ (2009) Mesenchymal stromal cells revert multiple myeloma cells to less differentiated phenotype by the combined activities of adhesive interactions and interleukin-6. Exp Cell Res 315(11):1904–1913. doi:S0014-4827(09)00129-3[pii]10.1016/j.yexcr.2009.03.016

Durie BG, Salmon SE (1975) A clinical staging system for multiple myeloma. Correlation of measured myeloma cell mass with presenting clinical features, response to treatment, and survival. Cancer 36(3):842–854

Evans CE, Galasko CS, Ward C (1989) Does myeloma secrete an osteoblast inhibiting factor? J Bone Joint Surg Br 71(2):288–290

Fizazi K, Lipton A, Mariette X, Body JJ, Rahim Y, Gralow JR, Gao G, Wu L, Sohn W, Jun S (2009) Randomized phase II trial of denosumab in patients with bone metastases from prostate cancer, breast cancer, or other neoplasms after intravenous bisphosphonates. J Clin Oncol 27(10):1564–1571. doi:JCO.2008.19.2146[pii]10.1200/JCO.2008.19.2146

Fulciniti M, Tassone P, Hideshima T, Vallet S, Nanjappa P, Ettenberg SA, Shen Z, Patel N, Tai YT, Chauhan D, Mitsiades C, Prabhala R, Raje N, Anderson KC, Stover DR, Munshi NC (2009) Anti-DKK1 mAb (BHQ880) as a potential therapeutic agent for multiple myeloma. Blood 114(2):371–379. doi:blood-2008-11-191577[pii]10.1182/blood-2008-11-191577

Giuliani N, Morandi F, Tagliaferri S, Lazzaretti M, Bonomini S, Crugnola M, Mancini C, Martella E, Ferrari L, Tabilio A, Rizzoli V (2007a) The proteasome inhibitor bortezomib affects osteoblast differentiation in vitro and in vivo in multiple myeloma patients. Blood 110(1):334–338. doi:blood-2006-11-059188[pii]10.1182/blood-2006-11-059188

Giuliani N, Morandi F, Tagliaferri S, Lazzaretti M, Donofrio G, Bonomini S, Sala R, Mangoni M, Rizzoli V (2007b) Production of Wnt inhibitors by myeloma cells: potential effects on canonical Wnt pathway in the bone microenvironment. Cancer Res 67(16):7665–7674. doi:67/16/7665[pii]10.1158/0008-5472.CAN-06-4666

Glass DA 2nd, Bialek P, Ahn JD, Starbuck M, Patel MS, Clevers H, Taketo MM, Long F, McMahon AP, Lang RA, Karsenty G (2005) Canonical Wnt signaling in differentiated osteoblasts controls osteoclast differentiation. Dev Cell 8(5):751–764. doi:S1534-5807(05)00097-3[pii]10.1016/j.devcel.2005.02.017

Guenther A, Gordon S, Tiemann M, Burger R, Bakker F, Green JR, Baum W, Roelofs AJ, Rogers MJ, Gramatzki M (2010) The bisphosphonate zoledronic acid has antimyeloma activity in vivo by inhibition of protein prenylation. Int J Cancer 126(1):239–246. doi:10.1002/ijc.24758

Gunn WG, Conley A, Deininger L, Olson SD, Prockop DJ, Gregory CA (2006) A crosstalk between myeloma cells and marrow stromal cells stimulates production of DKK1 and interleukin-6: a potential role in the development of lytic bone disease and tumor progression in multiple myeloma. Stem Cells 24(4):986–991. doi:2005-0220[pii]10.1634/stemcells.2005-0220

Gunn WG, Krause U, Lee N, Gregory CA (2011) Pharmaceutical inhibition of glycogen synthetase kinase-3beta reduces multiple myeloma-induced bone disease in a novel murine plasmacytoma xenograft model. Blood 117(5):1641–1651. doi:blood-2010-09-308171[pii]10.1182/blood-2010-09-308171

Guo J, Liu M, Yang D, Bouxsein ML, Saito H, Galvin RJ, Kuhstoss SA, Thomas CC, Schipani E, Baron R, Bringhurst FR, Kronenberg HM (2010) Suppression of Wnt signaling by Dkk1 attenuates PTH-mediated stromal cell response and new bone formation. Cell Metab 11(2):161–171. doi:S1550-4131(09)00405-7[pii]10.1016/j.cmet.2009.12.007

Haaber J, Abildgaard N, Knudsen LM, Dahl IM, Lodahl M, Thomassen M, Kerndrup GB, Rasmussen T (2008) Myeloma cell expression of 10 candidate genes for osteolytic bone disease. Only overexpression of DKK1 correlates with clinical bone involvement at diagnosis. Br J Haematol 140(1):25–35. doi:BJH6871[pii]10.1111/j.1365-2141.2007.06871.x

Han JH, Choi SJ, Kurihara N, Koide M, Oba Y, Roodman GD (2001) Macrophage inflammatory protein-1alpha is an osteoclastogenic factor in myeloma that is independent of receptor activator of nuclear factor kappaB ligand. Blood 97(11):3349–3353

Heider U, Kaiser M, Muller C, Jakob C, Zavrski I, Schulz CO, Fleissner C, Hecht M, Sezer O (2006) Bortezomib increases osteoblast activity in myeloma patients irrespective of response to treatment. Eur J Haematol 77(3):233–238. doi:EJH692[pii]10.1111/j.1600-0609.2006.00692.x

Henry DH, Costa L, Goldwasser F, Hirsh V, Hungria V, Prausova J, Scagliotti GV, Sleeboom H, Spencer A, Vadhan-Raj S, von Moos R, Willenbacher W, Woll PJ, Wang J, Jiang Q, Jun S,

Dansey R, Yeh H (2011) Randomized, double-blind study of denosumab versus zoledronic Acid in the treatment of bone metastases in patients with advanced cancer (excluding breast and prostate cancer) or multiple myeloma. J Clin Oncol 29(9):1125–1132. doi:JCO.2010.31. 3304[pii]10.1200/JCO.2010.31.3304

Hurt EM, Wiestner A, Rosenwald A, Shaffer AL, Campo E, Grogan T, Bergsagel PL, Kuehl WM, Staudt LM (2004) Overexpression of c-maf is a frequent oncogenic event in multiple myeloma that promotes proliferation and pathological interactions with bone marrow stroma. Cancer Cell 5(2):191–199. doi:S1535610804000194[pii]

Jakob C, Sterz J, Liebisch P, Mieth M, Rademacher J, Goerke A, Heider U, Fleissner C, Kaiser M, von Metzler I, Muller C, Sezer O (2008) Incorporation of the bone marker carboxy-terminal telopeptide of type-1 collagen improves prognostic information of the International Staging System in newly diagnosed symptomatic multiple myeloma. Leukemia 22(9):1767–1772. doi:leu2008159[pii]10.1038/leu.2008.159

Karsenty G (2008) Transcriptional control of skeletogenesis. Annu Rev Genomics Hum Genet 9:183–196. doi:10.1146/annurev.genom.9.081307.164437

Keller H, Kneissel M (2005) SOST is a target gene for PTH in bone. Bone 37(2):148–158. doi: S8756-3282(05)00117-1[pii]10.1016/j.bone.2005.03.018

Kulkarni NH, Halladay DL, Miles RR, Gilbert LM, Frolik CA, Galvin RJ, Martin TJ, Gillespie MT, Onyia JE (2005) Effects of parathyroid hormone on Wnt signaling pathway in bone. J Cell Biochem 95(6):1178–1190. doi:10.1002/jcb.20506

Kulkarni NH, Onyia JE, Zeng Q, Tian X, Liu M, Halladay DL, Frolik CA, Engler T, Wei T, Kriauciunas A, Martin TJ, Sato M, Bryant HU, Ma YL (2006) Orally bioavailable GSK-3alpha/beta dual inhibitor increases markers of cellular differentiation in vitro and bone mass in vivo. J Bone Miner Res 21(6):910–920. doi:10.1359/jbmr.060316

Kulkarni NH, Wei T, Kumar A, Dow ER, Stewart TR, Shou J, N'Cho M, Sterchi DL, Gitter BD, Higgs RE, Halladay DL, Engler TA, Martin TJ, Bryant HU, Ma YL, Onyia JE (2007) Changes in osteoblast, chondrocyte, and adipocyte lineages mediate the bone anabolic actions of PTH and small molecule GSK-3 inhibitor. J Cell Biochem 102(6):1504–1518. doi:10.1002/jcb.21374

Kyle RA, Yee GC, Somerfield MR, Flynn PJ, Halabi S, Jagannath S, Orlowski RZ, Roodman DG, Twilde P, Anderson K (2007) American Society of Clinical Oncology 2007 clinical practice guideline update on the role of bisphosphonates in multiple myeloma. J Clin Oncol 25(17): 2464–2472. doi:JCO.2007.12.1269[pii]10.1200/JCO.2007.12.1269

Lentzsch S, Gries M, Janz M, Bargou R, Dorken B, Mapara MY (2003) Macrophage inflammatory protein 1-alpha (MIP-1 alpha) triggers migration and signaling cascades mediating survival and proliferation in multiple myeloma (MM) cells. Blood 101(9): 3568–3573. doi:10.1182/blood-2002-08-23832002-08-2383[pii]

Li X, Pennisi A, Yaccoby S (2008) Role of decorin in the antimyeloma effects of osteoblasts. Blood 112(1):159–168. doi:blood-2007-11-124164[pii]10.1182/blood-2007-11-124164

Li X, Ominsky MS, Warmington KS, Morony S, Gong J, Cao J, Gao Y, Shalhoub V, Tipton B, Haldankar R, Chen Q, Winters A, Boone T, Geng Z, Niu QT, Ke HZ, Kostenuik PJ, Simonet WS, Lacey DL, Paszty C (2009) Sclerostin antibody treatment increases bone formation, bone mass, and bone strength in a rat model of postmenopausal osteoporosis. J Bone Miner Res 24(4): 578–588. doi:10.1359/jbmr.081206

Lotinun S, Pearsall RS, Davies MV, Marvell TH, Monnell TE, Ucran J, Fajardo RJ, Kumar R, Underwood KW, Seehra J, Bouxsein ML, Baron R (2010) A soluble activin receptor Type IIA fusion protein (ACE-011) increases bone mass via a dual anabolic-antiresorptive effect in Cynomolgus monkeys. Bone 46(4):1082–1088. doi:S8756-3282(10)00376-5[pii]10.1016/j.bone.2010.01.370

McCloskey EV, Dunn JA, Kanis JA, MacLennan IC, Drayson MT (2001) Long-term follow-up of a prospective, double-blind, placebo-controlled randomized trial of clodronate in multiple myeloma. Br J Haematol 113(4):1035–1043. doi:bjh2851[pii]

Melton LJ 3rd, Kyle RA, Achenbach SJ, Oberg AL, Rajkumar SV (2005) Fracture risk with multiple myeloma: a population-based study. J Bone Miner Res 20(3):487–493. doi:10.1359/JBMR.041131

Mitsiades CS, McMillin DW, Klippel S, Hideshima T, Chauhan D, Richardson PG, Munshi NC, Anderson KC (2007) The role of the bone marrow microenvironment in the pathophysiology of myeloma and its significance in the development of more effective therapies. Hematol Oncol Clin North Am 21(6):1007–1034. doi:S0889-8588(07)00115-3[pii]10.1016/j.hoc.2007.08.007 vii-viii

Morgan GJ (2011) Can bisphosphonates improve outcomes in patients with newly diagnosed multiple myeloma? Crit Rev Oncol Hematol 77(Suppl 1):S24–30. doi:S1040-8428(11) 70005-1[pii]10.1016/S1040-8428(11)70005-1

Morgan GJ, Davies FE, Gregory WM, Cocks K, Bell SE, Szubert AJ, Navarro-Coy N, Drayson MT, Owen RG, Feyler S, Ashcroft AJ, Ross F, Byrne J, Roddie H, Rudin C, Cook G, Jackson GH, Child JA (2010) First-line treatment with zoledronic acid as compared with clodronic acid in multiple myeloma (MRC Myeloma IX): a randomised controlled trial. Lancet 376(9757): 1989–1999. doi:S0140-6736(10)62051-X[pii]10.1016/S0140-6736(10)62051-X

Moschetta M, Di Pietro G, Ria R, Gnoni A, Mangialardi G, Guarini A, Ditonno P, Musto P, D'Auria F, Ricciardi MR, Dammacco F, Ribatti D, Vacca A (2010) Bortezomib and zoledronic acid on angiogenic and vasculogenic activities of bone marrow macrophages in patients with multiple myeloma. Eur J Cancer 46(2):420–429. doi:S0959-8049(09)00777-1 [pii]10.1016/j.ejca.2009.10.019

Mukherjee S, Raje N, Schoonmaker JA, Liu JC, Hideshima T, Wein MN, Jones DC, Vallet S, Bouxsein ML, Pozzi S, Chhetri S, Seo YD, Aronson JP, Patel C, Fulciniti M, Purton LE, Glimcher LH, Lian JB, Stein G, Anderson KC, Scadden DT (2008) Pharmacologic targeting of a stem/progenitor population in vivo is associated with enhanced bone regeneration in mice. J Clin Invest 118(2):491–504. doi:10.1172/JCI33102

Neri P, Kumar S, Fulciniti MT, Vallet S, Chhetri S, Mukherjee S, Tai Y, Chauhan D, Tassone P, Venuta S, Munshi NC, Hideshima T, Anderson KC, Raje N (2007) Neutralizing B-cell activating factor antibody improves survival and inhibits osteoclastogenesis in a severe combined immunodeficient human multiple myeloma model. Clin Cancer Res 13(19): 5903–5909. doi:13/19/5903[pii]10.1158/1078-0432.CCR-07-0753

Pennisi A, Ling W, Li X, Khan S, Wang Y, Barlogie B, Shaughnessy JD Jr, Yaccoby S (2010) Consequences of daily administered parathyroid hormone on myeloma growth, bone disease, and molecular profiling of whole myelomatous bone. PLoS One 5(12):e15233. doi: 10.1371/journal.pone.0015233

Qiang YW, Chen Y, Stephens O, Brown N, Chen B, Epstein J, Barlogie B, Shaughnessy JD Jr (2008) Myeloma-derived Dickkopf-1 disrupts Wnt-regulated osteoprotegerin and RANKL production by osteoblasts: a potential mechanism underlying osteolytic bone lesions in multiple myeloma. Blood 112(1):196–207. doi:blood-2008-01-132134[pii]10.1182/blood-2008-01-132134

Qin L, Qiu P, Wang L, Li X, Swarthout JT, Soteropoulos P, Tolias P, Partridge NC (2003) Gene expression profiles and transcription factors involved in parathyroid hormone signaling in osteoblasts revealed by microarray and bioinformatics. J Biol Chem 278(22):19723–19731. doi:10.1074/jbc.M212226200M212226200[pii]

Raje N, Roodman GD (2011) Advances in the biology and treatment of bone disease in multiple myeloma. Clin Cancer Res 17(6):1278–1286. doi:17/6/1278[pii]10.1158/1078-0432.CCR-10-1804

Robbiani DF, Chesi M, Bergsagel PL (2004) Bone lesions in molecular subtypes of multiple myeloma. N Engl J Med 351(2):197–198. doi:10.1056/NEJM200407083510223351/2/197[pii]

Roodman GD (2004) Mechanisms of bone metastasis. N Engl J Med 350(16):1655–1664. doi:10.1056/NEJMra030831350/16/1655[pii]

Rosen LS, Gordon D, Kaminski M, Howell A, Belch A, Mackey J, Apffelstaedt J, Hussein M, Coleman RE, Reitsma DJ, Seaman JJ, Chen BL, Ambros Y (2001) Zoledronic acid versus pamidronate in the treatment of skeletal metastases in patients with breast cancer or osteolytic lesions of multiple myeloma: a phase III, double-blind, comparative trial. Cancer J 7(5):377–387

Schmidmaier R, Simsek M, Baumann P, Emmerich B, Meinhardt G (2006) Synergistic antimyeloma effects of zoledronate and simvastatin. Anticancer Drugs 17(6):621–629. doi:10.1097/01.cad.0000215058.85813.0200001813-200607000-00003[pii]

Shaugnessy J, Zhan F, Kordsmeier B, Randolph C, McCastlain K, Barlogie B (2002) Gene expression profiling (GEP) after short term in vivo treatment identifies potential mechanisms of action of current drugs used to treat multiple myeloma. Blood (ASH Meeting Abstracts) 100:1

Shimazaki C, Uchida R, Nakano S, Namura K, Fuchida SI, Okano A, Okamoto M, Inaba T (2005) High serum bone-specific alkaline phosphatase level after bortezomib-combined therapy in refractory multiple myeloma: possible role of bortezomib on osteoblast differentiation. Leukemia 19(6):1102–1103. doi:2403758[pii]10.1038/sj.leu.2403758

Shipman CM, Rogers MJ, Apperley JF, Russell RG, Croucher PI (1997) Bisphosphonates induce apoptosis in human myeloma cell lines: a novel anti-tumour activity. Br J Haematol 98(3):665–672

Spencer GJ, Utting JC, Etheridge SL, Arnett TR, Genever PG (2006) Wnt signalling in osteoblasts regulates expression of the receptor activator of NFkappaB ligand and inhibits osteoclastogenesis in vitro. J Cell Sci 119(Pt 7):1283–1296. doi:jcs.02883[pii]10.1242/jcs.02883

Tai YT, Li XF, Breitkreutz I, Song W, Neri P, Catley L, Podar K, Hideshima T, Chauhan D, Raje N, Schlossman R, Richardson P, Munshi NCAnderson KC (2006) Role of B-cell-activating factor in adhesion and growth of human multiple myeloma cells in the bone marrow microenvironment. Cancer Res 66(13):6675–6682. doi:66/13/6675[pii]10.1158/0008-5472.CAN-06-0190

Tassone P, Forciniti S, Galea E, Morrone G, Turco MC, Martinelli V, Tagliaferri P, Venuta S (2000) Growth inhibition and synergistic induction of apoptosis by zoledronate and dexamethasone in human myeloma cell lines. Leukemia 14(5):841–844

Terpos E, Heath DJ, Rahemtulla A, Zervas K, Chantry A, Anagnostopoulos A, Pouli A, Katodritou E, Verrou E, Vervessou EC, Dimopoulos MA, Croucher PI (2006) Bortezomib reduces serum dickkopf-1 and receptor activator of nuclear factor-kappaB ligand concentrations and normalises indices of bone remodelling in patients with relapsed multiple myeloma. Br J Haematol 135(5):688–692. doi:BJH6356[pii]10.1111/j.1365-2141.2006.06356.x

Terpos E, Dimopoulos MA, Sezer O (2007) The effect of novel anti-myeloma agents on bone metabolism of patients with multiple myeloma. Leukemia 21(9):1875–1884. doi:2404843[pii] 10.1038/sj.leu.2404843

Tian E, Zhan F, Walker R, Rasmussen E, Ma Y, Barlogie B, Shaughnessy JD Jr (2003) The role of the Wnt-signaling antagonist DKK1 in the development of osteolytic lesions in multiple myeloma. N Engl J Med 349(26):2483–2494. doi:10.1056/NEJMoa030847349/26/2483[pii]

Ural AU, Yilmaz MI, Avcu F, Pekel A, Zerman M, Nevruz O, Sengul A, Yalcin A (2003) The bisphosphonate zoledronic acid induces cytotoxicity in human myeloma cell lines with enhancing effects of dexamethasone and thalidomide. Int J Hematol 78(5):443–449

Uy GL, Trivedi R, Peles S, Fisher NM, Zhang QJ, Tomasson MH, DiPersio JF, Vij R (2007) Bortezomib inhibits osteoclast activity in patients with multiple myeloma. Clin Lymphoma Myeloma 7(9):587–589

Vallet S, Raje N, Ishitsuka K, Hideshima T, Podar K, Chhetri S, Pozzi S, Breitkreutz I, Kiziltepe T, Yasui H, Ocio EM, Shiraishi N, Jin J, Okawa Y, Ikeda H, Mukherjee S, Vaghela N, Cirstea D, Ladetto M, Boccadoro M, Anderson KC (2007) MLN3897, a novel CCR1 inhibitor, impairs osteoclastogenesis and inhibits the interaction of multiple myeloma cells and osteoclasts. Blood 110(10):3744–3752. doi:blood-2007-05-093294[pii]10.1182/blood-2007-05-093294

Vallet S, Mukherjee S, Vaghela N, Hideshima T, Fulciniti M, Pozzi S, Santo L, Cirstea D, Patel K, Sohani AR, Guimaraes A, Xie W, Chauhan D, Schoonmaker JA, Attar E, Churchill M, Weller E, Munshi N, Seehra JS, Weissleder R, Anderson KC, Scadden DT, Raje N (2010) Activin A promotes multiple myeloma-induced osteolysis and is a promising target for myeloma bone disease. Proc Natl Acad Sci U S A 107(11):5124–5129. doi:0911929107 [pii]10.1073/pnas.0911929107

Vallet S, Pozzi S, Patel K, Vaghela N, Fulciniti MT, Veiby P, Hideshima T, Santo L, Cirstea D, Scadden DT, Anderson KC, Raje N (2011) A novel role for CCL3 (MIP-1alpha) in myeloma-induced bone disease via osteocalcin downregulation and inhibition of osteoblast function. Leukemia. doi:leu201143[pii]10.1038/leu.2011.43

Vij R, Horvath N, Spencer A, Taylor K, Vadhan-Raj S, Vescio R, Smith J, Qian Y, Yeh H, Jun S (2009) An open-label, phase 2 trial of denosumab in the treatment of relapsed or plateau-phase multiple myeloma. Am J Hematol 84(10):650–656. doi:10.1002/ajh.21509

von Metzler I, Krebbel H, Hecht M, Manz RA, Fleissner C, Mieth M, Kaiser M, Jakob C, Sterz J, Kleeberg L, Heider U, Sezer O (2007) Bortezomib inhibits human osteoclastogenesis. Leukemia 21(9):2025–2034. doi:2404806[pii]10.1038/sj.leu.2404806

Walker R, Barlogie B, Haessler J, Tricot G, Anaissie E, Shaughnessy JD Jr, Epstein J, van Hemert R, Erdem E, Hoering A, Crowley J, Ferris E, Hollmig K, van Rhee F, Zangari M, Pineda-Roman M, Mohiuddin A, Yaccoby S, Sawyer J, Angtuaco EJ (2007) Magnetic resonance imaging in multiple myeloma: diagnostic and clinical implications. J Clin Oncol 25(9):1121–1128. doi:JCO.2006.08.5803[pii]10.1200/JCO.2006.08.5803

Westendorf JJ, Kahler RA, Schroeder TM (2004) Wnt signaling in osteoblasts and bone diseases. Gene 341:19–39. doi:S0378-1119(04)00385-3[pii]10.1016/j.gene.2004.06.044

Wu P, Walker BA, Brewer D, Gregory WM, Ashcroft J, Ross FM, Jackson GH, Child AJ, Davies FE, Morgan GJ (2011) A gene expression-based predictor for myeloma patients at high risk of developing bone disease on bisphosphonate treatment. Clin Cancer Res 17(19):6347–6355

Yaccoby S (2005) The phenotypic plasticity of myeloma plasma cells as expressed by dedifferentiation into an immature, resilient, and apoptosis-resistant phenotype. Clin Cancer Res 11(21):7599–7606. doi:11/21/7599[pii]10.1158/1078-0432.CCR-05-0523

Yaccoby S (2010) Advances in the understanding of myeloma bone disease and tumour growth. Br J Haematol 149(3):311–321. doi:BJH8141[pii]10.1111/j.1365-2141.2010.08141.x

Yaccoby S, Wezeman MJ, Henderson A, Cottler-Fox M, Yi Q, Barlogie B, Epstein J (2004) Cancer and the microenvironment: myeloma-osteoclast interactions as a model. Cancer Res 64(6):2016–2023

Yaccoby S, Wezeman MJ, Zangari M, Walker R, Cottler-Fox M, Gaddy D, Ling W, Saha R, Barlogie B, Tricot G, Epstein J (2006) Inhibitory effects of osteoblasts and increased bone formation on myeloma in novel culture systems and a myelomatous mouse model. Haematologica 91(2):192–199

Yaccoby S, Ling W, Zhan F, Walker R, Barlogie B, Shaughnessy JD Jr (2007) Antibody-based inhibition of DKK1 suppresses tumor-induced bone resorption and multiple myeloma growth in vivo. Blood 109(5):2106–2111. doi:blood-2006-09-047712[pii]10.1182/blood-2006-09-047712

Zangari M, Esseltine D, Lee CK, Barlogie B, Elice F, Burns MJ, Kang SH, Yaccoby S, Najarian K, Richardson P, Sonneveld P, Tricot G (2005) Response to bortezomib is associated to osteoblastic activation in patients with multiple myeloma. Br J Haematol 131(1):71–73. doi:BJH5733[pii] 10.1111/j.1365-2141.2005.05733.x

Zavrski I, Krebbel H, Wildemann B, Heider U, Kaiser M, Possinger K, Sezer O (2005) Proteasome inhibitors abrogate osteoclast differentiation and osteoclast function. Biochem Biophys Res Commun 333(1):200–205. doi:S0006-291X(05)01075-2[pii]10.1016/j.bbrc.2005.05.098

Zhan F, Huang Y, Colla S, Stewart JP, Hanamura I, Gupta S, Epstein J, Yaccoby S, Sawyer J, Burington B, Anaissie E, Hollmig K, Pineda-Roman M, Tricot G, van Rhee F, Walker R, Zangari M, Crowley J, Barlogie B, Shaughnessy JD Jr (2006) The molecular classification of multiple myeloma. Blood 108(6):2020–2028. doi:blood-2005-11-013458[pii]10.1182/blood-2005-11-013458

Zipori D (2010) The hemopoietic stem cell niche versus the microenvironment of the multiple myeloma-tumor initiating cell. Cancer Microenviron 3(1):15–28. doi:10.1007/s12307-009-0034-7

Zwolak P, Manivel JC, Jasinski P, Kirstein MN, Dudek AZ, Fisher J, Cheng EY (2010) Cytotoxic effect of zoledronic acid-loaded bone cement on giant cell tumor, multiple myeloma, and renal cell carcinoma cell lines. J Bone Joint Surg Am 92(1):162–168. doi:92/1/162[pii]10.2106/JBJS.H.01679

Combinations of Bisphosphonates and Classical Anticancer Drugs: A Preclinical Perspective

Dr. Maria Michailidou and Dr. Ingunn Holen

Abstract

Bone metastases are frequent complications in advanced breast and prostate cancer among others, resulting in increased risk of fractures, pain, hypercalcaemia of malignancy and a reduction in patient independence and mobility. Bisphosphonates (BPs) are in wide clinical use for the treatment of cancer-induced bone disease associated with advanced cancer, due to their potent ability to reduce skeletal-related events (SREs) and improve quality of life. Despite the profound effect on bone health, the majority of clinical studies have failed to demonstrate an overall survival benefit of BP therapy. There is increasing preclinical evidence to suggest that inclusion of the most potent nitrogen-containing BPs (NBPs) in combination therapy results in increased antitumour effects and improved survival, but that the particular schedules used are of key importance to achieve optimal benefit. Recent clinical data have suggested that there may be effects of adjuvant NBP therapy on breast tumours outside the skeleton. These findings have led to renewed interest in the use of BPs in cancer therapy, in particular how they can be included as part of adjuvant protocols. Here we review the key data reported from preclinical model systems investigating the effects of combination therapy including BPs with particular emphasis on breast and prostate cancer.

Dr. M. Michailidou · Dr. I. Holen (✉)
Academic Unit of Clinical Oncology, DU39 Medical School,
University of Sheffield, Beech Hill Road,
Sheffield, S10 2RX, UK
e-mail: I.Holen@Sheffield.ac.uk

Abbreviations

ANZAC	AdditioN of Zoledronic Acid to neo-adjuvant Combination chemotherapy
AZURE	Adjuvant Zoledronic acid redUce Recurrence
bFGF	basic Fibroblast Growth Factor
BP	BisPhosphonate
DMC	Dorsal Microcirculation Chamber
EC	Endothelial Cells
ER	Estrogren Receptor
FEC	5-Fluorouracil + Epirubicin + Cyclophosphamide
HER2	Human Epidermal growth factor Receptor 2
HuDMEC	Human Dermal Microvascular Endothelial Cells
HUVEC	Human Umbilical Vein Endothelial Cells
GGOH	GeranylGeraniol
µCT analysis	micro-Computed Tomography
NBP	Nitrogen-containing BisPhosphonate
NSCLC	Non-Small Cell Lung Cancer
PDGF	Platelet-Derived Growth Factor
PSA	Prostate Specific Antigen
SCID	Severe Combined ImmunoDeficiency
SCLC	Small Cell Lung Cancer
SRE	Skeletal Related Event
UFT	TegaFur-Uracil
VEGF	Vascular Endothelial Growth Factor
ZANTE	Zoledronic acid ANd TaxoterE

Contents

1 Molecular Mechanism of Action of BPs.. 147
2 BPs-Proposed Mechanisms Behind Their Potential Antitumour Effects......................... 148
    2.1 In Vitro Models... 148
    2.2 In Vivo Models.. 148
3 BPs in Combination Therapy.. 149
    3.1 In Vitro Studies–The Foundation for BPs as Part of Combination Therapy........... 150
    3.2 In Vivo Studies–Further Evidence of Benefits of BPs in Combination Therapy ... 153
4 Combination Therapy with BPs-Effects on Tumour Growth in Bone............................ 153
    4.1 Summary–Effects on Tumour Growth in Bone 158
5 Combination Therapy with BPs-Effects on Peripheral Tumour Growth........................ 158
    5.1 Summary–Effects on Peripheral Tumour Growth....................................... 160
6 Sequential Combination Therapy with BPs in the Clinical Setting................................ 161
7 BPs in Combination Therapy–Effects on Normal Cells.. 162

7.1 Antiangiogenic Effects of BPs as Single Agents.. 162
 7.2 Antiangiogenic Effects of BPs in Combination Therapy 164
8 Conclusions.. 165
References.. 166

1 Molecular Mechanism of Action of BPs

Metastatic bone disease is a frequent skeletal complication in advanced breast and prostate cancer, as well as multiple myeloma. Bone metastases are associated with skeletal-related events (e.g. pathological fractures, spinal cord compression, hypercalcaemia, bone pain), leading to increased morbidity and mortality, and with severe implications for the quality of life of patients. Current therapy includes radiation therapy, surgery, chemotherapy, analgesics and anti-resorptive bisphosphonates. Bisphosphonates (BPs) are analogues of pyrophosphate with high affinity in binding to hydroxyapatite bone mineral surfaces with a preference for active metabolic sites of osteolysis (reviewed by Rogers et al. 2000). BPs are potent inhibitors of osteoclastic bone resorption, a key process involved in the formation of both lytic and blastic bone lesions associated with bone metastases (Rogers 2003). Due to the high affinity to bone, the osteoclast is the main cell type exposed to toxic doses of BPs through active resorption of bone. The molecular mechanism of action of BPs is now well established; simple BPs (like clodronate) act by incorporation into non-hydrolysable ATP analogues (Rogers et al. 1996), whereas the more potent NBPs inhibit key enzymes in the mevalonate pathway (Luckman et al. 1998). This pathway is responsible for cholesterol synthesis, and is therefore essential for viability of all nucleated cells. In addition, many proteins rely on this pathway for their post-translational modifications (prenylation), which is essential for their correct intracellular localisation and function (Brown et al. 2009b). By targeting this basic biochemical pathway, NBPs therefore have the potential to affect any cell type that takes up sufficient levels of the drugs, including tumour cells. In particular, tumour cells within bone metastases may be exposed to a 'high-BP' environment, resulting in reduced viability. However, there is little direct evidence supporting that tumour cells take up BPs within the bone microenvironment. BPs may also inhibit cancer cell growth indirectly, by reducing the osteoclast-mediated release of tumour growth factors from bone matrix (Rogers et al. 2000). Although outside the scope of this chapter, there is a large body of evidence supporting that this is a key mechanism whereby tumour growth in bone is modified by BP therapy (Clezardin et al. 2005; Fournier et al. 2010; Russell 2007). BPs reduce bone pain, pathological fractures and hypercalcaemia (Kohno 2008; Walkington and Coleman 2011) thus reducing skeletal-related morbidity, but do not convey a substantial increase in survival. There is also mounting experimental and clinical evidence showing that BPs can be used as effective prevention and treatment strategy against bone metastases in adjuvant therapy (reviewed by Coleman 2007). It is however important to bear in mind that even when bone resorption is virtually completely shut down by BPs, tumour progression in bone is only delayed. This indicates that tumours do reach a point when they become independent of bone growth factors/cytokines for their progression, and that targeting bone alone is not sufficient to eliminate tumour growth. An increasing number of patients live for several years following the diagnosis of bone metastasis, and this has led to a large body of research into the effects of BPs on tumour development and progression. In the following sections, we review some of the key studies investigating the potential antitumour effects of BPs, using both in vitro and in vivo model systems.

2 BPs-Proposed Mechanisms Behind Their Potential Antitumour Effects

2.1 In Vitro Models

A multitude of in vitro and in vivo studies have demonstrated that BPs induce apoptotic cell death in a variety of cancer types, including breast (Senaratne et al. 2002), prostate (Lee et al. 2001; Virtanen et al. 2002), myeloma (Shipman et al. 1997), lung (Koshimune et al. 2007), osteosarcoma (Kubista et al. 2006) and pancreatic cancer cell lines (Tassone et al. 2003; Märten et al. 2007). In particular, zoledronic acid has been found to cause dose- and time-dependent inhibition of various aspects of cellular function such as cell proliferation (Lee et al. 2001; Ory et al. 2007), adhesion (van der Plujim et al. 2005) and invasion (Boissier et al. 1997) into cellular matrix components (reviewed by Neville-Webbe et al. 2002 and Clezardin 2011). Although only briefly mentioned here, a large body of in vitro evidence supports that BPs may have direct antitumour effects, but that high concentrations and repeated/prolonged treatment is required to induce significant levels of tumour cell death. The clinical relevance of the in vitro studies is therefore limited to demonstrating a proof of principle, i.e. the fact that tumour cells could be negatively affected by BPs in vivo if they are exposed to sufficient doses of the drugs. However, the high affinity of BPs to bone and their short half-life in the circulation suggests that tumour cells may not be exposed to sufficient concentrations of BPs to be directly affected during standard clinical dosing.

2.2 In Vivo Models

Following on from the many reports of antitumour effects of BPs from in vitro models, this was further explored using in vivo models of tumour growth in bone, in particular focussing on zoledronic acid due to its widespread clinical application in the treatment of cancer-induced bone disease (reviewed by Brown and Holen 2009a). Effects on tumour growth following both prevention protocols (BP administered prior to tumour cell implantation) (Thudi et al. 2008; van der Pluijm 2005) and treatment protocols (Corey et al. 2003; Daubine et al. 2007) have been described. In summary, these studies have demonstrated that BP therapy leads to good control of bone disease in both settings, but that prevention protocols result in a better outcome compared to when treatment is commenced once tumour growth is well established. By administering BPs at early stages of tumour development in bone, cancer cells are targeted while they potentially still depend on the bone microenvironment for their colonisation and expansion. Once bone lesions develop, the disease is progressing fast and is less dependent on tumour-derived factors due to the increased tumour capacity for autocrine growth. These data suggest that the current clinical use of BPs in the treatment of established metastatic disease with confirmed radiological bone lesions is perhaps not optimal, and that earlier intervention may be required in order to improve patient outcome. The main problem with this change in strategy would be how to determine which patients are most at risk of developing bone metastases, as well as the diagnosis of early progression in bone (before the appearance of overt lesions). Research to identify reliable biomarkers for early detection of bone metastases is ongoing (Coleman et al. 2008), and if successful will improve our ability to move metastatic bone disease further into the realms of chronic diseases.

The in vivo studies confirmed the ability of BPs to inhibit the development of bone lesions, but also demonstrated that this is at best causing a *delay* rather than leading to complete prevention of skeletal tumour progression (reviewed by Brown and Holen 2009a). This reflects the experiences from the clinical setting where, although achieving good control of the bone disease, cancers do eventually progress despite continued BP therapy (Walkington and Coleman 2011). It is therefore clear that in order to eliminate tumour growth in bone, BPs must be used in combination with agents that target the tumour cells directly.

3 BPs in Combination Therapy

After more than a decade of research dedicated to detailed genetic analysis of the cancer cell, researchers are now turning their attention to elucidating the role of the host microenvironment in tumour development and progression (Mbeunkui and Johann 2009). Cells other than cancer cells are increasingly considered to be key therapeutic targets, e.g. the cells of the tumour vasculature (Heath and Bicknell 2009). The potential for inhibiting tumour growth through modification of the host microenvironment has long been recognised in the field of bone metastases, where the standard therapy includes BPs that specifically target the normal cells (osteoclasts) responsible for regulating bone turnover. Combining agents that directly affect tumour cells (cytotoxic drugs, targeted biological agents) with drugs that modify the tumour microenvironment (vasculature, immune system, bone) is likely to be required for successful eradication of tumours. In the following sections, we will summarise some of the key studies from in vitro and in vivo model systems that have provided support for a new role of NBPs as an integral part of combination therapy.

3.1 In Vitro Studies-The Foundation for BPs as Part of Combination Therapy

3.1.1 BPs Alone

With the discovery that the mechanism of action of NBPs involves inhibition of key enzymes in a basic metabolic pathway came the realisation that the effects of these agents may not be limited to the osteoclast (Rogers et al. 1996). Any cell that is exposed to and takes up sufficient levels of the drugs can in principle be initiated to undergo apoptotic cell death. This led to studies where a range of cancer cell types were treated with different NBPs for prolonged periods of time in culture, resulting in inhibition of proliferation and increased levels of cell death (Lee et al. 2001; Riebeling et al. 2002; Senaratne et al. 2002; Kuroda et al. 2004; Neville-Webbe et al. 2005; Kubista et al. 2006; Koshimune et al. 2007; Li et al. 2008). Although supporting that NBPs have the potential for inducing tumour cell death, these studies had several key limitations. The doses and exposure times used were often high and prolonged (mM doses for several days), far exceeding the levels of BPs achieved in the clinical situation in humans. If we take zoledronic acid as an example, this drug is administered every 3–4 weeks at a standard 4 mg infusion for the treatment of cancer-induced bone disease. The maximum level of circulating zoledronic acid is between 1–2 µM for around 2 h, as the drug rapidly binds to bone and the excess is excreted. The many in vitro reports of antitumour effects of BPs must be interpreted in the context of what is clinically relevant or at least potentially achievable. There are only a few reports of pulse treatment experiments, where cancer cells have been exposed to BPs for short time periods, the drug removed and effects on apoptotic cell death assessed at later time points. Using this approach, PC3 prostate cancer cells were shown to undergo similar levels of apoptotic cell death following exposure to 25 µM zoledronic acid for 2 h as those obtained following 72 h exposure to 5 µM (Clyburn et al. 2010). These data demonstrate that uptake of BPs by tumour cells can be relatively rapid in vitro, and that prolonged exposure to the drugs is perhaps not required for the initiation of cellular effects. It is therefore possible that the short period of drug exposure following a clinical infusion of zoledronic acid may be sufficient to affect tumour cells. However, the current standard of a single monthly administration is unlikely to cause levels of tumour cell death that have a significant impact on total tumour burden.

3.1.2 BPs as Part of Combination Treatment Regimens

Once it was established that BPs could affect tumour cells, Jagdev et al. carried out a pioneering study combining zoledronic acid with the chemotherapy agent paclitaxel, in order to determine whether this would increase the level of breast cancer cell apoptosis in vitro (Jagdev et al. 2001). MCF-7 breast cancer cells were exposed to 10 µM zoledronic acid and 2 nM paclitaxel, alone and in combination, and the level of apoptosis assessed at 72 h. There was a significant, synergistic increase in the level of apoptotic cell death following exposure to a combination of the two drugs, compared to that observed in cells treated with the single agents.

This study was the first to demonstrate that breast cancer cell death may be substantially increased by simultaneous administration of an anticancer agent and an NBP. Perhaps it was time to reconsider the view that BPs only function in bone, and only target the osteoclast? Could there be an increased benefit for patients by combining these agents? Following on from this initial report, several studies investigating the effects of combination therapy emerged, adding zoledronic acid to standard chemotherapy agents in different tumour cell types in vitro (Yoneda et al. 2000; Neville-Webbe et al. 2005 , 2006; Horie et al. 2007; Duivenvoorden et al. 2007). A significant new development was provided by a study comparing the antitumour effects of sequential drug administration to that of simultaneous exposure to the agents (Neville-Webbe et al. 2005). Neville-Webbe and colleagues clearly demonstrated that the order in which drugs are given has a major impact on treatment activity, with exposure to chemotherapy *prior* to treatment with zoledronic acid inducing the highest levels of breast cancer cell apoptosis compared to the reverse sequence, the drugs combined, or the single agents. Clinically achievable concentrations of the commonly used anthracyclin doxorubicin (0.05 µM for 24 h) followed by zoledronic acid (1 µM for 1 h) induced high levels of apoptosis both in MCF7 and MDA-MB-436 breast cancer cells, as well as in the prostate cancer cell line PC3. The effect was sequence-specific, in all cases the chemotherapy agent had to be given first to induce maximum levels of tumour cell death. Similar experiments combining doxorubicin with the less potent agent clodronate (simple BP) or alendronate (NBP) did not cause increased levels of apoptosis, supporting that this is a property of the more potent agent zoledronic acid. The synergistic increase in apoptosis was reversed by the addition of an intermediary of the mevalonate pathway, demonstrating that apoptosis was mediated through the specific molecular mechanisms of action of zoledronic acid. Intriguingly, the sequential treatment did not induce apoptosis of the non-malignant 3T3 cell line, suggesting that the effect is somehow tumour cell specific. Although unable to identify the precise molecular mechanisms responsible for the sequence-specific effects of doxorubicin and zoledronic acid, this study did convincingly demonstrate the importance of drug sequencing for optimising the antitumour effects. This was further supported by a subsequent study by the same team, this time using a sequence of paclitaxel followed by zoledronic acid in breast cancer cells (Neville-Webbe et al. 2006). The earlier study by Jagdev explored the effects of high doses of these two agents added simultaneously and exposing cells for up to 72 h (Jagdev et al. 2001), conditions not achievable in the clinical setting. As a result, it was crucial to study short-term effects of the treatments. Neville-Webbe et al. exposed MCF7 cells to 2nM paclitaxel for 4 h followed by 25 µM zoledronic acid for a brief period of just 1 h, and compared this to the reverse sequence, adding both agents at the same time, or giving the single agents (Neville-Webbe et al. 2006). As was the case for doxorubicin, the highest levels of tumour cell apoptosis at 72 h were induced when the cells were exposed to paclitaxel prior to zoledronic acid. The non-malignant breast epithelial cell line MCF10A was insensitive to the sequential treatment, again supporting a tumour cell-specific effect. Comparing the effects in BRCA1$^+$ (HCC1-BR116) and

BRCA1⁻ (HC1937) breast cancer cell lines, the highest levels of apoptotic cell death were induced by sequential treatment with paclitaxel followed by zoledronic acid in cells that carry BRCA1.

That the sequence of exposure is important for apoptotic cell death is further supported by a recent study using prostate cancer cells (Clyburn et al. 2010). PC3, DU145 and LNCaP cells were treated with 0.05 μM doxorubicin (24 h) and 5 μM zoledronic acid (4 h) alone, in combination and in sequence, and the level of apoptosis was measured at 72 h. As was seen for breast cancer cells, both hormone-responsive and non-responsive prostate cancer cells were most sensitive to sequential exposure to doxorubicin followed by zoledronic acid, compared to all other treatments. The effect was attributed largely to zoledronic acid, as it could be reversed by the addition of the mevalonate pathway intermediary GGOH. Although doxorubicin is not commonly used in the treatment of prostate cancer, this study is important as it demonstrates that the sequence-specific effects of combination therapy with doxorubicin and zoledronic acid is not limited to breast cancer cell lines. The potential for the inclusion of BPs in sequential treatment schedules in advanced prostate cancer would require the expansion of these studies to include chemotherapy agents currently used to treat this group of patients.

Although the reports discussed above have demonstrated that the highest levels of tumour cell apoptosis are generated when the cells are exposed to the chemotherapy agent followed by zoledronic acid, simultaneous drug administration was also found to be superior to single agent therapy in all cases. This is in agreement with reports from studies combining docetaxel and zoledronic acid in prostate cancer cells in vitro (Fabbri et al. 2008, Ullen et al. 2005). Ullen and colleagues reported that combination treatment of two prostate cancer cell lines, PC3 and DU145, with zoledronic acid and docetaxel, reduced cell viability compared to single agent treatments (Ullen et al. 2005). However, there was a differential response of these two cell lines, with combination treatment having a synergistic interaction in DU145 cells, whereas increased cell death in PC3 cells was suggested to result from increased sensitivity of the cell line to the BP. In a similar study, the effects of sequential combination regimes were investigated by Fabbri et al. (2008), who compared the effects of combination treatment with docetaxel and zoledronic acid in the hormone-sensitive prostate cancer cell line LNCaP, using two different sequential treatment schedules. In both cases, cells were exposed to short-term simultaneous treatment with zoledronic acid and docetaxel (1 h) followed or preceded by prolonged exposure to zoledronic acid (72, 96 and 120 h). It was reported that a priori treatment with the cytotoxic agent profoundly affected cell viability in a synergistic manner, compared to the treatment regimen where zoledronic acid was given first. Taken together, the data from the in vitro models clearly show that combining BPs with anticancer agents results in a significant increase in tumour cell death, although the precise mechanism of action remains to be identified.

3.2 In Vivo Studies–Further Evidence of Benefits of BPs in Combination Therapy

As demonstrated in the in vitro studies summarised in the previous section, addition of BPs to other anticancer agents results in increased antitumour effects. There was thus a strong rationale for exploring the potential of the inclusion of BPs into combination therapy using in vivo models. These focussed on elucidating potential benefits of zoledronic acid in models of tumour growth in bone, as this is the agent of choice in the clinical management of cancer-induced bone disease (reviewed by Brown and Holen 2009a). There have also been reports of increased antitumour effects following inclusion of zoledronic acid in the treatment of tumours growing outside the skeleton (Giraudo et al. 2004; Ottewell et al. 2008b). Key findings from both types of studies will be discussed in the following sections.

4 Combination Therapy with BPs-Effects on Tumour Growth in Bone

Most studies exploring whether the addition of BPs to chemotherapy results in improved antitumour effects have been performed in breast cancer models, with a limited number of reports using models of prostate cancer (Brubaker et al. 2006; Kim et al. 2005) and small cell lung cancer (Matsumoto et al. 2005; Yano et al. 2003). Research on the antitumour activity of BPs in animal models of tumourigenesis and metastasis is reviewed by Clézardin et al. (2011). We will first turn our attention to studies of how combination therapy impacts tumour growth in bone.

In one of the earliest reports in this field, Hiraga and colleagues aimed to establish the effect of UFT (tegafur–uracil) in combination with zoledronic acid on the development of bone metastases in the syngeneic 4T1/luc model (Hiraga et al. 2004). The murine breast cancer cell line 4T1/luc was injected in the mammary fat pad of female BALB/c mice, resulting in dissemination of tumour cells to bone and subsequent development of bone metastases. A single injection of zoledronic acid (250 µg/kg, day 7) or oral administration of UFT (20 mg/kg/day, days 14–21) resulted in a significant reduction in the area of bone metastases, and this was further decreased following combination therapy. The therapeutic effect was found to be site-specific, as the primary tumour burden in the mammary fat pad was not affected, while tumour growth in bone was significantly decreased. The results indicate that tumour cells in bone may be exposed to higher concentrations of BPs compared to tumours at other sites, explaining why they are preferentially affected by the treatment.

Whereas the initial in vivo effects were seen following high dosing of BPs to obtain a therapeutic effect on bone metastases, more recent research has aimed to determine whether clinically achievable BP schedules are effective. Using the bone-specific B02 cell model, Ottewell and colleagues investigated whether the addition of a single dose of zoledronic acid (100 µg/kg, equivalent to the 4 mg clinical dose) to weekly doxorubicin treatment (2 mg/kg) caused a reduction in tumour burden compared to giving doxorubicin alone (Ottewell et al. 2008a). Following i.v. injection of B02 cells in female BALB/c nu/nu mice, treatment was initiated once tumour growth in bone was confirmed on day 18. Mice were administered saline, doxorubicin (2 mg/kg), zoledronic acid (100 µg/kg), zoledronic acid and doxorubicin simultaneously, or doxorubicin followed 24 h later by zoledronic acid. A second administration of doxorubicin was given to the appropriate groups on day 25. The experiment was terminated on day 32, and bone lesions as well as tumour volume, tumour cell proliferation and apoptosis were assessed on histological sections. The area of lytic bone lesions was determined, and bone structure/integrity assessed by CT analysis. As expected, zoledronic acid, alone, in sequence or combination with doxorubicin, caused a significant reduction in osteolytic lesions and increase bone volume. However, tumour volume was only reduced in the group receiving doxorubicin followed by zoledronic acid, and only the intra-osseous part of the tumour was affected by the treatment. This differential therapeutic effect between the intra- and extra-osseous parts of the same tumour was mirrored by the number of apoptotic and actively proliferating tumour cells in the different regions of the tumour. Detailed analysis demonstrated that in the parts of the tumour that had expanded outside the bone marrow, there was only a minor increase in the number of apoptotic tumour cells caused by the sequential therapy, and tumour cell proliferation was unaffected. These results support the hypothesis that not only does tumour growth become independent of the bone microenvironment in the advanced stage, but also that distinct regions of the same tumour respond differently to therapy, depending on the microenvironment. Despite this complication, administration of a single dose of zoledronic acid in addition to doxorubicin did result in improved bone quality, reduced expansion of lytic lesions and decreased tumour burden compared to single agent therapy. It is possible that early combination treatment, initiated before the tumours cause bone lesions, may further increase the antitumour effect.

Another way to improve outcome is to administer repeated sequential treatment, as was investigated in a second study by Ottewell et al. (2009). Using intratibial implantation of MDA-MB-436 breast cancer cells that grow slowly in bone, effects of a 6-week schedule of weekly doxorubicin (2 mg/kg) followed 24 h later by zoledronic acid (100 µg/kg) on tumour growth and bone integrity were determined. Bone tumours were isolated from each treatment group, allowing the comparison of alterations in tumour gene expression caused by the different schedules. Compared to the saline control, there was a moderate reduction in tumour volume following 6 weeks of zoledronic acid, whereas doxorubicin had no effect. In contrast, sequential administration of doxorubicin followed by zoledronic acid resulted in decreased bone tumour burden, accompanied by activation of intrinsic and extrinsic apoptotic pathways in the tumours. Decreased expression of several cyclins and cyclin-dependent kinases regulating cell progression through G1, G1/S, G2 and G2/M phases of the cell cycle were specifically detected. This was the first report showing that in vivo administration of clinically achievable doses of doxorubicin followed by zoledronic acid caused schedule-specific inhibition of breast tumour growth in bone. The reduction in bone tumour burden was associated with a complex combination of induction of pro-apoptotic proteins and suppression of proteins regulating cell cycle progression. Although this study identified some of the molecular mechanisms mediating the anti-tumour effects of combination therapy with doxorubicin and zoledronic acid, the reasons for the sequence specificity remain to be established. Repeated sequential treatment did reduce both tumour burden and bone disease in this model, but tumours were not completely eliminated, suggesting that further optimisation of therapy (e.g. giving several cycles of repeated sequential treatment) should be explored.

Studies of combination therapy for bone metastases are not limited to using doxorubicin and zoledronic acid, but effects of other anticancer agents and different NBPs have also been investigated. Combining the antibiotic doxycycline with zoledronic acid was tested in a model where intracardiac injection of MDA-MB-231 human breast cancer cells in 5-week-old Balb/c nu/nu mice was used to initiate tumour growth in bone (Duivenvoorden et al. 2007). Pellets releasing doxycycline ($\sim$15 mg/kg/day) or placebo pellets were implanted s.c. 3 days prior to tumour cell inoculation, and zoledronic acid treatment (0.2 ug/mouse every 2 days) commenced on the same day and continued until day 28. As expected, there was a significant positive effect of zoledronic acid on bone density, whether this was given as a single agent or combined with doxycycline. One of the intriguing results from this study was that treatment with zoledronic acid alone resulted in a 93% reduction of tumour area in soft tissue adjacent to the affected bones, and in a 73% reduction in total tumour burden. The authors suggest that this supports a direct effect of the drug on tumour cells outside the bone microenvironment. However, the report does not specify whether suppression of tumour growth in bone was associated with a reduction in extra-osseous tumour growth in these animals. An alternative explanation for these results could therefore be that due to good tumour control in bone caused by zoledronic acid, there is less expansion of tumour to extra-skeletal sites. Compared to the single agents, combination therapy with doxycycline and zoledronic acid was superior, causing a decrease in tumour burden in bone and surrounding soft tissues, as well as reduced osteolysis. As a note of caution, treatment in the latter study was initiated prior to tumour cell injection, potentially targeting the very early stages of tumour cell colonisation in the bone. To strengthen the case for clinical relevance, the effects of this regimen should also be investigated in a model where tumour growth is established prior to the initiation of treatment.

Effects of combining docetaxel with risedronate on tumour growth in bone have been investigated following direct intratibial implantation of MDA-MB-231-B/luc$^+$ cells in female BALB/c nu/nu mice (van Beek et al. 2009). Treatment commenced on day 2, and animals were administered risedronate (150 µg/kg, 5x/week), docetaxel (2, 4, or 8 mg/kg, 2x/week) or a combination of docetaxel (4 mg/kg, 2x/week and risedronate (150 µg/kg, 5x/week) for a period of 5 weeks. In one set of experiments, animals were administered saline, zoledronic acid (37.5, 75 or 150 µg/kg) or risedronate (150 µg/kg) both 5x/week for 5 weeks. Bone integrity and tumour burden were assessed at the end of the protocol. Both BPs prevented tumour-induced bone destruction of the tibia, but did not affect tumour burden as measured by bioluminescence. Histological analysis confirmed that administration of BPs did not reduce tumour growth outside the bone marrow, in accordance with the findings of Ottewell (Ottewell 2008a). Docetaxel was able to completely suppress tumour growth at the highest dose tested (8 mg/kg), and a suboptimal dose of 4 mg/kg was therefore used in the combination experiments with risedronate. The combination therapy eliminated tumour growth and preserved bone in 6/7 animals, whereas docetaxel alone reduced tumour growth in 2/5 animals and risedronate alone had no effect on tumour growth. These results suggest that by combining risedronate and docetaxel, a lower dose of the chemotherapy agent is needed to achieve an antitumour response as compared to single agent therapy. As metastatic bone disease is increasingly considered to be a long-term chronic condition, careful monitoring of the risk of future treatment-induced side effects will become an integral part of clinical management. The opportunity to use low doses of chemotherapy in combination with BPs may therefore be a new way to manage patients with bone metastases, but this must be established in clinical studies.

Although the majority of the studies of BPs in combination therapy have been performed in breast cancer models, there are a limited number of reports from other tumour types that frequently metastasise to bone. Effects of zoledronic acid, paclitaxel and STI571 (Imatinib mesylate, Gleevec) have been investigated using a prostate cancer model (Kim et al. 2005). PC-3MM2 prostate cancer cells were implanted into the tibia of nude mice, leading to tumour growth in bone and the development of lymph node metastases. Animals were treated three days after implantation of PC-3MM2 cells for a total of 5 weeks with paclitaxel (8 mg/kg, 1x/week), STI571 (50 mg/kg, daily) and zoledronic acid (25 µg/kg, 2x/day), or they received combinations of two or three of the drugs. Treatment with zoledronic acid and/or paclitaxel did not decrease bone tumour burden or lymph node metastases. STI571 administration resulted in a reduced incidence of bone and lymph node tumors, and reduced tumour weight. The latter effect was also observed after treatment with zoledronic acid, probably as a result of the very high cumulative dose in this study (animals receiving the equivalent of the clinical 4 mg dose given every 2 days for 5 weeks). The combined administration of all three agents was found to be most effective at reducing bone tumour burden, tumour weight, inhibition of bone loss and also caused a significant decrease in lymph node metastases. The anti-metastatic effects were associated with reduced osteoclast activity, increased tumour cell apoptosis and a decrease in tumour cell proliferation, suggesting that both direct and indirect (via bone) mechanisms were involved. The data indicate that a treatment regimen designed to target different stages of the heterogenic tumour growth and dissemination might be a possible new therapeutic approach for prostate cancer patients with a high risk of tumour spread to the bones. However, the effects of clinically achievable doses of zoledronic acid as part of this schedule needs to be determined.

The potential benefits of combining zoledronic acid with docetaxel in prostate cancer growth in bone have been explored in a model of using established, intratibial LNCaP prostate cancer xenografts in male SCID mice (Brubaker et al. 2006). In this model, tumour growth is associated with significant new bone growth and a periosteal reaction, mimicking the osteoblastic nature of prostate cancer bone lesions. Animals were administered a 7-week schedule of zoledronic acid (100ug/kg, 2x/week), docetaxel (20 mg/kg every 2 weeks) or a combination of both drugs, and effects on bone and tumour growth were evaluated by histology and measurement of bone mineral density. Compared to controls, tumour volume and osteoclast numbers were reduced and bone volume increased in animals receiving zoledronic acid, both alone and in combination with docetaxel. In contrast, osteoblast numbers were unaffected by all treatments. Tumour burden as assessed by the measurement of serum levels of prostate specific antigen (PSA) revealed that only the combination of both drugs significantly reduced PSA levels. However, when intra-osseous tumour volume was assessed by bone histomorphometry, zoledronic acid, given alone and in combination, induced a reduction in tumour volume. This apparent discrepancy between the two different measurements of tumour burden may be explained by the technical challenges associated with measuring tumour volume in bone (3D) by the analysis of 2D histological sections. In addition, tumour growth outside the bone marrow may have contributed to PSA levels, but would not be captured if only intra-osseous tumour is included in the histomorphometry analysis. The authors suggest that zoledronic acid sensitizes prostate cancer cells to docetaxel, resulting in additive antitumour effects of the two drugs. However, no direct evidence in support of this hypothesis has been published so far, and alternative explanations for the increased antitumour effect of combination therapy should be considered. It is possible that the reduced tumour burden is a result of two independent effects, with zoledronic acid reducing tumour growth by affecting bone (by inhibiting the release of tumour growth factors), whereas docetaxel inhibits tumour cell proliferation (and indirectly dampens cancer-induced bone disease). Regardless of the precise mechanism, the data do support the potential for this combination to be tested in patients with advanced prostate cancer.

Yano and colleagues have carried out a study investigating the effects of a BP in combination with VP-16 on bone metastasis from lung cancer (Yano et al. 2003). Human SCLC SBC-5 cells were injected intravenously in natural killer cell-depleted SCID mice, resulting in bone and visceral metastases, including lung, liver and kidney. The topoisomerase II inhibitor VP-16 (200 µg, days 2, 3, 9, 10), the BP minodronate (0.2 µg on day 7), or a combination of the two drugs, were administered for a total of up to 5 weeks. Minodronate treatment significantly reduced tumour burden in bone, associated with a decrease in osteoclast numbers, whereas visceral tumour burden was unaffected. In contrast, administration of VP-16 resulted in a reduction of the number of metastases in lungs and liver, and in a reduced number of metastatic foci in bone, but had no effect on tumour growth in kidneys or lymph nodes. Combination treatment enhanced the anti-metastatic effect in bone, accompanied by reduced osteoclast numbers and reduced lung and liver metastases (compared to control and single treatments), resulting in a significantly improved survival. These data support the hypothesis that treatment with a BP in combination with a classical anticancer drug does have the potential to cause a significant reduction of tumour progression in bone; however, visceral metastases that commonly are the most fatal, remain unaffected. This underscores the importance of early intervention for the subsequent outcome of anti-cancer therapy, because current treatment is very limited once tumour cells spread to multiple organs.

4.1 Summary-Effects on Tumour Growth in Bone

The studies discussed above all support that there is added benefit by the inclusion of BPs into modern treatment regimens of bone metastasis, regardless of cancer or lesion type. The most potent BP in clinical use, zoledronic acid, offers the greatest benefit, in line with its superior ability to inhibit osteoclast activity. By adding a BP to anticancer therapy, there is a clear positive effect on bone integrity, the number and progression of bone lesions are reduced and there is a significant reduction of tumour growth within the bone marrow. However, several key questions remains unanswered, e.g. whether BPs are taken up by the tumour cells within bone metastatic foci, and, if so, whether the cells are directly modified by the drugs. Alternatively, the effects of BPs may exclusively be mediated through the inhibition of bone resorption. The studies described above were not designed to distinguish between direct and indirect antitumour effects, and most investigators would probably agree that both mechanisms contribute to the ability of BPs to reduce tumour growth in bone. Despite many reports convincingly demonstrating increased antitumour effects following combination therapy, tumour growth was never entirely abolished in these models. Eventually, there is still the potential for improving combination regimens, e.g. by including the latest biological anticancer agents in addition to the standard chemotherapy drugs and antiresorptive agents.

5 Combination Therapy with BPs-Effects on Peripheral Tumour Growth

Whereas there is a clear rationale for the combination of BPs and anticancer agents in the treatment of bone metastases, their high affinity for bone and rapid clearance from the circulation suggest that therapeutic doses of BPs are unlikely to be achieved in peripheral tumours. There has long been the consensus that BPs would have little or no effect on tumour growth outside the skeleton. However, a number of published reports have shown that BPs, in particular zoledronic acid, can reduce growth of peripheral tumours in models from a range of tumour types, including non small cell lung cancer (NSCLC) (Li et al. 2008), small-cell lung cancer (SCLC) (Matsumoto et al. 2005), cervical carcinoma (Giraudo et al. 2004), breast cancer (Hiraga et al. 2004; Michigami et al. 2002) and mesothelioma (Wakchoure et al. 2006) Although frequently using high and repeated dosing of the BP, the data suggest these drugs to have the capacity to modify tumour growth outside the skeleton. It remains unclear whether this is caused by a direct uptake of the drug by the tumour cells, or is mediated through effects in bone.

The suggested effect of BPs on peripheral tumours led Ottewell and colleagues to carry out a definitive study on the effects of clinically relevant doses of zoledronic acid, alone or in combination with doxorubicin, on subcutaneous tumor growth of MDA-MB-436 xenografts (Ottewell et al. 2008b). There is no direct bone involvement in this model, and no evidence of tumour spread to the skeleton from subcutaneous primary tumours. Cells were injected s.c. into female MF1 nu/nu mice, and once tumours were palpable, animals were treated 1x/week for 6 weeks with saline, doxorubicin (2 mg/kg), zoledronic acid (100 μg/kg), zoledronic acid and doxorubicin together, doxorubicin followed 24 h later by zoledronic acid, and the reverse sequence. No significant effect on tumour size was seen in animals receiving single agent therapy compared to saline control, whereas simultaneous drug administration resulted in approximately a 50% reduction of tumour size when compared to tumours treated with doxorubicin alone. Sequential treatment with doxorubicin followed by zoledronic acid caused almost complete inhibition of tumour growth, but administration of the reverse drug sequence had no effect. Detailed histological analysis of the tumours revealed that treatment with doxorubicin followed by zoledronic acid, as well as simultaneous drug treatment, caused increased levels of cancer cell apoptosis and reduced proliferation, in agreement with the effects on tumour burden. In comparison, single agent treatment and sequential administration of zoledronic acid followed by doxorubicin had no effect. Pathway-specific gene array analysis was performed to elucidate changes in gene expression induced by sequential treatment. This showed that 30 genes involved in cell cycle regulation and apoptosis were specifically changed by more than twofold in tumours from animals receiving doxorubicin followed by zoledronic acid. The reduction of tumour growth was also associated with a reduction in tumour vascularisation. Taken together, the results in this study support the hypothesis that zoledronic acid exhibits significant antitumour effects when given in combination with doxorubicin, even in tumours located outside the bone. As seen in the models of bone metastases (Ottewell et al. 2008b; Yano et al. 2003; Kim et al. 2005), the effect was sequence-specific, with reversal of the drugs resulting in complete loss of the effect. This particular result may provide some clues as to the mechanisms involved. If BPs act by binding rapidly to bone and subsequently mediating an effect on peripheral tumours, one would expect that the sequence of exposure would be irrelevant. We know that BPs stay in the skeleton for prolonged periods of time (years) and are able to suppress bone resorption for at least several weeks. Could it be that the antitumour effect of zoledronic acid in this model is independent of the inhibition of bone resorption? This possibility can be investigated by adding another agent (e.g. high-dose clodronate) prior to the administration of doxorubicin followed by zoledronic acid. This would ensure the suppression of osteoclastic bone resorption, and any antitumour effects of subsequent treatment would therefore be independent of the anti-resorptive actions of zoledronic acid. Still, the hypothesis that zoledronic acid acts on peripheral tumours exclusively through the modification of bone cannot be disproven. However, it is possible that at least some of the treatment effect is caused by a reduction in the release of bone-derived factors into the circulation, with subsequent effects in the tumour. But would this not happen regardless of the order of drug administration? The reason for any sequence-specificity has to be elucidated in future studies.

In a subsequent study, the same team investigated whether the antitumour effect of sequential doxorubicin and zoledronic acid therapy persists once treatment is withdrawn after 6 weeks (Ottewell et al. 2010). Using the same model as described above, groups of animals with established subcutaneous tumours were divided into 5 different groups, receiving saline, 2 mg/kg doxorubicin, 100 µg/kg zoledronic acid, and 2 groups receiving doxorubicin followed 24 h later by zoledronic acid for either 6 weeks or weekly until the experiment was terminated (day 169). All animals in the control or single treatment groups were sacrificed once tumour volume reached a predefined threshold. In contrast, animals receiving sequential therapy were not sacrified before the end of the study. Most important was the finding that there was no tumour re-growth following the withdrawal of treatment, and no significant difference was seen in residual tumour volume between the group receiving continuous weekly treatment compared to those that had only received a 6-week course. These data are very promising, demonstrating that once tumour burden is reduced as a result of sequential therapy, there is no evidence for a rebound of tumor growth.

5.1 Summary–Effects on Peripheral Tumour Growth

The breast cancer studies described above, although providing strong evidence for a beneficial antitumour effect of BPs combined with chemotherapy on tumours outside the skeleton, have so far not been confirmed in other cancer cell types. This would be required in order to validate these data, and to convincingly demonstrate that the effects are not particular to the cell lines or models used. As far as breast cancer is concerned, sequential administration of clinically relevant doses of doxorubicin followed by zoledronic acid reduces the growth of both early (just palpable) as well as established subcutaneous tumours. Studies in neo-adjuvant breast cancer have indicated that adding zoledronic acid following anthracycline also adds on the clinical activity on the primary tumor, supporting a potential antitumour effect of BPs outside the skeleton (Coleman et al. 2010; Winter et al. 2010 abstr).

6 Sequential Combination Therapy with BPs in the Clinical Setting

This chapter sumarizes our current knowledge obtained from preclinical studies of BPs in combination therapy, and we will only briefly touch on their implications for clinical cancer management. It is important to bear in mind that in clinical studies, BPs are always added to any other appropriate treatment patients receive, so all studies will in fact be combination studies, and single agent control groups are most often not included. However, the frequency of BP administration (every 3–4 weeks for zoledronic acid) and the temporal separation from chemotherapy is not optimized to mirror the specific schedules used in the in vivo models. Separating treatments by 24 h was found to be particularly effective at inhibiting tumour growth in the breast cancer models. However, such an approach requires additional consultations with the oncologist, and therefore is considered rather inconvenient. As a result, patients are currently likely to receive the zoledronic acid infusion immediately following chemotherapy. However, two clinical studies that have adapted the 24 h separation between chemotherapy and zoledronic acid warrant our special attention.

The first of these is the ANZAC study, investigating AdditioN of Zoledronic Acid to neo-adjuvant Combination chemotherapy (Winter et al. 2010 abstr.) A total of 40 breast cancer patients (without evidence of bone metastases) were randomised to receive zoledronic acid (4 mg i.v.) or not, 24 h after the first cycle of FEC100 chemotherapy. Patients were stratified according to stage, ER and HER2 status, menopausal status and time since diagnosis. All patients had a core biopsy taken on day 5 (three days post zoledronic acid infusion), prior to the second cycle of chemotherapy, an optional core biopsy on day 21 followed by completion of neo-adjuvant chemotherapy and appropriate surgery. The primary objective in ANZAC was to determine whether the addition of zoledronic acid to neo-adjuvant chemotherapy causes an increase in the levels of tumour cell apoptosis between the diagnostic and the 5-day core biopsy, compared to neo-adjuvant chemotherapy alone. Whether the addition of zoledronic acid causes a reduction in the levels of tumour cell proliferation between the preoperative core biopsy, a day 5 interim biopsy ($\pm$ day 21) and the tumour specimen at final surgery will also be assessed. The data from this study are expected to be published in 2011, and will reveal whether the addition of a single administration of zoledronic acid results in any increased effects on apoptosis and/or proliferation of cells in the primary tumour as compared to the standard chemotherapy. The main difference between ANZAC and the preclinical studies is that zoledronic acid is only added to the first cycle of chemotherapy, whereas a 6-week schedule of weekly treatment was used in the in vivo models that showed a reduction in peripheral tumour growth (Ottewell et al. 2008b).

The concept of sequence specificity is supported by a recent report from a phase I clinical trial in prostate cancer. The ZANTE study applied metronomic administration of Zoledronic acid ANd TaxoterE in 22 patients with castration-resistant prostate cancer who received either escalating doses of taxotere (day 1) followed by 2 mg zoledronic acid (day 2), or the reverse schedule, every 2 weeks (Facchini et al. 2010). The main objective of the study was to assess safety and tolerability, but the authors also report that whereas 6/9 patients in the group receiving taxotere prior to zoledronic acid achieved disease control, this was not observed in any of the 11 patients who received the reverse sequence. Although the results of small studies like this must be interpreted with caution, there is an indication that the order in which the drugs are given may make a difference for the outcome. These pilot data will need to be confirmed in a larger study powered to determine whether there is a significant difference in anti-tumour effects depending on the drug sequence. The ZANTE study has demonstrated that addition of zoledronic acid on a separate day to the chemotherapeutic drug is acceptable for patients, and that the combination with taxotere is well tolerated and safe, providing important new information for the design of future clinical studies.

7 BPs in Combination Therapy–Effects on Normal Cells

In the clinical setting, cancer patients may receive a combination of different therapies such as radiotherapy, chemotherapy, analgesics, bisphosphonates and endocrine agents among others. As discussed in the previous sections, the anti-tumour effects of BPs when added to chemotherapy have been comprehensively investigated. Less is known about the effects of combining BPs with anticancer agents on normal cells, as the majority of studies have focussed on therapeutic effects in the tumour. One exception is the reported reduction in subcutaneous breast tumour vascularisation following treatment with doxorubicin and zoledronic acid, indicating an antiangiogenic effect of this combination (Ottewell et al. 2008b). In the following section, we discuss the published evidence relating to BP combination therapy on cells of the normal vasculature, but it is important to bear in mind that a range of other normal cell types may also be affected, including macrophages, various bone marrow precursors and immune cells (reviewed by Holen and Coleman 2010).

7.1 Antiangiogenic Effects of BPs as Single Agents

Over the past decade, there have been increasing efforts to target tumour angiogenesis as a therapeutic approach against cancer (Heath and Bicknell 2009). Positive outcomes following combination treatment with a BP and cytotoxic agents at low doses suggested that this could be more effective than single agent therapy, and potentially also cause fewer or milder side effects, which are normally a result of the administration of high doses of a single agent. Could the combination of a BP with other anticancer agents have similar effects on the tumour vasculature? In addition, as evidence of anti-tumour properties of combination treatment at clinically relevant concentrations accumulates, it is increasingly important to establish whether these schedules are detrimental to normal tissues.

Antiangiogenic effects of zoledronic acid have been previously demonstrated, through a reduction of angiogenic growth factor-induced vascularisation of normal tissue or subcutaneous implants in animal models (Fournier et al. 2002; Wood et al. 2002). Zoledronic acid has been shown to impede cell cycle progression causing accumulation in the S-phase in human umbilical vein EC (HUVEC) (Wood et al. 2002). This effect was associated with cyclin expression and upregulation of cyclin-related kinase inhibitors and accompanied by inhibition of HUVEC proliferation (Fournier et al. 2002; Wood et al. 2002) and induction of apoptosis (Wood et al. 2002). Effective dosing ranges and incubation periods in studies on HUVEC proliferation vary from 3–30 µM for 24 h (Wood et al. 2002) to 100 µM for 48 h (Fournier et al. 2002). We found an inhibitory effect on human dermal microvascular EC (HuDMEC) only at high concentrations (50 µM) and after prolonged incubation times (24–72 h), which was accompanied by cell cycle arrest at the S-phase after 48 and 72 h of treatment (Michailidou et al. 2010). These data suggest that there is a dose range of zoledronic acid that does not cause EC apoptosis but leads to cytostasis. An apoptosis-independent mechanism of action of zoledronic acid has previously been reported in tumour cells (Ory et al. 2007) independently of p53 status (Kuroda et al. 2004). BPs also have an impact on other normal cells in vitro, including fibroblasts (Walter et al. 2010). In a recent study by Yamada et al., zoledronic acid inhibited differentiation of endothelial progenitor cells derived from bone marrow at low doses, while induction of apoptosis was observed at higher doses (Yamada et al. 2009). This was supported by Ziebart et al. (2009), studying possible causes of BP-associated osteonecrosis of the jaw, one of the reported side effects of potent BPs. The study showed significant antiangiogenic effects of zoledronic acid, pamidronate, ibandronate (NBPs) and clodronate (non-NBP) on endothelial progenitor cells and HUVEC using a migration-, a 3D angiogenesis- and apoptosis assays (Ziebart et al. 2009). Many of the differences in the effective doses of BPs are likely to be caused by differences in the endocytic capacity of the cells used. Comparing uptake of zoledronic acid by HUVEC and HuDMEC, we found that there were distinct differences in the ability of cells to internalise the agent as measured by the accumulation of the unprenylated form of the GTPase Rap1a (Michailidou et al. 2010). Although we cannot directly link any of the effects of zoledronic acid to impaired prenylation of specific proteins, zoledronic acid affected Rap1a prenylation at 50 µM in HuDMEC, whereas lower doses are sufficient to cause a similar effect in tumour cells (Goffinet et al. 2006; Wakchure et al. 2006). In addition, zoledronic acid monotherapy has recently been shown to reduce tumour angiogenesis in a transgenic mouse mammary tumour model (Coscia et al. 2010). The reduced tumour burden was associated with a decrease in macrophage infiltration as well as lowering of local levels of pro-angiogenic VEGF. There were no obvious effects on vascularisation of normal tissues like kidney and colon in the zoledronic acid treated animals. In the clinical setting, where adverse vascular effects are a key concern, antiangiogenic effects of zoledronic acid have been reported in studies of patients with advanced cancer. The effect was identified as a reduction in the levels of circulating angiogenic factors such as VEGF, PDGF (Santini et al. 2003) and FGF (Zimering, 2002). No vascular side effects were recorded in these studies, most likely due to specific targeting of rapidly growing tumour vessels, leaving normal tissues with established vasculature unaffected.

7.2 Antiangiogenic Effects of BPs in Combination Therapy

Following on from studies showing increased antitumour effects caused by combinations of paclitaxel and zoledronic acid (Jagdev et al. 2001; Neville-Webbe et al. 2006), we used in vitro and in vivo models to explore whether these two agents would also modify the normal vasculature and hence potentially cause adverse effects (Michailidou et al. 2010). As summarised above, there are several reports demonstrating that BPs modify angiogenesis, whereas surprisingly few studies have investigated the effects of paclitaxel on the vasculature. Paclitaxel is a cytotoxic microtubule-interfering agent (Belotti et al. 1996), and has been reported to induce apoptotic cell death in endothelial cells at doses lower than those required to affect tumour cells via an apoptosis-independent mechanism (Pasquier et al. 2004; Pasquier et al. 2005). High doses of paclitaxel have been shown to have anti-angiogenic effects in vitro, compared to the clinically relevant concentrations (Bezzi et al. 2003; Pasquier et al. 2004, 2005). Our investigation, the first to determine the combined effects of zoledronic acid and paclitaxel, showed induced accumulation of endothelial cells in S phase and caused failure of their ability to form tubules on Matrigel surfaces. In breast cancer cells, the highest levels of apoptosis were induced when the cytotoxic agent preceded treatment with zoledronic acid, whereas in EC, simultaneous treatment with both agents induced the highest levels of apoptosis (Michailidou et al. 2010).

Zoledronic acid and paclitaxel disrupted basic cytoskeletal-related functions of EC tubule formation when used as single agents, following 24 h of treatment, however increased sensitivity was demonstrated following combination treatment. Our data suggest that cytoskeletal-dependent processes of EC are primarily sensitive to zoledronic acid with increased effects following the combination regimen with paclitaxel, whereas viability-related processes such as apoptotic cell death, cell cycle progression or proliferation were more resistant to treatments. These data are in contrast to studies in breast cancer cells where sequential drug exposure (zoledronic acid followed by paclitaxel) was the most effective schedule (Neville-Webbe et al. 2006). The molecular mechanisms responsible for this differential response remain to be identified, but may be linked to differences in metabolic activity and uptake of the agents, as tumour cells are generally characterised by rapid proliferation rates in contrast to relatively slowly propagating EC. Our study on EC migration showed inhibitory effects only at high doses (100 μM) of zoledronic acid, and it is unlikely that EC would be affected during standard therapy. Paclitaxel, due to its microtubule blocking effect, is reported to cause antimigratory effects of HUVEC at doses ranging between 10 pM (Belotti et al. 1996) and 0.1–10 nM (Grant et al. 2003; Hotchkiss et al. 2002).

Following in vitro studies that showed modulation of antiangiogenic effects on normal microvascular EC, we determined the effects of combined treatment with zoledronic acid and paclitaxel in vivo (Michailidou et al. 2010). For this, we used the dorsal microcirculation chamber (DMC) model that allows assessment of the acute treatment responses of the normal vasculature. In vivo studies of testosterone-induced angiogenesis in castrated rats have shown a 35% reduction in prostate weight compared to control animals caused by inhibition of vascularisation of the ventral prostate, following daily subcutaneous administration with 20 μg/kg of zoledronic acid (Fournier et al. 2002). In an angiogenesis model using fibroblast and vascular endothelial growth factor-induced vascularised implants, zoledronic acid inhibited angiogenesis following daily subcutaneous administration of 10 and 100 μg/kg for 6 days (Wood et al. 2002). Although we used 100 μg/kg zoledronic acid, which corresponds to the clinical monthly dose of 4 mg (Daubine et al. 2007), the treatment frequency is much more intensive and in agreement with our in vitro data that suggest low sensitivity of EC to zoledronic acid (Michailidou et al. 2010). Animals were treated with increasing doses of zoledronic acid (50, 100 and 150 μg/kg, subcutaneously), or paclitaxel (10, 20 and 30 mg/kg, intravenously). No detrimental effects were detected in arteries or venules, and only minor transient decreases in arteriolar diameters were noted. In combination experiments, where animals were administered 100 μg/kg of zoledronic acid followed by 20 mg/kg paclitaxel, there were no significant effects on arteriolar or venular diameters, and no treatment morbidity was detected. This lack of adverse vascular effects was further supported by the histological assessment that showed normal cell and tissue morphology and vascularisation in muscle, liver, brain, spleen and lungs. Following this detailed investigation, there is no indication that combined therapy with zoledronic acid and paclitaxel is associated with deleterious vascular side effects, precluding clinical testing of this schedule.

8   Conclusions

The preclinical evidence included in this review suggests that there is a strong rationale for including bisphosphonates in combination therapy, in particular in the advanced cancer setting. There is a clear benefit of BPs in a range of in vivo models of cancer-induced bone disease, showing a decrease in tumour progression and improved bone quality. Whether there could also be increased antitumour effects following inclusion of BPs in the treatment of tumours that have spread to extra-osseous sites remains to be confirmed in animal models other than breast cancer. Importantly, the addition of BPs to other therapies is not associated with increased adverse events, indicating that these schedules are well tolerated and would not cause major complications for patients. Clinical studies are ongoing that will clarify whether the positive indications from preclinical models are also valid in the clinic.

References

Belotti D, Vergani V, Drudis T et al (1996) The microtubule-affecting drug paclitaxel has antiangiogenic activity. Clin Cancer Res 2:1843–1849

Bezzi M, Hasmim M, Bieler G et al (2003) Zoledronate sensitizes endothelial cells to tumor necrosis factor-induced programmed cell death: evidence for the suppression of sustained activation of focal adhesion kinase and protein kinase B/Akt. J Biol Chem 278:43603–43614

Boissier S, Magnetto S, Frappart L et al (1997) Bisphosphonates inhibit prostate and breast carcinoma cell adhesion to unmineralized and mineralized bone extracellular matrices. Cancer Res 57:3890–3894

Brown HK, Holen I (2009a) Anti-tumour effects of bisphosphonates-what have we learned from in vivo models? Curr Can Drug Targets 9(7):807–823

Brown HK, Ottewell PD, Coleman RE et al. (2009b) The kinetochore protein Cenp-F is a potential novel target for zoledronic acid in breast cancer cells. J Cell Mol Med 8 [Epub ahead of print]

Brubaker KD, Brown LG, Vessella RL et al (2006) Administration of zoledronic acid enhances the effects of docetaxel on growth of prostate cancer in the bone environment. BMC Cancer 6:15

Clezardin P (2011) Bisphosphonates' antitumor activity: An unraveled side of a multifaceted drug class. Bone 48(1):71–79

Clézardin P, Benza I, Croucher PI (2011) Bisphosphonates in preclinical bone oncology. Bone 49(1):66–70

Clezardin P, Ebetino FH, Fournier PGJ (2005) Bisphosphonates and cancer-induced bone disease: beyond their anti-resorptive activity. Cancer Res 65(12):4971–4974

Clyburn RD, Reid P, Evans CA et al (2010) Increased anti-tumour effects of doxorubicin and zoledronic acid in prostate cancer cells in vitro: supporting the benefits of combination therapy. Cancer Chemother Pharmacol 65:969–978

Coleman RE (2007) Emerging strategies in bone health management for the adjuvant patient. Semin Oncol 34(Suppl 4):S11–S16

Coleman RE, Brown J, Terpos E et al (2008) Bone markers and their prognostic value in metastatic bone disease: clinical evidence and future directions. Cancer Treat Rev 34(7):629–639

Coleman RE, Winter MC, Cameron D et al (2010) The effects of adding zoledronic acid to neoadjuvant chemotherapy on tumour response: explanatory evidence for direct anti-tumour activity in breast cancer. Brit J Cancer 102:1099–1105

Corey E, Brown LG, Quinn JE et al (2003) Zoledronic Acid exhibits inhibitory effects on osteoblastic and osteolytic metastases of prostate cancer. Clin Cancer Res 9:295–306

Coscia M, Quaglino E, Iezzi M et al (2010) Zoledronic acid repolarizes tumour-associated macrophages and inhibits mammary carcinogenesis by targeting the mevalonate pathway. J Cell Mol Med 14(12):2803–28015

Daubine F, Le Gall C, Gasser J et al (2007) Antitumour effects of clinical dosing regimens of bisphosphonates in experimental breast cancer bone metastasis. J Natl Cancer Inst 99:322–330

Duivenvoorden WC, Vukmirović-Popović S, Kalina M et al (2007) Effect of zoledronic acid on the doxycycline-induced decrease in tumour burden in a bone metastasis model of human breast cancer. Brit J Cancer 96(10):1526–1531

Fabbri F, Brigliadori G, Carloni S et al (2008) Zoledronic acid increases docetaxel cytotoxicity through pMEK and Mcl-1 inhibition in a hormone-sensitive prostate carcinoma cell line. J Transl Med 6:43

Facchini G, Caraglia M, Morabito A et al (2010) Metronomic administration of Zoledronic acid and taxotere combination in castration resistant prostate cancer patients: Phase I ZANTE trial. Cancer Biol Ther 10(6):543–548

Fournier P, Boissier S, Filleur S et al (2002) Bisphosphonates inhibit angiogenesis in vitro and testosterone-stimulated vascular regrowth in the ventral prostate in castrated rats. Cancer Res 62:6538–6544

Fournier PG, Stresing V, Ebetino FH et al (2010) How do bispshosphonates inhibit bone metastasis in vivo? Neoplasia 12(7):571–578

Giraudo E, Inoue M, Hanahan D (2004) An amino-bisphosphonate targets MMP-9-expressing macrophages and angiogenesis to impair cervical carcinogenesis. J Clin Invest 114:623–633

Goffinet M, Thoulouzan M, Pradines A et al (2006) Zoledronic acid treatment impairs protein geranyl-geranylation for biological effects in prostatic cells. BMC Cancer 6:60

Grant DS, Williams TL, Zahaczewsky M et al (2003) Comparison of antiangiogenic activities using paclitaxel (taxol) and docetaxel (taxotere). Int J Cancer 104:121–129

Heath VL, Bicknell R (2009) Anticancer strategies involving the vasculature. Nat Rev Clin Oncol 6(7):395–404

Hiraga T, Williams PJ, Ueda A et al (2004) Zoledronic acid inhibits visceral metastases in the 4T1/luc mouse breast cancer model. Clin Cancer Res 10:4559–4567

Holen I, Coleman RE (2010) Anti-tumour activity of bisphosphonates in preclinical models of breast cancer. Breast Cancer Res 12:214

Horie N, Murata H, Kimura S et al (2007) Combined effects of a third-generation bisphosphonate, zoledronic acid with other anticancer agents against murine osteosarcoma. Br J Cancer 96:255–261

Hotchkiss KA, Ashton AW, Mahmood R et al (2002) Inhibition of endothelial cell function in vitro and angiogenesis in vivo by docetaxel (Taxotere): association with impaired repositioning of the microtubule organizing center. Mol Cancer Ther 1:1191–1200

Jagdev SP, Coleman RE, Shipman CM et al (2001) The bisphosphonate, zoledronic acid, induces apoptosis of breast cancer cells: evidence for synergy with paclitaxel. Br J Cancer 84(8):1126–1134

Kim SJ, Uehara H, Yazici S et al (2005) Modulation of bone microenvironment with zoledronate enhances the therapeutic effects of STI571 and paclitaxel against experimental bone metastasis of human prostate cancer. Cancer Res 65(9):3707–3715

Kohno N (2008) Treatment of breast cancer with bone metastasis: bisphosphonate treatment - current and future. Int J Clin Oncol 13(1):18–23

Koshimune R, Aoe M, Toyooka M et al (2007) Anti-tumor effect of bisphosphonate (YM529) on non-small cell lung cancer cell lines. BMC Cancer 7:8

Kuroda J, Kimura S, Segawa H et al (2004) p53-independent anti-tumor effects of the nitrogen-containing bisphosphonate zoledronic acid. Cancer Sci 95:186–192

Kubista B, Trieb K, Sevelda F et al (2006) Anticancer effects of zoledronic acid against human osteosarcoma cells. J Orthop Res 24(6):1145–1152

Lee MV, Fong EM, Singer FR et al (2001) Bisphosphonate treatment inhibits the growth of prostate cancer cells. Cancer Res 61:2602–2608

Li Y–Y, Chang JW, Chou WC et al (2008) Zoledronic acid is unable to induce apoptosis, but slows tumor growth and prolongs survival for non-small-cell lung cancers. Lung Cancer 59(2):180–191

Luckman SP, Hughes DE, Coxon FP et al (1998) Nitrogen-containing bisphosphonates inhibit the mevalonate pathway and prevent post-translational prenylation of GTP-binding proteins, including Ras. J Bone Miner Res 13(4):581–589

Märten A, Lilienfeld-Toal M, Büchler MW et al (2007) Zoledronic acid has direct antiproliferative and antimetastatic effect on pancreatic carcinoma cells and acts as an antigen for delta2 gamma/delta T cells. J Immunother 30(4):370–377

Matsumoto S, Kimura S, Segawa H et al (2005) Efficacy of the third-generation bisphosphonate, zoledronic acid alone and combined with anti-cancer agents against small cell lung cancer cell lines. Lung Cancer 47(1):31–39

Mbeunkui F, Johann DJ Jr (2009) Cancer and the tumour microenvironment: a review of an essential relationship. Cancer Chemother Pharmacol 63(4):571–582

Michailidou M, Brown HK, Lefley DV et al (2010) Microvascular endothelial cell responses in vitro and in vivo: modulation by zoledronic acid and paclitaxel? J Vasc Res 47:481–493

Michigami T, Hiraga T, Williams PJ et al (2002) The effect of the bisphosphonate ibandronate on breast cancer metastasis to visceral organs. Breast Cancer Res Treat 75:249–258

Neville-Webbe HL, Holen I, Coleman RE (2002) The anti-tumour activity of bisphosphonates. Cancer Treat Rev 28:305–319

Neville-Webbe HL, Rostami-Hodjegan A, Evans CA et al (2005) Sequence- and schedule-dependent enhancement of zoledronic acid induced apoptosis by doxorubicin in breast and prostate cancer cells. Int J Cancer 113:364–371

Neville-Webbe HL, Evans CA, Coleman RE et al (2006) Mechanisms of the synergistic interaction between the bisphosphonate zoledronic acid and the chemotherapy agent paclitaxel in breast cancer cells in vitro. Tumour Biol 27:92–103

Ottewell PD, Deux B, Mönkkönen H et al (2008a) Differential effect of doxorubicin and zoledronic acid on intraosseous versus extraosseus breast tumour growth in vivo. Clin Cancer Res 14:4658–4666

Ottewell PD, Mönkkönen H, Jones M et al (2008b) Antitumor effects of doxorubicin followed by zoledronic acid in a mouse model of breast cancer. J Natl Cancer Inst 100(16):1167–1178

Ottewell PD, Woodward JK, Lefley DV et al (2009) Anticancer mechanisms of doxorubicin and zoledronic acid in breast cancer tumor growth in bone. Mol Cancer Ther 8(10):2821–2832

Ottewell PD, Lefley DV, Cross SS et al (2010) Sustained inhibition of tumor growth and prolonged survival following sequential administration of doxorubicin and zoledronic acid in a breast cancer model. Int J Cancer 126(2):522–532

Ory B, Blanchard F, Battaglia S et al (2007) Zoledronic acid activates the DNA S-phase checkpoint and induces osteosarcoma cell death characterized by apoptosis-inducing factor and endonuclease-G translocation independently of p53 and retinoblastoma status. Mol Pharmacol 71(1):333–343

Pasquier E, Carre M, Pourroy B et al (2004) Antiangiogenic activity of paclitaxel is associated with its cytostatic effect, mediated by the initiation but not completion of a mitochondrial apoptotic signaling pathway. Mol Cancer Ther 3:1301–1310

Pasquier E, Honore S, Pourroy B et al (2005) Antiangiogenic concentrations of paclitaxel induce an increase in microtubule dynamics in endothelial cells but not in cancer cells. Cancer Res 65:2433–2440

Riebeling C, Forsea A-M, Raisova M et al (2002) The bisphosphonate pamidronate induces apoptosis in human melanoma cells in vitro. Br J Cancer 87:366–371

Rogers MJ et al (2003) New insights into the molecular mechanisms of action of bisphosphonates. Curr Pharm Des 9(32):2643–2658

Rogers MJ, Brown RJ, Hodkin V et al (1996) Bisphosphonates are incorporated into adenine nucleotides by human aminoacyl-tRNA synthetase enzymes. Biochem Biophys Res Commun 224(3):863–869

Rogers MJ, Gordon S, Benford HL et al (2000) Cellular and molecular mechanisms of action of bisphosphonates. Cancer 88(suppl 12):2961–2978

Russell RGG (2007) Bisphosphonates: mode of action and pharmacology. Pediatrics 119:S150–S162

Santini D, Gentilucci UV, Vincenzi B et al (2003) The antineoplastic role of bisphosphonates: from basic research to clinical evidence. Ann Oncol 14:1468–1476

Senaratne SG, Colston KW (2002) Direct effects of bisphosphonates on breast cancer cells. Breast Cancer Res 4:18–23

Shipman CM, Rogers MJ, Apperley JF et al (1997) Bisphosphonates induce apoptosis in human myeloma cell lines: a novel anti-tumour activity. Br J Haematol 98(3):665–672

Tassone P, Tagliaferri P, Viscomi C et al (2003) Zoledronic acid induces antiproliferative and apoptotic effects in human pancreatic cancer cells in vitro. Br J Cancer 88:1971–1978

Thudi NK, Martin CK, Nadella MV et al (2008) Zoledronic acid decreased osteolysis but not bone metastasis in a nude mouse model of canine prostate cancer with mixed bone lesions. Prostate 68(10):1116–1125

Ullén A, Lennartsson L, Harmenberg U et al (2005) Additive/synergistic antitumoral effects on prostate cancer cells in vitro following treatment with a combination of docetaxel and zoledronic acid. Acta Oncol 44(6):644–650

van Beek ER, Lowik CW, van Wijngaarden J et al (2009) Synergistic effect of bisphosphonate and docetaxel on the growth of bone metastasis in an animal model of established metastatic bone disease. Breast Cancer Res Treat 118(2):307–313

van der Pluijm G, Que I, Sijmons B et al (2005) Interference with the microenvironmental support impairs the de novo formation of bone metastases in vivo. Cancer Res 65(17): 7682–7690

Virtanen SS, Väänänen HK, Härkönen PL et al (2002) Alendronate inhibits invasion of PC-3 prostate cancer cells by affecting the mevalonate pathway. Cancer Res 62:2708–2714

Wakchoure S, Merrell MA, Aldrich W et al (2006) Bisphosphonates inhibit the growth of mesothelioma cells in vitro and in vivo. Clin Cancer Res 12:2862–2868

Walkington L, Coleman RE (2011) Advances in management of bone disease in breast cancer. Bone 48(1):80–87

Walter C, Klein MO, Pabst A et al (2010) Influence of bisphosphonates on endothelial cells, fibroblasts, and osteogenic cells. Clin Oral Investig 14(1):35–41

Winter MC, Syddal SP, Cross SS et al. (2010) ANZAC: A randomised neoadjuvant biomarker study investigating the anti-tumour activity of the AdditioN of Zoledronic Acid to Chemotherapy in breast cancer. Abstract Presented at the 33rd Annual San Antonio Breast Cancer Symposium Dec 8–12, San Antonio, TX, USA

Wood J, Bonjean K, Ruetz S et al (2002) Novel antiangiogenic effects of the bisphosphonate compound zoledronic acid. J Pharmacol Exp Ther 302:1055–1061

Yamada J, Tsuno NH, Kitayama J et al (2009) Anti-angiogenic property of zoledronic acid by inhibition of endothelial progenitor cell differentiation. J Surg Res 151(1):115–120

Yano S, Zhang H, Hanibuchi M et al (2003) Combined therapy with a new bisphosphonate, minodronate (YM529), and chemotherapy for multiple organ metastases of small cell lung cancer cells in severe combined immunodeficient mice. Clin Cancer Res 9(14):5380–5385

Yoneda T, Michigami T, Yi B et al (2000) Actions of bisphosphonate on bone metastasis in animal models of breast carcinoma. Cancer 88:2979–2988

Ziebart T, Pabst A, Klein MO et al. (2009) Bisphosphonates: restrictions for vasculogenesis and angiogenesis: inhibition of cell function of endothelial progenitor cells and mature endothelial cells in vitro. Clin Oral Investig 15(1):105–111

Zimering MB (2002) Effect of intravenous bisphosphonates on release of basic fibroblast growth factor in serum of patients with cancer-associated hypercalcemia. Life Sci 70(16):1947–1960

Perspectives in the Elderly Patient: Benefits and Limits of Bisphosphonates and Denosumab

Daniele Santini, Maria Elisabetta Fratto and Matti Aapro

Abstract

Skeletal metastases affect a large percentage of the cancer population and contribute to a marked decrease in their quality of life and survival, in particular in elderly population. A future end-point of bone-protecting therapy is the demonstration of its ability to prevent or improve results in the treatment of metastatic disease, enlarging their clinical indications in metastatic and osteoporotic setting with different schedules. In this chapter we will discuss on pharmacokinetic and pharmacodynamic interactions of bisphosphonates in elderly, and the preclinical and clinical evidences of anticancer activity of bone-targeted therapies will be critically described. The clinical results of new targeted therapies (such as rank/rankl/OPG inhibition) will be reported both in bone metastatic and in adjuvant settings. Finally, the prevention of cancer treatment-induced bone loss (CTIBL) represents both in young and more in old patients an emerging issue in the bone health care. For this reason, this chapter will discuss the results of current therapies in this clinical setting.

Contents

1	Introduction..	172
2	Bisphosphonates and Safety Profile: Pharmacokinetic and Pharmacodynamic Interactions...	173

D. Santini (✉) · M. E. Fratto
Medical Oncology, University Campus Bio-Medico, Via Alvaro del Portillo, 200, 00128 Rome, Italy
e-mail: d.santini@unicampus.it

M. Aapro
Institut Multidisciplinaire d'Oncologie, IMO Clinique de Genolier, Genolier, Switzerland

3	Preclinical Data on the Antitumoral Efficacy of Bisphosphonates to Prevent Bone Metastases	174
4	The Evolving Role of Zoledronic Acid in Reducing the Risk of Breast Cancer Recurrence in Elderly Patients	174
5	Bisphosphonates and the Risk of Postmenopausal Breast Cancer	176
6	Prospective Trials of Zoledronic Acid in the Adjuvant Setting	176
7	Ongoing Adjuvant Phase III Trials	178
8	Denosumab in the Elderly: Efficacy in Metastatic Disease and New Perspectives in the Adjuvant Setting	180
9	Conclusions	182
	References	183

1 Introduction

Skeletal metastases affect a large percentage of the cancer population and contribute to a marked decrease in their quality of life and survival. Furthermore, the median age of cancer patients is growing and the incidence of osteoporosis and fractures parallels this fact. Osteoporosis is a common disease, that is inherently related to age,but might also be treatment-related. The main consequence of osteoporosis is an increased incidence of fractures. The increase of age-related osteoporotic fractures associated with the increase of bone metastases-related fractures results not only in an increase of morbidity, but also in a decrease of survival and an increase of the consumption of health resources (Barkin et al. 2005). Impaired mobility and bone pain, and associated treatment may lead to several complications, such as deep vein thrombosis, pulmonary embolism and pneumonia, constipation. Bone metastases cause considerable morbidity, including pain, impaired mobility, hypercalcemia, pathologic fractures, spinal cord or nerve root compression and bone marrow infiltration (Coleman 1997). All these clinical conditions increase the incidence of Skeletal-Related Events (SREs), which are defined for study purposes as bone pain, fractures, radiation to bone, surgery to bone (including cementoplasty) and spinal cord compression with consequent impairment of quality of life and a decrease of overall survival as shown by Saad et al. (2007) in patients with multiple myeloma and patients with bone metastases from breast and prostate cancer, both in young and elderly patients. For all these reasons, preserving bone health in the elderly cancer patient by e.g. treatment with bone-protecting agents may provide meaningful quality of life benefits and may avoid SRE and possibly improve overall survival (OS) of these patients. In addition to the prevention of SREs, emerging evidence suggests that the new-generation bisphosphonates may also provide additional benefits including delayed disease progression in bone and a potential increase in survival through a direct and indirect antitumor activity (Saad 2008). For these considerations, a future end-point of bone-protecting therapy is to demonstrate the ability to prevent or improve results in the treatment of metastatic disease, extending their clinical indications in the metastatic and osteoporotic setting.

2 Bisphosphonates and Safety Profile: Pharmacokinetic and Pharmacodynamic Interactions

Although the benefits of bisphosphonates are well documented in elderly patients with osteoporosis, no randomized trials have been conducted specifically in elderly patients with metastatic bone disease (MBD) to date (Gridelli 2007). Without these data, it is not possible to predict the exact effects of bisphosphonates in this population in terms of efficacy, safety and potential impact on clinical outcome. A single-institution report has demonstrated the efficacy of zoledronic acid on pain and quality of life in elderly patients with bone metastases from solid tumors (Addeo et al. 2008). A retrospective study has suggested that multiple myeloma patients are more likely to experience renal impairment with zoledronic acid than with ibandronate (Weide et al. 2010). For these reasons, age-related conditions and co-morbidities must be taken into consideration before using bisphosphonates to treat bone metastases in elderly cancer patients. Even if there is no evidence for the pharmacokinetics and pharmacodynamics of bisphosphonates to be markedly different in elderly patients with normal renal function, the use of bisphosphonates to prevent SREs warrants special consideration in the elderly patient, due to a physiologic decline of organ function and co-morbidities that require the use of several concomitant drugs (Pillai et al. 2006). Elderly patients may have impaired renal function or renal insufficiency as a result of age-related kidney function decline. Furthermore, they may have underlying renal impairment related to their disease (especially in case of multiple myeloma) (Goldschmidt et al. 2000). Concomitant medications for the treatment of the primary cancer (Patterson and Reams 1992) may also be nephrotoxic (Tanvetyanon and Stiff 2006). Moreover, elderly patients are at higher risk to develop renal impairment due to reduced hydration, overuse of non-steroidal anti-inflammatory drugs for analgesic purposes and concomitant treatment with antihypertensive, anti-diabetic drugs and lipid-lowering agents. For all these reasons, elderly patients may be at a higher risk for renal toxicity. To prevent renal toxicity, the International Society for Geriatric Oncology (SIOG), in its clinical practice recommendations for the use of bisphosphonates in elderly patients, strongly recommends the assessment and optimization of hydration status and monitoring of creatinine clearance in elderly cancer patients before each bisphosphonate administration (Body et al. 2007). In non-metastatic patients, the use of zoledronic acid is an attractive perspective to prevent fractures in the elderly, due to the often low adherence to oral osteoporosis medications. A recent trial (HORIZON) has demonstrated the efficacy and safety of once-yearly intravenous zoledronic acid 5 mg in elderly postmenopausal women with osteoporosis age 75 or older. At 3 years, the incidence of vertebral and nonvertebral fractures was significantly lower in the zoledronic acid group than in the placebo group. The incidence of adverse events was higher with zoledronic acid, although the rate of serious adverse events and deaths was comparable between the two groups (Boonen et al. 2010).

3 Preclinical Data on the Antitumoral Efficacy of Bisphosphonates to Prevent Bone Metastases

Bisphosphonates are inhibitors of osteoclast-mediated bone resorption and have shown clinical utility in the treatment of disease metastatic to the bones (Santini et al. 2006). There is increasing in vivo preclinical evidence that bisphosphonates can reduce skeletal tumor burden and inhibit the formation of bone metastases in animal models (Clézardin et al. 2005). In fact, bisphosphonates may render the bone a less favorable microenvironment for tumor cell colonization by reducing osteoclast-mediated bone resorption which, in turn, would deprive tumor cells of bone-derived growth factors released from the bone matrix (Santini et al. 2003). In addition, bisphosphonates appear to have direct antitumor effects, shown both in vitro and in animal models. In fact recent trials have demonstrated that bisphosphonates inhibit tumor cell adhesion, invasion, proliferation and induce apoptosis in several human tumor cell lines in vitro (Santini et al. 2007). Bisphosphonates have also demonstrated indirect antitumor effects targeting the tumor-stroma-lymphocyte cross-talk. In particular, several in vitro and in vivo data have shown that bisphosphonates have effects on angiogenesis and on the stimulation of gamma/delta T lymphocytes (Caraglia et al. 2006). It has been debated that the experimental conditions used to study the efficacy of bisphosphonates in tumor-bearing animals are different from the conditions in patients with bone metastases. Indeed, bisphosphonate doses employed in animal studies to demonstrate antitumor effects are 10–40 times higher than the dosing regimens that have been approved for the treatment of cancer patients with skeletal metastases. Recently, Daubinè et al. used a mouse model of human breast cancer with bone metastasis to examine the effects of different dosing regimens of two bisphosphonates, zoledronic acid and clodronate, on osteolysis and skeletal tumor growth. They demonstrated that clinically relevant doses of bisphosphonates produced meaningful antitumor effects, in terms of tumor reduction and prevention (Daubiné et al. 2007). All these findings represent the base to translate preclinical studies to clinical trials of bisphosphonates in the prevention of bone metastases.

4 The Evolving Role of Zoledronic Acid in Reducing the Risk of Breast Cancer Recurrence in Elderly Patients

A large number of studies (Diel et al. 1998; Powles et al. 2006; Saarto et al. 2006; Jaschke et al. 2004; Ha and Li 2007) suggest that both oral and intravenous bisphosphonates may reduce breast cancer recurrence and may also reduce locoregional recurrence (Eidtmann et al. 2008; Aapro 2006). Clinical trials with clodronate, an orally administered non-nitrogen bisphosphonate, as adjuvant treatment for breast cancer strongly suggested a potential role of clodronate in the prevention of bone metastasis. Specifically, Diel et al. randomized 302 patients with primary breast cancer and tumor cells in the bone marrow (BM) to receive clodronate (1600 mg/day for two years) or standard follow-up. They demonstrated that clodronate can reduce the incidence and number of new bone and visceral metastases in these women with breast cancer who were at high risk for distant metastases (Diel et al. 1998). Similarly, Powles et al. showed that clodronate (1,600 mg/day) is effective to prevent bone metastases in patients with early breast cancer (Powles et al. 2006). On the contrary, Saarto et al. showed that clodronate had no effect on OS, initially reporting a reduction in disease-free survival and an increase in extra-skeletal metastases with clodronate. However, a marked imbalance in patient characteristics between the two groups weakens the findings of that particular study (Saarto et al. 2006). Jaschke et al. also demonstrated a significant reduction of bone metastases in breast cancer patients with micrometastases to the BM when treated with oral clodronate versus placebo after 3 years median follow-up (Jaschke et al. 2004). Recently, a meta-analysis did not find a statistically significant survival benefit in patients receiving adjuvant clodronate therapy. Furthermore, no differences were found in the elderly subgroup population (Ha and Li 2007). Accordingly, oral clodronate was not registered as adjuvant treatment in patients with early breast cancer, still bisphosphonates may play a role in preventing bone metastases when using optimized treatment schedules or the more potent nitrogen-containing bisphosphonates. These data however led to the development of the ongoing NSABP-B-34 placebo-controlled phase III trial that will recruit 4200 patients with Stage I/II breast cancer. Patients are randomized to receive standard treatment (chemotherapy, hormonal therapy, both, or neither) plus clodronate (1600 mg/day) for three years versus standard therapy alone. Patients are stratified by age (under 50 vs. 50 and over), number of positive lymph nodes (0 vs. 1–3 vs. 4 or more), and hormone receptor status (estrogen receptor and progesterone receptor negative vs. positive). The primary end-point of this study is to evaluate if daily clodronate is effective in preventing bone metastases, comparing time to bone and distant metastasis in the two arms. Time to first SREs and OS will be evaluated as secondary end-points.

Although the mechanism of zoledronic acid-mediated inhibition of Cancer Treatment Induced Bone Loss (CTIBL) depends on the inhibition of osteoclast-mediated bone resorption, the mechanisms underlying the significant improvements in disease-free survival observed in some patients with early breast cancer are likely to be multifactorial. Several large, randomized, multicenter trials have evaluated whether upfront or delayed zoledronic acid therapy can decrease BMD loss in postmenopausal breast cancer patients undergoing treatment with aromatase inhibitors. These trials are Z-FAST, with 602 patients enrolled, ZO-FAST, with 1066 patients enrolled and E-ZO-FAST, with 527 patients enrolled (Gnant et al. 2009a). The primary objective of these studies was to compare the change in lumbar spine BMD. Secondary objectives include disease recurrence rate and time to disease recurrence. Patients had a median age of 58 years. Even if further follow up is needed, promising results seem to indicate that zoledronic acid can reduce disease recurrence. In fact, the 36-months analysis of ZO-FAST has demonstrated that upfront zoledronic acid reduces the risk of disease recurrence at local and distant sites by 45%, with 2 versus 10 local recurrences and 20 versus 30 distant recurrences (Eidtmann et al. 2010). The 48-months follow-up analysis of the ZO-FAST study produced some exciting data on disease-free survival, with 29 events in the upfront group versus 49 events in the delayed group ($p = 0.018$). (Coleman et al. 2009). In ABCSG-12, patients receiving endocrine therapy plus zoledronic acid experienced fewer disease events (disease recurrence or death) than those receiving endocrine therapy alone. In this setting, zoledronic acid not only reduced the number of patients with bone metastases, but also reduced distant recurrence, locoregional recurrence and contralateral breast cancer (Gnant et al. 2009b). This evidence suggests that zoledronic acid may improve disease-free survival by exerting antitumor effects both in and outside the bones. Although these data are not specific to the elderly population, there is no reason to believe that the same proportional risk reduction would not be observed in patients above the age of 70.

5 Bisphosphonates and the Risk of Postmenopausal Breast Cancer

Recently, the association between oral bisphosphonate use and invasive breast cancer was examined in postmenopausal women enrolled into the Women's Health Initiative (WHI). Of the 154,768 participants, 2,816 were oral bisphosphonate users at entry. Patients between 50 and 80 years of age were enrolled. After a mean follow-up time of 7.8 years, invasive breast cancer incidence was lower in bisphosphonate users ($P < 0.01$), as was the incidence of estrogen receptor (ER)–positive invasive cancers ($P = 0.02$). A similar but not significant trend was seen for ER-negative-invasive cancers (Chlebowski et al. 2010). Another trial has evaluated the correlation between bisphosphonates and the risk of postmenopausal breast cancer. More specifically, the use of bisphosphonates was assessed in 4,039 postmenopausal patients (median age: 63,6 years) and controls (median age: 65,6 years). The use of bisphosphonates for more than 1 year was associated with a significantly reduced relative risk of breast cancer (28% reduced risk). Breast tumors identified in bisphosphonates users were more often ER-positive and less often poorly differentiated (Rennert et al. 2010). The results suggest that bisphosphonate therapy is associated with a reduced risk of developing breast cancer in elderly patients. Moreover, bisphosphonates may favorably influence the risk profile of incident breast cancer.

6 Prospective Trials of Zoledronic Acid in the Adjuvant Setting

Prospective studies have been designed and are ongoing with the aim to evaluate the role of zoledronic acid and other bisphosphonates as adjuvant therapy in different tumors. The AZURE study (Zoledronic Acid for the Prevention of Bone Metastases in Breast Cancer) was designed for patients with stage II/III breast cancer (3,360 patients). The primary endpoint was disease-free survival. Time to bone and distant metastasis, SREs and OS were also evaluated as secondary endpoints. Patients have been stratified according to lymph node status (N+/N−), tumor stage, estrogen receptor status, adjuvant systemic therapy and pre-/postmenopausal status. Patients were randomized to receive standard chemotherapy plus zoledronic acid versus standard chemotherapy alone. The investigators first reported on the neo-adjuvant treatment results. The mean residual invasive tumor size in the chemotherapy versus the chemotherapy plus zoledronic acid group was 27.4 and 15.5 mm, respectively, a difference that was statistically significant ($P = 0.006$). The pathological complete response rate was 6.9% in the chemotherapy group and 11.7% in the chemotherapy plus zoledronic acid group ($P = 0.15$). There was no difference in axillary nodal involvement ($P = 0.63$). These data suggest a potential direct anti-tumor effect of zoledronic acid in combination with chemotherapy, with the need to perform validating prospective studies (Coleman et al. 2010). At SISABCS 2010, Coleman et al. presented the results of the AZURE study. Patient characteristics including stage, number of positive axillary nodes, chemotherapy type, ER status, menopausal status and concomitant use of statins were well balanced. 3208 patients (96%) received (neo) adjuvant chemotherapy (93% anthracyclines, 23% taxanes), while 152 patients received endocrine treatment only. In the zoledronic acid arm, 752 patients were premenopausal, 244 patients were postmenopausal for <5 years, 519 patients were postmenopausal for >5 years. In the control arm, 751 patients were premenopausal, 247 patients were postmenopausal for <5 years, 519 patients were postmenopausal for >5 years. As of October 2010, with a median follow up of 59 months, there have been 752 DFS events (ZOL 377; control 375; $p = 0.79$). A subgroup analysis of premenopausal, ER+ patients ($n = 1185$) gave no indication of any benefit from adding zoledronic acid. However, a highly significant heterogeneity was found for the effect of zoledronic acid by menopausal status (the analysis for the treatment effect in postmenopausal patients was a preplanned analysis and the study was powered for this aim). Actually, the addition of zoledronic acid improved DFS ($p = 0,001$) and OS ($p = 0.017$) in women postmenopausal for >5 years or >60 years of age (Coleman RE et al. [S4-5] Adjuvant Treatment with Zoledronic Acid in Stage II/III Breast Cancer. The AZURE Trial (BIG 01/04). Presented at: SABCS 2010). These data suggest some benefit of adding zoledronic acid to standard adjuvant treatment, at least in postmenopausal patients with early breast cancer.

To further address whether the use of bisphosphonates in the adjuvant setting of breast cancer might have any effect on the natural course of the disease in more general terms, a meta-analysis has been conducted including published and unpublished randomized controlled trials. The analysis included data from 13 eligible trials involving 6886 patients randomized to treatment with bisphosphonates ($n = 3414$) or either placebo or no treatment ($n = 3472$). The addition of bisphosphonates to standard adjuvant breast cancer treatment did not reduce the overall number of deaths ($P = 0.079$), bone metastases ($P = 0.413$), overall disease recurrences ($P = 0.321$), distant relapse ($P = 0.453$), visceral recurrences ($P = 0.820$), or local relapses ($P = 0.756$). However, subgroup analyses showed that already at that time, the use of zoledronic acid was associated with a significantly lower risk for disease recurrence ($P = 0.025$). The use of zoledronic acid was not associated with any significant difference in death ($P = 0.085$) and the occurrence of bone metastases (Mauri et al. 2010).

7 Ongoing Adjuvant Phase III Trials

S0307 is a joint SWOG/Intergroup/NSABP trial of 6000 stage I–III breast cancer patients randomized to receive one of three different bisphosphonates in addition to standard systemic therapy. Patients receive either oral clodronate 1600 mg daily for 3 years ($n = 2000$), oral ibandronate 50 mg daily ($n = 2000$) for 3 years, or i.v. zoledronic acid 4 mg monthly for the first 6 months and every 3 months for 2.5 years ($n = 2000$). The primary endpoint for the trial is disease-free survival. Secondary endpoints include OS, distribution of sites of first recurrence, adverse events and serum/tumor markers as predictors for disease recurrence in the bone. Safety assessments include monitoring for ONJ and renal function. Recruitment started in 2005, and the trial is now closed for accrual and awaiting publication of results.

The German trial SUCCESS (primary end point disease-free survival) has completed the enrolment of 3700 early high risk breast cancer patients, receiving zoledronic acid therapy for 2 or 5 years following adjuvant chemotherapy. Also in Germany, a recently closed phase III clinical trial (ICE Trial) has evaluated the effects of adjuvant treatment with ibandronate with or without capecitabine in elderly patients (>64 years of age) with early breast cancer. Patients have been stratified according to: lymph node status (N+/N−), estrogen receptor status and adjuvant systemic therapy. 1400 patients will be accrued. The primary endpoint of this study is event-free survival (EFS).

Regarding prostate cancer patients, Mason et al. showed that adjuvant clodronate did not improve bone-metastasis free survival and OS when compared with placebo. Overall, median patient age was 70 years (49–85). The authors concluded that adjuvant clodronate does not modify the natural history of non-metastatic prostate cancer (median follow-up time 10 years) (Mason et al. 2007). The EAU-ZEUS study was designed to evaluate if the early administration of zoledronic acid in high risk patients (Gleason score >8 and/or presence of positive lymph nodes and/or PSA >20 at diagnosis) can prevent or delay the appearance of bone metastases. 1420 patients have been accrued, and the key endpoints of the study are time to bone metastases, OS, PSA doubling time and sub-studies on bone markers. Patients have been randomized to receive i.v. zoledronic acid 4 mg every 3 months for 48 months compared with a control group (no zoledronic acid treatment). The RADAR trial also included high risk prostate cancer patients (pT2b-4 or pT2a with Gleason score ≥ 7 and PSA ≥ 10). It was designed to evaluate if 18 months of androgen deprivation therapy in conjunction with radiotherapy is superior to 6 months androgen deprivation therapy prior to and during radiotherapy, and if 18 months of zoledronic acid therapy is effective to prevent bone loss caused by androgen deprivation therapy and reduce the risk of

Table 1 Some randomized prospective trials of zoledronic acid in the adjuvant setting

Study	Treatment design	Pts enrolled/planned	Pts Characteristics	End-points
NSABP B-34	Standard TP ± Clodronate	4200 planned	Stage I/II breast cancer	DFS; time to bone and distant metastasis, SREs, OS
Intergroup S037	Standard TP + ZA vs Standard TP + Oral Ibandronate vs Standard TP vs Clodronate	6000 planned	Stage I-III breast cancer	DFS, OS, distribution of sites of first recurrence, adverse events, serum/tumor markers as predictors of bone recurrence
SUCCESS	ZA 2 years vs 5 years	3700 enrolled	High risk breast cancer	DFS
EAU-ZEUS	ZA vs Control Group	1420 planned	High risk prostate cancer	Time to bone metastasis, OS, PSA doubling time, sub-studies on bone markers
RADAR	LH-RH analogue prior to and during first month of radiation treatment +/ZA	1000 planned	High risk prostate cancer	PSA relapse- free survival, Changes in OPF, loss of BMD, OS, time to local and bone metastases free survival
2419	ZA vs Control Group	292/446	Stage IIIA-IIIB NSCLC	Time to bone metastases, rate of bone metastasis at 6, 12, 18, and 24 months, SREs, OS
ANZAC	FEC vs FEC + ZA	Not reported	Stage II/III breast cancer Neo-adjuvant setting	Effects of treatment on apoptosis, proliferation, angiogenesis

Abbreviations BMD bone mineral density, DFS Disease-Free Survival, EFS Event-Free Survival, NSCLC Non-Small Cell Lung Cancer, OPF osteoporotic fractures, OS Overall Survival; Pts: patients; SREs: Skeletal-Related Events TP Therapy, ZA Zoledronic Acid; FEC: 5-Fluorouracil, epirubicin, cyclophosphamide bone metastases. The recruitment has been completed with 1300 patients. In the active comparator arm, patients will receive LH-RH analogs for 5 months prior to and during the first month of radiotherapy (for a total of 6 months) with or without zoledronic acid. In the two experimental arms, patients will receive LH-RH analog for 18 months with or without zoledronic acid. The main endpoints are PSA relapse-free survival, changes in osteoporotic fractures, loss of BMD, treatment-related toxicity, quality of life, progression-free survival and OS. Two interim analyses will be performed five and ten years after the recruitment of the last patient. The 2419 trial was designed to evaluate zoledronic acid treatment in the prevention or delay of bone metastasis in Non-Small-Cell Lung Cancer (NSCLC) patients. The key endpoints to be evaluated will be time to bone metastases, rate of bone metastasis at 6, 12, 18 and 24 months, number of SREs and OS. This study will recruit 446 patients with stage IIIa or IIIb NSCLC. The inclusion criteria are patients who have completed primary treatment, no progression after primary treatment, no more than 8 months from diagnosis to randomization. Patients are randomized to zoledronic acid 4 mg every 3–4 weeks vs. no zoledronic acid, with all patients receiving 500 mg calcium and 400–500 UI of vitamin D per day. Treatment duration was established at 24 months from study entry. The results of these ongoing trials on the impact of bisphosphonates will be of high interest in defining the clinical benefit and role of bisphosphonates as adjuvant therapy in tumor patients. Table 1 summarizes the ongoing prospective adjuvant trials of bisphosphonates in preventing bone metastases in cancer patients.

8 Denosumab in the Elderly: Efficacy in Metastatic Disease and New Perspectives in the Adjuvant Setting

Receptor Activator of nuclear Factor-kB Ligand (RANKL), the Receptor Activator of Nuclear Factor-kB (RANK) and the decoy receptor Osteoprotegerin (OPG) are members of the TNF and TNF receptor superfamily able to induce proliferation, differentiation, activation and apoptosis of osteoclasts. Bone remodeling is mediated by the interaction between RANKL expressed on the osteoclasts, RANK expressed on the osteoclast surface and OPG, the decoy receptor for RANKL that prevents osteoclast activation. The RANK/RANKL/OPG pathway displays a key role in the growth of bone metastases: RANKL activates osteoclast-mediated bone resorption with a consequent release of matrix growth factors. The release of these factors can further induce the growth of tumor cells, establishing a positive feedback mechanism. There is increasing evidence for a direct role of the RANK/RANKL interaction in the development of bone metastases (Guise 2000).

Denosumab (AMG 162), a fully humanized IgG2 antibody, was developed to treat patients with skeletal pathologies mediated by osteoclasts, such as bone metastasis, multiple myeloma and CTIBL. On the basis of preclinical data, many clinical trials were conducted to investigate denosumab in metastatic bone disease. Recently, the results of a large clinical trial comparing denosumab versus zoledronic acid in breast cancer have been published. The study demonstrated that denosumab was superior to zoledronic acid and reduced the risk of a first on-study SRE by 18% (HR: 0.82, 95% CI:0.71, 0.95; P value was less than 0.0001 for non-inferiority and equal to 0.01 for superiority) and of first and subsequent SRE by 23% on multiple event analysis (HR: 0.77; 95% CI: 0.66, 0.89; $P = 0.001$) (Stopeck et al. 2010). At ASCO 2010, the results of the non-inferiority trial evaluating denosumab versus zoledronic acid in bone metastases from advanced cancer or multiple myeloma were presented. The time to first SRE or hypercalcemia of malignancy was significantly longer in the denosumab group (HR: 0.83 [95% CI: 0.71, 0.97], $p = 0.02$) as was time to first radiation to bone (HR: 0.78; 95% CI: 0.63, 0.97, $p = 0.03$). In the subgroup analysis of patients with multiple myeloma (10% of patients), mortality was higher for patients treated with denosumab compared with those treated with zoledronic acid. However, the limited number of patients in this subgroup precludes definite conclusions (Vadhan-Raj et al. 2010), and a prospective trial in multiple myeloma patients is ongoing. At ASCO 2010, the non-inferiority study evaluating denosumab compared with ZA for the treatment of bone metastases in patients with castration-resistant prostate cancer was presented. Denosumab significantly delayed the time to first on-study SRE compared to zoledronic acid, (HR: 0.82; 95% CI: 0.71, 0.95; $p = 0.008$). The median time to first on-study SRE was 20.7 months in patients receiving denosumab vs. 17.1 months in patients receiving zoledronic acid. Denosumab also significantly delayed the time to first and subsequent on-study SRE (multiple event analysis) (HR: 0.82; 95% CI: 0.71, 0.94; $p = 0.004$) (Fizazi et al. 2010). In view of these data, approval of denosumab 120 mg s.c. once a month for the prevention of skeletal-related events in patients with bone metastases from solid tumors was granted by the FDA in 2010, excluding patients with multiple myeloma.

There is also some information with regards to denosumab and CTIBL. In the pivotal trial of 7868 women between 60 and 90 years of age with osteoporosis, the incidence of vertebral fractures (2.3 vs. 7.2%; p: 0.001), nonvertebral fractures (6.5 vs. 8.0%; p: 0.01) and hip fractures (0.7 vs. 1.2%; p: 0.04) all were significantly reduced in the denosumab compared to the placebo group (Cummings et al. 2009). In a recent randomized phase III placebo-controlled trial of patients with ER-positive non-metastatic breast cancer and low bone mass who were on adjuvant aromatase inhibitor (AI) treatment, denosumab demonstrated significant activity in preventing AI-associated bone loss. In fact, denosumab resulted in a significant and rapid increase in lumbar spine BMD both at 12 months (5.5%; p: 0.0001) and 24 months (7.6%; p: 0.0001). In subgroup analyses at 12 and 14 months, denosumab therapy was associated with larger gains in BMD compared to placebo across multiple skeletal sites, regardless of age, body mass index, time since menopause, duration or type of AI treatment or baseline T-score (Ellis et al. 2009). Ongoing phase III trials are examining this novel agent for the management of bone loss in patients receiving AI treatment for breast cancer, among others in Austria (ABCSG-18) (National Institutes of Health 2010).

A recent trial evaluated patients with prostate cancer and CTIBL receiving denosumab every 6 months or placebo. Mean patient age in this study was 75 years, and 83% of patients were 70 years of age or older. At 24 months, bone mineral density of the lumbar spine had increased by 5.6% in the denosumab group as compared with a loss of 1.0% in the placebo group ($P < 0.001$). Administration of denosumab was also associated with a significant increase of BMD at the total hip, femoral neck and distal third of the radius at all time points. Finally, patients who received denosumab had a decreased incidence of new vertebral fractures at 36 months (1.5%, vs. 3.9% with placebo) (relative risk 0.38; 95% confidence interval 0.19–0.78; $P = 0.006$) (Smith et al. 2009). To date, denosumab 60 mg s.c. every 6 months is approved by the EMA and FDA for the indication of osteoporosis and CTIBL in patients with prostate cancer, and registration also allows for the use of denosumab for aromatase inhibitor (AI)-Induced Bone Loss (AIBL).

A phase III study has evaluated the efficacy of denosumab (120 mg every 4 weeks) versus placebo in patients with prostate cancer without bone metastases. The primary endpoint of this study is the time to first occurrence of bone metastases or death for any cause. Final results are expected for 2011, and an Amgen Press Release (http://www.amgen.com/media-_pr_detail.jsp?releaseID=1507379) announced that the study has reached the primary end-point regarding bone metastasis-free survival. In fact, denosumab has shown to increase bone-metastasis-free survival by 4.2 months compared with placebo (HR $= 0.85$; $P = 0.03$), without improvement of OS. Moreover, a randomized, double-blind, placebo-controlled phase 3 study is evaluating denosumab as adjuvant treatment for women with early-stage breast cancer at high risk of recurrence. Main eligibility criteria include histologically confirmed breast cancer stage II or III at high risk of recurrence, indication for adjuvant chemotherapy and/or endocrine therapy and/or HER-2 targeted therapy, performance status <2, age≥ 18 years and adequate organ function. 3600 patients will be randomized to receive denosumab versus placebo every four weeks. The primary endpoint is disease-free survival [45].

9 Conclusions

The aging of the population has been associated with an increased prevalence of chronic diseases and cancer. Accordingly, the management of older patients is a high priority of current medical practice. Bisphosphonates are an important option in this group of patients. To date, preclinical and clinical studies are evaluating effects of bisphosphonates and denosumab on survival in the adjuvant and advanced setting. First data suggest that bisphosphonates may prolong the survival in some subgroups of cancer patients, and the elderly patient might derive some extra benefit of bone-targeted treatments. Currently, there are limited data from randomized clinical trials on the effects of bisphosphonates specifically in elderly cancer patients. However, there have been a number of clinical trials with bisphosphonates that have included substantial numbers of elderly patients. Moreover, further clinical trials to assess the role of bisphosphonates and denosumab in indications such asthe prevention of CTIBL are currently in progress. The existing data suggest that bisphosphonates could be considered anticancer drugs at least in the elderly, even if the results of large randomized phase III trials designed for elderly patients are unavailable [45]. New molecules are under evaluation for the treatment of bone metastases from malignant tumors, and this is also true for the elderly. Denosumab is the compound which is in most advanced clinical development, and presently available approved indications include the elderly, where the drug might have an advantage as there is no need to monitor renal function. However caution about potential hypocalcemia are needed for denosumab and osteonecrosis of the jaw prevention is mandatory for most bone-directed therapies mentioned. Targeting the bone by preventing SREs and bone metastases in the elderly patient has potential for improving survival and quality of life in many patients with cancer.

References

Barkin RL, Barkin SJ, Barkin DS (2005) Perception, assessment, treatment, and management of pain in the elderly. Clin Geriatr Med 21(3):465–490

Coleman RE (1997) Skeletal complications of malignancy. Cancer 80(8 Suppl):1588–1594

Saad F, Lipton A, Cook R, Chen YM, Smith M, Coleman R (2007) Pathologic fractures correlate with reduced survival in patients with malignant bone disease. Cancer 110(8):1860–1867

Saad F (2008) New research findings on zoledronic acid: Survival, pain, and anti-tumour effects. Cancer Treat Rev 34(2):183–192

Gridelli C (2007) The use of bisphosphonates in elderly cancer patients. Oncologist 12(1):62–71

Addeo R, Nocera V, Faiola V, Vincenzi B, Ferraro G, Montella L, Guarrasi R, Rossi E, Cennamo G, Tonini G, Capasso E, Santini D, Caraglia M, Del Prete S (2008) Management of pain in elderly patients receiving infusion of zoledronic acid for bone metastasis: a single-institution report. Support Care Cancer 16(2):209–214 Epub 2007 Aug 14

Weide R, Koppler H, Antras L, Smith M, Chang MP, Green J, Wintfeld N, Neary MP, Duh MS (2010) Renal toxicity in patients with multiple myeloma receiving zoledronic acid vs. ibandronate: a retrospective medical records review. J Cancer Res Ther 6(1):31–35

Pillai G, Gieschke R, Goggin T, Barrett J, Worth E, Steimer JL (2006) Population pharmacokinetics of ibandronate in Caucasian and Japanese healthy males and postmenopausal females. Int J Clin Pharmacol Ther 44(12):655–667

Goldschmidt H, Lannert H, Bommer J, Ho AD (2000) Multiple myeloma and renal failure. Nephrol Dial Transplant 15:301–304

Patterson WP, Reams GP (1992) Renal toxicities of chemotherapy. Semin Oncol 19:521–858

Tanvetyanon T, Stiff PJ (2006) Management of the adverse effects associated with intravenous bisphosphonates. Ann Oncol 17:897–907

Body JJ, Coleman R, Clezardin P, Ripamonti C, Rizzoli R, Aapro M (2007) International society of geriatric oncology (SIOG) clinical practice recommendations for the use of bisphosphonates in elderly patients. Eur J Cancer 43:852–858

Boonen S, Black DM, Colón-Emeric CS, Eastell R, Magaziner JS, Eriksen EF, Mesenbrink P, Haentjens P, Lyles KW (2010) Efficacy and safety of a once-yearly intravenous zoledronic acid 5 mg for fracture prevention in elderly postmenopausal women with osteoporosis aged 75 and older. J Am Geriatr Soc 58(2):292–299 Epub 2010 Jan 8

Santini D, Fratto ME, Vincenzi B et al (2006) Zoledronic acid in the management of metastatic bone disease. Expert Opin Biol Ther 6(12):1333–1348

Clézardin P, Ebetino FH, Fournier PGJ (2005) Bisphosphonates and cancer induced bone disease: beyond their antiresorptive activity. Cancer Res 65:4971–4974

Santini D, Vespasiani Gentilucci U, Vincenzi B et al (2003) The antineoplastic role of bisphosphonates: from basic research to clinical evidence. Ann Oncol 14:1468–1476

Santini D, Galluzzo S, Vincenzi B et al (2007) New developments of aminobisphosphonates: the double face of Janus. Ann Oncol 18(Suppl 6):vi164-7

Caraglia M, Santini D, Marra M et al (2006) Emerging anti-cancer molecular mechanisms of aminobisphosphonates. Endocr Relat Cancer 13:7–26

Daubiné F, Céline Le Gall C, Gasser J, Green J, Clézardin P (2007) Antitumor Effects of Clinical Dosing Regimens of Bisphosphonates in Experimental Breast Cancer Bone Metastasis. JNCI 99(4):322–330

Diel IJ, Solomayer EF, Costa SD et al (1998) Reduction in new metastases in breast cancer with adjuvant clodronate treatment. N Engl J Med 339:357–363

Powles T, McCroskey E, Paterson A (2006) Oral bisphosphonates as adjuvant therapy for operable breast cancer. Clin Cancer Res 12:6301s–6304s

Saarto T, Vehmanen L, Blomqvist C, Elomaa I (2006) 10-year follow-up of the efficacy of clodronate on bone mineral density (BMD) in early stage breast cancer. J Clin Oncol ASCO Annual Meeting Proceedings Part I 24(18 Suppl):Abstr 676

Jaschke A, Bastert G, Solomayer EF et al (2004) Adjuvant clodronate treatment improves the overall survival of primary breast cancer patients with micrometastases to bone marrow—a longtime follow-up. J Clin Oncol (Meeting Abstracts) 22:529

Ha TC, Li H (2007) Meta-analysis of clodronate and breast cancer survival. Br J Cancer 6: 1796–1801

Eidtmann H, Bundred NJ, DeBoer R et al. (2008) The effect of zoledronic acid on aromatase inhibitor associated bone loss in postmenopausal women with early breast cancer receiving adjuvant letrozole: 36 months follow-up of ZO-FAST. 31st Annual Meeting of the San Antonio Breast Cancer Symposium, December 10-14, 2008, San Antonio, TX (abstr 44)

Aapro M (2006) Improving bone health in patients with early breast cancer by adding bisphosphonates to letrozole: The Z-ZO-E-ZOFAST program. Breast 15(Suppl 1):S30–S40

Gnant M, Mlineritsch B, Schippinger W et al (2009a) Endocrine therapy plus zoledronic acid in premenopausal breast cancer. N Engl J Med 360:679–691

Eidtmann H, Bundred NJ, DeBoer R et al (2010) The effect of zoledronic acid on aromatase inhibitor associated bone loss in postmenopausal women with early breast cancer receiving adjuvant letrozole: 36 months follow-up of ZO-FAST. Ann Oncol 21(11):2188–2194

Coleman R et al. (2009) Impact of Zoledronic Acid in Postmenopausal Women with Early Breast Cancer Receiving Adjuvant Letrozole: Z-FAST, ZO-FAST, and E-ZO-FAST. Presented at: 32nd SABCS; 2009. Abstract 4082

Gnant M, Mlineritsch B, Schippinger W, Luschin-Ebengreuth G, Pöstlberger S, Menzel C, Jakesz R, Seifert M, Hubalek M, Bjelic-Radisic V, Samonigg H, Tausch C, Eidtmann H, Steger G, Kwasny W, Dubsky P, Fridrik M, Fitzal F, Stierer M, Rücklinger E, Greil R, ABCSG-12 Trial Investigators, Marth C (2009b) Endocrine therapy plus zoledronic acid in premenopausal breast cancer. N Engl J Med 360(7):679–691 Erratum in: N Engl J Med. 2009 May 28;360(22):2379

Chlebowski RT, Chen Z, Cauley JA, Anderson G, Rodabough RJ, McTiernan A, Lane DS, Manson JE, Snetselaar L, Yasmeen S, O'Sullivan MJ, Safford M, Hendrix SL, Wallace RB (2010) Oral bisphosphonate use and breast cancer incidence in postmenopausal women. J Clin Oncol 28(22):3582–3590 Epub 2010 Jun 21

Rennert G, Pinchev M, Rennert HS (2010) Use of bisphosphonates and risk of postmenopausal breast cancer. J Clin Oncol 28(22):3577–3581 Epub 2010 Jun 21

Coleman RE, Winter MC, Cameron D, Bell R, Dodwell D, Keane MM, Gil M, Ritchie D, Passos-Coelho JL, Wheatley D, Burkinshaw R, Marshall SJ, Thorpe H, AZURE (BIG01/04) Investigators (2010) The effects of adding zoledronic acid to neoadjuvant chemotherapy on tumour response: exploratory evidence for direct anti-tumour activity in breast cancer. Br J Cancer 102(7):1099–1105 Epub 2010 Mar 16

Coleman RE, Thorpe HC, Cameron D, Dodwell D, Burkinshaw R, Keane M, Gil M, Houston SJ, Grieve RJ, Barrett-Lee PJ, Ritchie D, Davies C, Bell R[S4-5] Adjuvant Treatment with Zoledronic Acid in Stage II/III Breast Cancer. The AZURE Trial (BIG 01/04). Presented at: SABCS 2010

Mauri D, Valachis A, Polyzos NP et al (2010) Does Adjuvant Bisphosphonate in Early Breast Cancer Modify the Natural Course of the Disease? A Meta-Analysis of Randomized Controlled Trials. J Natl Compr Canc Netw 8:279–286

Mason MD, Sydes MR, Glaholm J et al (2007) Oral sodium clodronate for nonmetastatic prostate cancer–results of a randomized double-blind placebo-controlled trial: Medical Research Council PR04 (ISRCTN61384873). J Natl Cancer Inst 99(10):765–776

Guise TA (2000) Molecular mechanisms of osteolytic bone metastases. Cancer 88(12 Suppl): 2892–2898

Stopeck A, Lipton A, Body JJ et al (2010) Denosumab compared with zoledronic acid for the treatment of bone metastases in patients with advanced breast cancer: a randomized double-blind study. J Clin Oncol 28(35):5132–5139

Vadhan-Raj S, Henry DH, von Moos R et al (2010) Denosumab in the treatment of bone metastases from advanced cancer or multiple myeloma (MM): Analyses from a phase III randomized trial. J Clin Oncol 28(Suppl):15s [abstract 9042]

Fizazi K, Carducci MA, Smith MR et al (2010) A randomized phase III trial of denosumab versus zoledronic acid in patients with bone metastases from castration-resistant prostate cancer. J Clin Oncol 28(Suppl):18s [abstract LBA4507]

Cummings SR, San Martin J, McClung MR et al (2009) FREEDOM Trial. Denosumab for prevention of fractures in postmenopausal women with osteoporosis. N Engl J Med 361:756–765

Ellis GK, Bone HG, Chlebowski R et al (2009) Effect of denosumab on bone mineral density in women receiving adjuvant aromatase inhibitors for non-metastatic breast cancer: subgroup analyses of a phase 3 study. Breast Cancer Res Treat 118:81–87

National Institutes of Health. A randomised, double-blind, placebo-controlled, multi-centre phase 3 study to determine the treatment effect of denosumab in subjects with non-metastatic breast cancer receiving aromatase inhibitor therapy. Clinicaltrials.gov web site. Available at: http://clinicaltrials.gov/ct2/show/NCT00556374. Accessed August 6, 2010

Smith MR, Egerdie B, Hernández Toriz N, Feldman R, Tammela TL, Saad F, Heracek J, Szwedowski M, Ke C, Kupic A, Leder BZ, Goessl C, Denosumab HALT Prostate Cancer Study Group (2009) Denosumab in men receiving androgen-deprivation therapy for prostate cancer. N Engl J Med 361(8):745–755 Epub 2009 Aug 11

Denosumab: First Data and Ongoing Studies on the Prevention of Bone Metastases

Roger von Moos and Tomas Skacel

Abstract

Bone metastases are associated with a major patient and healthcare burden resulting from the impact and the management of associated skeletal-related events (including spinal cord compression, pathologic fracture and surgery or radiation to bone). In preclinical studies, RANK Ligand inhibition has been shown to prevent the development of bone and some visceral metastases. Clinical studies are ongoing to evaluate whether the fully human monoclonal antibody denosumab, which targets RANK Ligand, can prevent the development of bone metastases in high-risk patients. Findings from a phase 3 study in men with high-risk non-metastatic castration-resistant prostate cancer demonstrated that denosumab (120 mg every 4 weeks) significantly increased bone metastasis-free survival (primary endpoint) by 4.2 months (median) versus placebo (HR 0.85 [0.73, 0.98]; $P = 0.028$). This is the first study to demonstrate the clinical benefit of a bone-targeted agent in this setting. Further evaluation of denosumab in the prevention of metastatic disease is warranted and ongoing in other tumor types.

R. von Moos (✉)
Department Medical Oncology, Kantonsspital Graubuenden,
Loestrasse 170, 7000 Chur, Switzerland
e-mail: roger.vonmoos@ksgr.ch

T. Skacel
First Faculty of Medicine, Clinical Department of Haematology,
Charles University in Prague, Czeh Republic

T. Skacel
Amgen Switzerland, Zahlerweg 6, 6301 Zug, Switzerland

Contents

1 Introduction... 188
2 Denosumab 189
   2.1 Current Indications and Efficacy.. 189
   2.2 Safety 190
3 Denosumab: Prevention of Bone Metastases in Prostate Cancer................ 191
4 Denosumab: Prevention of Bone Metastases in Breast Cancer 192
5 Denosumab: Prevention of Bone Metastases in Other Tumors 194
References... 195

1 Introduction

Although the precise incidence of bone metastases is not known, it is estimated that they occur in approximately 65–75% of patients with advanced breast or prostate cancer and in 30–40% of patients with other solid tumors (Coleman 2001). Left untreated, the osteoclast-mediated 'vicious cycle' drives further tumor growth and bone destruction. Tumor cells release factors that directly or indirectly stimulate osteoclast activation (Fig. 1). These factors induce expression of RANK Ligand (RANKL; the key mediator of osteoclast formation, maturation and function), PTHrP, and also downregulates osteoprotegerin (an inhibitor of osteoclastic bone resorption) (Guise and Mundy 1998; Kitazawa and Kitazawa 2002; Mundy 2002; Roodman 2004). The resulting osteolysis by the activated osteoclasts releases further growth factors from within the bone matrix and tumor, thereby promoting further bone destruction (Roodman 2004). This interaction between the tumor cells, the surrounding bone microenvironment and the involvement of RANKL has been implicated in the development of bone metastases secondary to breast, prostate, thyroid, renal and lung cancer as well as neuroblastoma and multiple myeloma (Roodman 2004). RANK expression has also been observed on a number of cancer cell lines. Activation of RANK receptors on the tumor cells by the ligand (RANKL) causes an increase in cancer cell migration and invasion (Armstrong 2008). Furthermore, preclinical studies have shown that the presence of RANK on tumor cells enhances lung and bone metastasis (Gonzalez-Suarez et al. 2010; Jones 2006; Tan 2011). Although not an example of metastatic disease, these preclinical data are also supported by a clinical phase 2 trial in Giant Cell Tumor of the bone, a rare primary osteolytic bone tumor with substantial skeletal morbidity. Results of this study (Thomas et al. 2010) showed an impressive 86% response rate with 84% of patients experiencing a clinical benefit (including pain reduction requiring less analgesia, functional improvements, mobility and bone repair).

Metastatic bone disease can result in clinically significant skeletal morbidity, including the requirement of radiation to bone (as a means of pain palliation), occurrence of a pathological fracture, the need for surgery to stabilize bone or spinal cord compression. The negative impact of these skeletal-related events, both from a patient quality of life perspective and the healthcare resource burden,

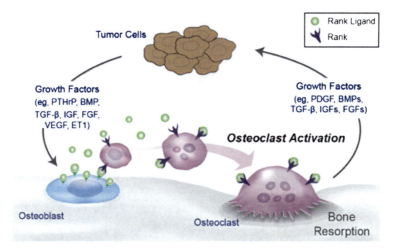

Fig. 1 The vicious cycle of bone destruction in metastatic bone disease (adapted from Clines and Guise (2008))

highlights the importance of preventing bone metastases as a means of preventing the later complications.

2 Denosumab

Denosumab is a fully human monoclonal antibody that binds specifically to RANKL and prevents it from binding with the RANK receptor. Thus, neutralizing RANKL with denosumab inhibits osteoclast formation, maturation, function and prevents osteolysis (Fig. 2).

2.1 Current Indications and Efficacy

Denosumab is available in two different dose forms for the management of two different oncological indications. A 60 mg subcutaneous dose every 6 months (Prolia®) is approved in the European Union for the treatment of bone loss associated with hormone ablation in men with prostate cancer at increased risk of fractures (European Medicines Agency 2010) and additionally for treatment of bone loss induced by aromatase inhibitors in women with breast cancer in Switzerland (Swiss Medic 2010) and the USA (United States Federal Drugs Agency 2011a). In a large phase 3 clinical trial in men with prostate cancer receiving androgen deprivation therapy, denosumab (60 mg every 6 months) significantly decreased the incidence of new vertebral fractures versus placebo (1.5 vs. 3.9%, respectively; RR 0.38; 95% CI 0.19, 0.78; $P = 0.006$) (Smith et al. 2009).

Denosumab (XGEVA®; 120 mg every 4 weeks) is also approved in the USA for the 'prevention of skeletal-related events in patients with bone metastases from

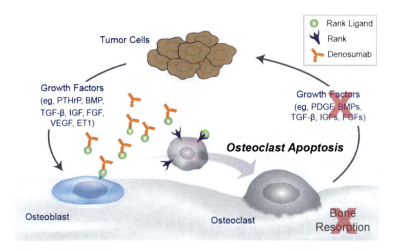

Fig. 2 Denosumab binds RANKL and interrupts the vicious cycle of bone destruction in metastatic bone disease

solid tumors' denosumab is not indicated for use in patients with multiple myeloma (United States Federal Drugs Agency 2011b) and in the European Union for the 'prevention of skeletal-related events (pathological fracture, radiation to bone, spinal cord compression or surgery to bone) in adults with bone metastases from solid tumors' (European Medicines Agency 2011). The efficacy and safety of the 120 mg dose was assessed in three identically designed randomised, double-blind, double-dummy, phase 3 trials where patients ($N = 5723$) with bone metastases/lesions secondary to prostate cancer, breast cancer, other solid tumors or multiple myeloma received either subcutaneous denosumab (120 mg every 4 weeks) with intravenous placebo ($N = 2862$) or intravenous zoledronic acid (4 mg every 4 weeks) with subcutaneous placebo ($N = 2861$). In a planned integrated analysis of the three studies, denosumab was superior to zoledronic acid in delaying the time to first on-study skeletal-related event (primary endpoint) by 17% (median 27.7 months vs. 19.5 months, respectively; HR 0.83; 95% CI 0.76, 0.90; $P < 0.0001$). Denosumab was also superior in delaying time to first and subsequent on-study skeletal-related events by 18% (HR 0.82; 95% CI 0.75, 0.89; $P < 0.0001$) (Lipton et al. 2010).

2.2 Safety

In the integrated analysis of the advanced cancer trials, adverse events were similar for denosumab (120 mg every 4 weeks) and zoledronic acid with 96.2% and 96.8% of patients reporting adverse events and 56.3 and 57.1% of patients reporting serious adverse events, respectively (Lipton et al. 2010). Incidence of osteonecrosis of the jaw was similar between treatment arms (1.8 vs. 1.3%, respectively; $P = 0.13$). Hypocalcaemia (mostly asymptomatic in both arms) was reported in more patients receiving denosumab (9.6%) than those receiving zoledronic acid (5.0%). Grade 3 hypocalcaemia was reported in 2.5% and 1.2% of patients, respectively. Grade 4 hypocalcaemia was only reported in 0.6% and 0.2% of patients. Denosumab does not require dose adjustments or withholding for renal function. Furthermore, incidence of adverse events potentially associated with renal toxicity was lower in the denosumab arm (9.2%) versus the zoledronic acid arm (11.8%). Similarly, adverse events with acute phase reactions reported within 3 days of treatment were reported for fewer patients in the denosumab arm than the zoledronic acid arm (8.7% vs. 20.2%) (Lipton et al. 2010).

3 Denosumab: Prevention of Bone Metastases in Prostate Cancer

Preclinical evidence suggests that RANKL inhibition reduces progression of established prostate cancer to the bone through inhibition of bone remodeling (Zhang et al. 2003). Furthermore, this reduction in bone resorption may prevent the outgrowth of marrow micrometastases (van der Pluijm et al. 2005). Results from other preclinical studies have also shown that activation of RANK on the surface of tumor cells leads to an increase in cancer cell migration and invasion (Armstrong 2008). Both of these mechanisms may play an important role in prevention of bone metastasis and progression of prostate cancer.

A recently reported global phase 3 study (NCT00286091) evaluated the effect of denosumab (120 mg every 4 weeks) on bone metastasis-free survival. Eligibility criteria included men with non-metastatic castrate-resistant prostate cancer at high risk for developing bone metastasis, characterized by a PSA value ≥ 8.0 ng/mL obtained ≤ 3 months before randomization and/or a PSA doubling time ≤ 10 months. Patients were randomised 1:1 to receive either subcutaneous denosumab ($N = 716$) or subcutaneous placebo ($N = 716$) every 4 weeks with recommended calcium (≥ 500 mg) and vitamin D (≥ 400 IU) supplementation. The primary efficacy endpoint was bone metastasis-free survival, defined as time to first bone metastasis (either symptomatic or asymptomatic) or death from any cause. Bone metastases were detected by routine bone scans and were confirmed by an independent central reading facility using a second imaging modality (radiography, computed tomography or magnetic resonance imaging). Time to first bone metastasis (either symptomatic or asymptomatic) and overall survival were also evaluated (Smith et al. 2011).

Smith et al. reported a significant treatment benefit with denosumab versus placebo in these patients. Bone metastasis-free survival was significantly increased by a median of 4.2 months versus placebo (HR 0.85; 95% CI 0.73, 0.98; $P = 0.028$). Time to symptomatic bone metastasis was also delayed (HR 0.67; 95% CI 0,49, 0,92; $P = 0.01$). Overall survival was similar between groups. Adverse events and serious adverse events were generally similar between the two treatment groups and the yearly cumulative incidence of osteonecrosis of the jaw was similar to the rates previously reported for this agent in the advanced cancer setting (cumulative incidence year 1, 1.1%; year 2, 2.9%; year 3, 4.2%) (Smith et al. 2011). This is the first large randomised study to demonstrate that targeting bone resorption prevents bone metastasis in men with castrate resistant prostate cancer.

The study did not plan for patient follow-up beyond the first bone metastasis. As such, it is unclear whether the delay of the first bone metastasis will translate into a later onset of and overall lower number of skeletal-related events. The study also does not provide a definitive answer about a potential survival benefit of denosumab in this patient population, which can only be seen later in the course of the disease. Denosumab given monthly at 120 mg prevents or delays bone metastasis in prostate cancer. It is an open question as to whether a similar outcome could potentially be achieved with other doses and schedules of denosumab. Additional trials in this high-risk prostate cancer population addressing these questions are of interest.

4 Denosumab: Prevention of Bone Metastases in Breast Cancer

Bone is the most common site of distant recurrence in women with early stage breast cancer, accounting for approximately 40% of first metastatic recurrences in this population (Coleman 2007). It has been shown in the preclinical setting that RANKL and RANK are expressed in human breast cancer tissue (Gonzalez-Suarez et al. 2010) and this increased RANK expression may be associated with an increased incidence of hyperplasia and adenocarcinoma (Gonzalez-Suarez et al. 2006). RANK expression in primary breast tumors is correlated with lymph node and bone metastases (Santini et al. 2011). It was also observed that RANKL knockout mice did not develop normal mammary epithelial glands as a response to pregnancy hormones. This observation suggests that RANK/RANKL could be the missing link between sex hormones and breast cancer (Koch 2011). In an experimental mouse model, Penninger's group found a markedly decreased incidence and delayed onset of breast cancer when RANK was inactivated in the mammary epithelium (Schramek et al. 2010). These findings were confirmed in a second study by Gonzalez-Suarez et al. published in Nature; use of pharmacological RANKL inhibition reduced the development of sex hormone-induced mammary cancer from 100 to 10% in wild-type mice (Gonzalez-Suarez et al. 2010). Similarly, in transgenic mice with overactive RANK functionality an increased and accelerated formation of mammary tumors was observed (Gonzalez-Suarez et al. 2010). Since RANKL/RANK has a key role in bone metabolism, it could be speculated that microcalcification as a sign of breast malignancy could be seen in this context (Koch 2011). Furthermore, in a mouse model, RANKL inhibition has significantly delayed de novo breast cancer skeletal metastases formation and improved survival (Canon et al. 2008a, b). Thus, inhibition of osteoclast activity via the RANK/RANKL pathway is a potential strategy for delaying and preventing the development of bone and visceral metastases.

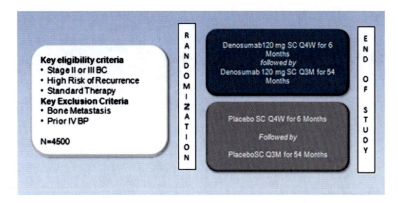

Fig. 3 Study design: Denosumab as adjuvant treatment for women with high risk early breast cancer receiving neoadjuvant or adjuvant therapy (D-CARE)

Two ongoing phase 3 randomized clinical trials may provide evidence regarding denosumab's potential role in preventing bone and visceral metastasis in breast cancer patients. A randomized double-blind, placebo-controlled, multicenter, international phase 3 study compares denosumab with placebo as adjuvant treatment for women with early stage breast cancer who are at high risk of disease recurrence (D-CARE, NCT01077154; Fig. 3).

Eligibility criteria are: women aged ≥ 18 years; ECOG performance status 0 or 1; histologically confirmed AJCC stage II or III breast cancer; high risk of breast recurrence; receiving or scheduled to receive concurrent standard of care systemic adjuvant or neoadjuvant chemotherapy and/or endocrine therapy and/or HER-2 targeted therapy. A total of 4,500 patients are planned to be randomised 1:1 to receive either subcutaneous denosumab (120 mg every 4 weeks) for 6 months followed by denosumab (120 mg every 3 months) for 54 months or subcutaneous placebo (every 4 weeks) for 6 months followed by placebo (every 3 months) for 54 months. Vitamin D (≥ 400 IU) and calcium (≥ 500 mg) supplementation is required unless patients develop hypercalcaemia. The primary endpoint is bone metastasis-free survival (BMFS). Secondary endpoints are disease-free survival, overall survival and distant recurrence-free survival. Safety, patient-reported outcomes (pain and health utilities) and breast density will also be assessed. Patients who develop a documented bone metastasis will discontinue treatment and enter follow-up. This trial is ongoing and recruiting patients; estimated completion of the trial is October 2016.

The second large phase 3 clinical trial (ABCSG-18) with more than 3400 patients is being conducted in Austria and other European countries (Fig. 4). Postmenopausal women treated with aromatase inhibitors are enrolled in this study. The primary endpoint is the time to first clinical fracture, the secondary endpoints include the incidence of new vertebral fractures, the incidence of new or worsening of pre-existing vertebral fractures and the percentage change in total lumbar spine, total hip and femoral neck bone mineral bone density. Exploratory

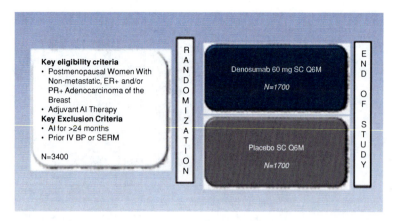

Fig. 4 Study design: Denosumab in patients with breast cancer receiving aromatase inhibitor therapy (ABCSG-18)

endpoints will provide information about the effect of denosumab on bone metastasis-free survival, disease-free survival and overall survival. The study is estimated to complete recruitment by November 2013.

Since the value of bisphosphonates in this breast cancer setting remains unclear, these two large phase 3 trials should provide additional evidence about the role of RANKL inhibition in the adjuvant setting.

5 Denosumab: Prevention of Bone Metastases in Other Tumors

Invasion of distant tissues by tumor cells is the primary cause of therapeutic failure in the treatment of lung cancer. In preclinical evaluations, RANKL inhibition has prevented tumor-associated osteolytic and osteoblastic disease and reduced skeletal tumor burden in all murine models of lung cancer that have been tested (Feeley et al. 2006). These data suggest that treatment of lung cancer patients with bone disease with a RANKL inhibitor may suppress tumor-induced bone destruction and the progression of the skeletal tumor. Although this remains to be evaluated in a prospective study, a recently presented post-hoc analysis of the lung cancer cohort from the phase 3 solid tumor study may provide some initial clinical evidence. The exploratory analysis was performed analyzing overall survival among the 801 patients with non-small cell or small cell lung cancer. In this cohort, a survival advantage was seen among those with lung cancer receiving denosumab versus those receiving zoledronic acid (median 8.9 months vs. 7.7 months, respectively; HR 0.80; 95% CI 0.67, 0.95; $P = 0.01$). Improved survival was also observed among patients with non-small cell lung cancer ($N = 702$), with a median survival of 9.5 months with denosumab versus 8.1 months with zoledronic acid (HR 0.78; 95% CI 0.65, 0.94; $P = 0.01$)

(Scagliotti et al. 2011). Although this analysis was not preplanned a strong signal in a direct survival benefit was observed. These initial data suggest further evaluation of the effect of denosumab on the prevention of bone metastases and survival in lung cancer is warranted.

RANKL plays a central role in normal and pathologic bone remodeling and probably an important role in cancer cell migration and invasion. RANK inhibition is a promising approach to prevent development of bone metastases in variety of solid tumors through improved bone integrity. It remains to be seen whether RANK/RANKL pathway inhibition possesses direct antitumor effect in human breast, prostate and lung cancer. Further intensive preclinical and clinical research is required and ongoing to answer these important questions.

Acknowledgments Editorial support was provided by Emma Thomas of Amgen (Europe) GmbH.

References

Armstrong AP (2008) RANKL Acts directly on RANK-expressing prostate tumor cells and mediates migration and expression of tumour metastatic genes. Prostate 68:92–104

Canon J et al (2008a) The RANKL inhibitor OPG-Fc delays the de novo establishment of breast cancer skeletal metastases in an MDA-MB-231 mouse model. Cancer Treat Rev 34:S60

Canon J et al (2008b) Inhibition of RANKL blocks skeletal tumor progression and improves survival in a mouse model of breast cancer bone metastasis. Clin Exp Metastasis 25(2): 119–129

Clines GA, Guise TA (2008) Molecular mechanisms and treatment of bone metastasis. Expert Rev Mol Med 10:e7

Coleman RE (2001) Metastatic bone disease: clinical features, pathophysiology and treatment strategies. Cancer Treat Rev 27(3):165–176

Coleman R (2007) Potential use of bisphosphonates in the prevention of metastases in early-stage breast cancer. Clin Breast Cancer 7(Suppl 1):S29–S35

European Medicines Agency (2010) Prolia (Denosumab) summary of product characteristics. http://www.ema.europa.eu/docs/en_GB/document_library/EPAR_Product_Informaion/human/001120/WC500093526.pdf

European Medicines Agency (2011) XGEVA (Denosumab) summary of product characteristics. http://www.ema.europa.eu/docs/en_GB/ocument_library/EPAR_Product_Information/human/002173/WC500110381.pdf

Feeley BT, Liu NQ et al (2006) Mixed metastatic lung cancer lesions in bone are inhibited by noggin overexpression and Rank:Fc administration. J Bone Miner Res 21(10):1571–1580

Gonzalez-Suarez E et al (2006) Overexpression of RANK in the Mouse mammary gland increases proliferation and susceptibility to chemically induced mammay tumors. Breast Cancer Res Treat 100:S23 (Abstract 24)

Gonzalez-Suarez E, Jacob AP et al (2010) RANK ligand mediates progestin-induced mammary epithelial proliferation and carcinogenesis. Nature 468(7320):103–107

Guise TA, Mundy GR (1998) Cancer and bone. Endocr Rev 19(1):18–54

Kitazawa S, Kitazawa R (2002) RANK ligand is a prerequisite for cancer-associated osteolytic lesions. J Pathol 198(2):228–236

Jones DH, Nakashima T et al (2006) Regulation of cancer cell migration and bone metastasis by RANKL. Nature 440(7084):692–696

Koch L (2011) Cancer: RANKL inhibition-a new weapon against breast cancer. Nat Rev Endocrinol 7(1):2

Lipton A et al (2010) Comparison of denosumab versus zoledronic acid (ZA) for treatment of bone metastases in advanced cancer patients: an integrated analysis of 3 pivotal trials (Abstract 1249P). Ann Oncol 21(Suppl 8): viii 379

Mundy GR (2002) Metastasis to bone: causes, consequences and therapeutic opportunities. Nat Rev Cancer 2(8):584–593

Roodman GD (2004) Mechanisms of bone metastasis. N Engl J Med 350(16):1655–1664

Santini D, Schiavon G et al (2011) Receptor activator of NF-kB (RANK) expression in primary tumors associates with bone metastasis occurrence in breast cancer patients. PLoS One 6:e19234

Scagliotti G, Hirsh V et al (2011) Overall survival improvement in patients with lung cancer treated with denosumab versus zoledronic acid: results from a randomised phase 3 study. J Thor Oncol 6 (6 (Suppl 2)): S273 (Abstract O01.01)

Schramek D, Leibbrandt A et al (2010) Osteoclast differentiation factor RANKL controls development of progestin-driven mammary cancer. Nature 468(7320):98–102

Smith MR, Egerdie B et al (2009) Denosumab in men receiving androgen-deprivation therapy for prostate cancer. N Engl J Med 361(8):745–755

Smith M, Saad F et al (2011) Denosumab to prolong bone metastasis-free survival in men with castrate-resistant prostate cancer: results of a global phase 3, randomized, double-blind trial. American Urological Association annual meeting. Washington, DC, USA

Swissmedic (2010) Authorised medicinal products. http://www.swissmedic.ch/zulassungen/00171/00181/01382/index.html?lang=en

Tan W, Zhang W et al (2011) Tumour-infiltrating regulatory T cells stimulate mammary cancer metastasis through RANKL-RANK signaling. Nature 470(7335):548–553

Thomas D, Henshaw R et al (2010) Denosumab in patients with giant-cell tumour of bone: an open-label, phase 2 study. Lancet Oncol 11(3):275–280

United States Federal Drugs Agency (2011a) Denosumab (Prolia) prescribing information USA. http://pi.amgen.com/united_states/prolia/prolia_pi.pdf

United States Federal Drugs Agency (2011b) Denosumab (XGEVA) Prescribing Information USA http://pi.augen.com/united.states/xgeva/xgeva.pi.pdf

van der Pluijm G, Que I et al (2005) Interference with the microenvironmental support impairs the de novo formation of bone metastases in vivo. Cancer Res 65(17):7682–7690

Zhang J, Dai J et al (2003) Soluble receptor activator of nuclear factor kappaB Fc diminishes prostate cancer progression in bone. Cancer Res 63(22):7883–7890

Diagnostic and Prognostic Use of Bone Turnover Markers

Markus Joerger and Jens Huober

Abstract

The use of bone turnover markers in oncology includes monitoring of anticancer treatment in patients with malignant disease metastatic to the bones (*therapeutic monitoring*), predicting the risk of bone relapse in patients with a first diagnosis of potentially curative, early-stage malignant tumors (*prognostic use*), and making an early diagnosis of (microscopic) malignant bone disease in patients with a known malignant tumor to start early bone-targeted treatment and avoid skeletal-related events (*diagnostic use*). Concerning *prognostic use*, there is limited evidence for bone turnover markers to predict the occurrence of metachronous bone metastases in patients with early-stage malignant tumors, with serum PINP (N-terminal propeptide of procollagen type 1), ICTP (Carboxyterminal cross-linked telopeptide of type I collagen), bone sialoprotein (BSP), and tumor immunoexpression of BSP being the most promising candidates. Concerning *diagnostic use*, serum bone-specific alkaline phosphatise (BSAP), PINP and osteoprotegerin (OPG) were repeatedly shown to be associated with synchronous bone metastases in patients with breast or lung cancer, but sensitivity of these markers was too low to suggest that they might be preferred over conventional bone scans for the diagnosis of bone metastases. A somewhat higher sensitivity for the diagnosis of bone metastases was found for urinary NTx (N-terminal cross-linked telopeptide of type I collagen) and serum ICTP in solid tumor patients, serum TRAcP-5b (Tartrate-resistant acid phosphatase type 5b) in patients with breast cancer and serum BSAP, PINP and OPG in prostate cancer patients. Both prognostic and diagnostic use of bone turnover markers are reviewed in this chapter.

M. Joerger (✉) · J. Huober
Department of Medical Oncology and Breast Centre,
Cantonal Hospital, St. Gallen, Switzerland
e-mail: markus.joerger@gmail.com; markus.joerger@kssg.ch

Contents

1	Introduction	198
2	Overview on Bone Markers	199
	2.1 Bone Formation Markers	199
	2.2 Bone Resorption Markers	201
	2.3 Osteoclast Regulators: Receptor Activator of Nuclear Factor-κB Ligand/ Osteoprotegerin	202
	2.4 Bone Sialoproteins	203
3	Prognostic Use of Bone Markers	204
	3.1 Prognostic Use of Bone Markers in Breast Cancer	208
	3.2 Prognostic Use of Bone Markers in Prostate Cancer	209
	3.3 Prognostic Use of Bone Markers in Lung Cancer	209
	3.4 Prognostic Use of Bone Markers in Multiple Myeloma	210
4	Diagnostic Use of Bone Markers	211
	4.1 Diagnostic Use of Bone Markers in Various Tumors	212
	4.2 Diagnostic Use of Bone Markers in Breast Cancer	213
	4.3 Diagnostic Use of Bone Markers in Prostate Cancer	214
	4.4 Diagnostic Use of Bone Markers in Lung Cancer	216
5	Conclusions	217
	5.1 Prognostic Use of Bone Turnover Markers	217
	5.2 Diagnostic Use of Bone Turnover Markers	218
References		218

1 Introduction

The majority of solid malignant tumors have a strong propensity to spread to the bone. The mechanisms involved in cancer dissemination to bone are complex, and the changes in bone metabolism are very profound, once bony metastases have occurred. The use of bone markers in oncology covers mainly three topics. The first is monitoring of anticancer treatment in patients with established malignant disease metastatic to the bones. However, this is not the topic of the present chapter. The second application is to use bone turnover markers as a prognostic tool for patients with a first diagnosis of potentially curative, early-stage malignant disease, to predict the risk of disease relapse in the bones, and potentially apply preventive measures such as adjuvant chemotherapy or bisphosphonates. The third application is to use bone markers for an early diagnosis of (microscopic) malignant bone disease in patients with a known malignant tumor, and potentially start early bone-targeted treatment to delay overt malignant bone disease with subsequent complications such as pain, fractures and immobility.

Diagnostic procedures for metastatic bone disease traditionally focus on the localization and characterization of the lesion, using different imaging techniques such as radiographs, computed tomography, magnetic resonance imaging (MRI),

^{99}technecium bone scans and positron-emission tomography (PET) scans. These diagnostic tools have been proven to be effective in identifying established metastatic spread. However, earlier (microscopic) stages of malignant bone disease cannot be diagnosed with conventional radiological or radionuclide imaging. In such cases, bone markers might be of particular value to enable early diagnosis of malignant bone disease, or even provide some information on the future risk of developing bone metastases in patients with early malignant disease. Under normal conditions, bone remodeling is a balanced, lifelong continuum of resorption of old bone (through the action of osteoclasts) and replacing the removed tissue by an equal amount of newly formed bone (through the action of osteoblasts). The presence of bone metastases greatly perturbs this balance. Driven by a number of tumor-derived factors, the osteoclasts surrounding cancer metastases become activated and start resorbing bone substance. By contrast, bone formation may be increased or decreased, but is usually inadequate to compensate for the increase in bone resorption. Radiographically, this results in predominantly lytic or mixed lytic–sclerotic lesions, as typically seen in breast cancer metastases to bone. By contrast, sclerotic lesions are typically found in prostate cancer, characterized at the cellular level by a relative excess of bone formation as compared to bone resorption. However, even the skeletal metastases of prostate cancer are characterized by an increased rate of both bone resorption and formation. Therefore, high bone turnover is a general feature of metastatic bone disease, and is accompanied by a respective increase of both markers of bone formation and bone resorption.

There are some practical and important issues for the analysis and interpretation of bone markers, including diurnal variation of serum concentrations, that might reach 20% of the absolute values, potential seasonal variation and gender differences. These various reasons for diagnostic variability have recently been reviewed by Coleman et al. (2008). Although bone markers may have the potential as diagnostic or prognostic tools in cancer patients, the available data do not allow final conclusions regarding the accuracy and validity of any of the presently used markers in the primary or secondary prevention of bone metastases. Still, available data allow to give an overview on the potential diagnostic and prognostic use of bone markers in patients with solid malignancies or multiple myeloma, as outlined in this chapter.

2 Overview on Bone Markers

2.1 Bone Formation Markers

By-products of osteogenesis or osteoblast-secreted factors can provide insight into the activity of bone formation (Table 1).

2.1.1 Bone-Specific Alkaline Phosphatase

Bone-specific alkaline phosphatase (BSAP) hydrolyses pyrophosphates, thereby removing an inhibitor of osteogenesis while creating the inorganic phosphate that is required for generation and deposition of hydroxyapatite. BSAP is secreted from

Table 1 Markers of bone formation

Marker	Specimen	Normal range	Diagnostic use for bone metastases	Prognostic use for bone metastases
BSAP	Serum	PreM. women: 2.9–14.5 µg/L (Coleman et al. 2008) PostM. women: 3.8–22.6 µg/L (Coleman et al. 2008) Men: 3.7–20.9 µg/L (Coleman et al. 2008)	High values associated with bone metastases in 200 cancer patients (Oremek et al. 2003) High values associated with bone metastases in 295 prostate cancer patients (Lorente et al. 1999)	
OC	Serum	PreM. women: 1.0–36 µg/L (Heuck and Wolthers 1998) Men: 1.0–35 µg/L (Heuck and Wolthers 1998)	Low values associated with bone metastases in lung cancer patients (Karapanagiotou et al. 2010)	Low values predict relapse in bone in 79 patients with newly diagnosed NSCLC (Terpos et al. 2009)
PICP	Serum	Women: 50–170 µg/L (Caillot-Augusseau et al. 1998; Puistola et al. 1993) Men: 38–202 µg/L (Caillot-Augusseau et al. 1998; Puistola et al. 1993)	High values associated with bone metastases in 200 cancer patients (Oremek et al. 2003) High values associated with bone metastases in 276 cancer patients (Koizumi et al. 2003)	High values predict tumor relapse in bone in 373 early breast cancer (Jukkola et al. 2001)
PINP	Serum	Women: 31.7–70.7 µg/L (Bauer et al. 2006) Men: 21–78 µg/L (Nguyen et al. 2007)	High values associated with bone metastases in breast cancer patients (Luftner et al. 2005) High values associated with bone metastases in prostate cancer patients (Koizumi et al. 2001; Thurairaja et al. 2006; Koopmans et al. 2007)	

BSAP bone-specific alkaline phosphatase, *OC* osteocalcin, *PICP* C-terminal propeptide of procollagen type 1, *PINP* N-terminal propeptide of procollagen type 1, *PreM* premenopausal, *PostM* postmenopausal osteoblasts to the bone matrix to allow for bone mineralization. There are different alkaline phosphatase isoforms secreted by various organs into the serum, with predominant isoforms originating from the bone, liver or intestines. The bone-specific isoform (BSAP) is a relatively specific marker for osteogenesis. However, elevated serum concentrations of BSAP might also be found in patients with liver dysfunction, as BSAP is normally cleared from the serum by the liver.

2.1.2 Osteocalcin

Osteocalcin (Bauer et al. 2006) is the major non-collagen protein in the bone matrix, and is produced by osteoblasts among other cells. Osteocalcin serum or urinary concentrations reflect both osteolysis and osteogenesis, and concentrations can also be increased in patients with renal dysfunction or hyperlipidemia. Multiple isoforms of osteocalcin are found in the serum or in urine, and current assays might not detect them all (Ivaska et al. 2005).

2.1.3 Propeptides of Procollagen Type I

Collagen type I comprises approximately 90% of the organic bone matrix. After extracellular excretion of the N-terminal propeptide of procollagen type 1 (PINP) and C-terminal propeptide of procollagen type 1 (PICP), these peptides are coupled to collagen and released into the serum. Therefore, levels of PINP and PICP reflect the activity of osteogenesis. Both PINP and PICP are removed by the liver. Other than PICP, PINP can also be deposited directly into the bone matrix, and has been found to constitute 5% of the non-collagenous protein in bone. Data from the literature suggest that PINP has a greater diagnostic validity as compared to PICP (Brasso et al. 2006).

2.2 Bone Resorption Markers

By-products of osteolysis or osteoclast-secreted factors can provide insight into the activity of bone resorption (Table 2).

2.2.1 Pyridinoline and Deoxypyridinoline

Pyridinoline (PYD) and deoxypyridinoline (DPD) are products of the posttranslational modification of lysine and hydroxylysine. They stabilize mature type-1 collagen in bone, cross-linking the telopeptide domain of a collagen fibril to the helical region of an adjacent collagen fibril. Bone resorption results in a release of PYD and DPD into the blood, followed by renal excretion. DPD is found almost exclusively in bone. The contribution from soft tissues to the systems pool of PYD might make the latter less accurate than other bone markers.

2.2.2 C-telopeptide and N-telopeptide of Type I Collagen

C-terminal cross-linked telopeptide of type I collagen (CTx) and N-terminal cross-linked telopeptide of type I collagen (NTx) are the carboxyterminal and aminoterminal peptides, respectively, of mature type I collagen, and both are released during bone resorption. Degradation products of collagen are of various sizes, i.e. osteoclast-derived fragments are different from those formed in non-skeletal tissues. The CTx peptide exists as α or β-isoforms, with β-isoforms found more often in mature bone. Both CTx and NTx can be analyzed in serum or urine, but urinary concentrations must be adjusted for urine dilution, which may add to the analytical error. Because CTx levels were less elevated in patients with Paget's disease as compared to NTx, and more elevated in patients with hyperthyroidism (Calvo et al. 1996), serum concentrations of NTx might be more specific to processes in the bone as compare to CTx.

2.2.3 Carboxyterminal Cross-Linked Telopeptide of Type I Collagen

Carboxyterminal cross-linked telopeptide of type I collagen generated by metalloproteinases (ICTP) is another metabolic product of mature type I collagen resorption, that is usually detected by immunoassays against the telopeptide portion of the collagen fragment between the two α1-chains. Increased levels of serum ICTP correlate with bone resorption. Importantly, cathepsin K-mediated bone resorption by osteoclasts cleaves the collagen at the antigenic site, and the resulting ICTP fragment is not detected by conventional immunoassays (Sassi et al. 2000). This might explain why ICTP is less sensitive for more physiological changes in bone turnover such as those accompanied by treatment with estrogen or bisphosphonates (Coleman et al. 2008).

2.2.4 Tartrate-Resistant Acid Phosphatase Type 5b

Tartrate-resistant acid phosphatase type 5b (TRAcP-5b) is secreted primarily by activated osteoclasts and is one of two isoforms detected in human serum. Activated macrophages secrete the TRAcP-5a isoform. Osteoclasts secrete the active enzyme TRAcP-5b, before it enters the circulation, where it is inactivated. Serum TRAcP-5b levels are analyzed by immunoassays, and they have been shown to be a good surrogate for bone resorption.

2.3 Osteoclast Regulators: Receptor Activator of Nuclear Factor-κB Ligand/Osteoprotegerin

Receptor activator of nuclear factor-κB (RANK) and its ligand (RANKL) are required for osteoclastogenesis. RANKL (also referred to as OPGL, TRANCE or ODF) is a member of the tumor necrosis factor (TNF) family of cytokines that binds to its receptor RANK to control osteoclast differentiation, activation and survival (Jones et al. 2006). Osteoprotegerin (OPG) is a soluble decoy receptor for RANKL that blocks ligand binding to RANK, thereby preventing the signaling required for osteoclast differentiation and activation (Teitelbaum 2000). In preclinical models of bone metastases secondary to melanoma or prostate cancer, neutralization of RANKL by OPG resulted in a marked reduction in tumor burden in bones, but not in other organs (Jones et al. 2006). These data revealed that local differentiation factors, such as RANKL, play an important role in cell migration in a metastatic tissue-specific manner (*reviewed in* Mori et al. 2009). In a retrospective analysis, Santini et al. analyzed RANK immunoexpression in tissue from bone metastases from 74 patients with solid tumors, and found a high concordance between RANK immunoexpression in bone metastases and the corresponding primary tumor (Santini et al. 2011). These data support the central role of the RANK/RANKL/OPG pathway in the development of bone metastases in solid tumor patients.

Serum levels of OPG and both soluble and total RANKL are assessed by immunoassay. Elevated levels of either protein alone or increases in the ratio of RANKL to OPG have been investigated as a prognostic tool in patients with bone metastases, with rather controversial results (Jung et al. 2004; Leeming et al. 2006).

2.4 Bone Sialoproteins

Histological studies have shown that the two sialoproteins, bone sialoprotein (BSP) and osteopontin (OPN) are induced in multiple types of cancer, and that serum concentrations of BSP and OPN are significantly higher in patients with various solid tumors as compared to healthy controls (Fedarko et al. 2001). BSP is a member of the Small Integrin-Binding Ligand N-linked Glycoprotein (SIBLING) family of proteins that also includes OPN, dentin matrix protein 1 (DMP1), dentin sialophosphoprotein, and matrix extracellular phosphoglycoprotein (Fisher and Fedarko 2003). BSP is a non-collagenous bone matrix protein secreted by osteoclasts, and is present in all mineralized tissues. Recent evidence suggests that—in the presence of RANKL—BSP might synergistically induce osteoclastogenesis (Valverde et al. 2005). BSP contributes to osteoclast survival and decreased apoptosis. Regulation of BSP activity is achieved through dephosphorylation by TRAcP (Ek-Rylander et al. 1994). Serum BSP levels are measured by immunoassays. Elevated serum BSP levels have been reported in patients with various solid malignancies (Jung et al. 2004; Fedarko et al. 2001) and in multiple myeloma (Woitge et al. 2001). Although many of the SIBLING proteins are predominately expressed in bone, several of these proteins have been shown to be aberrantly expressed in a variety of malignant tumors (Fisher et al. 2004), and expression of BSP in these tumors has been proposed to play a role in the homing of tumor cells to the bone, and in the enhanced survival of tumor cells in the bone microenvironment (Jain et al. 2002). Bone sialoprotein is expressed by many malignant tissues, including breast, prostate (Waltregny et al. 2000), lung (Bellahcene et al. 1997) and several other cancer types (Fisher et al. 2004), and BSP expression is markedly lower in visceral metastases as compared to bone metastases in human breast and prostate cancers, suggesting some role of BSP in the pathogenesis of bone metastases (Waltregny et al. 2000). BSP-integrin interactions are important to stimulate the migration of tumor-derived cells. Although the specific mechanisms by which BSP stimulates migration are not known, it has been reported that BSP can increase the invasiveness of cancer cells by forming a trimolecular complex with integrins and the matrix metalloproteinase MMP-2 (gelatinase A), increasing localized matrix degradation (Karadag et al. 2004). While BSP may play an important role as an adaptor molecule participating in the attachment of proteins to the cell surface of migrating cells, the protein may also play a more direct role, stimulating molecular signals at the focal adhesion resulting in expression of pro-metastatic factors.

Serum concentrations of BSP have been shown to correlate with markers of bone resorption in malignant bone disease and are often elevated in patients with tumors metastatic to bone (Seibel et al. 1996). Of particular interest, the highest levels seemed to occur in patients with bone metastases from cancers that are known to express BSP ectopically, such as breast, prostate or thyroid cancers (Bellahcene et al. 1996).

3 Prognostic Use of Bone Markers

There are accumulating data describing the association between specific bone markers and the outcome with respect to skeletal-related events (SRE) in patients with bone metastases from malignant tumors. At the same time, there are only limited data on the prognostic value of bone markers in patients with early-stage cancer where no metastatic spread to the bones has been diagnosed. The term "prognostic markers" is used here for clinical studies that focus on the clinical outcome in patients receiving either no or standard anticancer treatment, in contrast to "predictive markers" that look at the clinical outcome with respect to a well-defined, often newer or experimental treatment. In 2005, Brown et al. studied 441 patients with bone metastases from various solid malignancies, and found high levels of urinary N-telopeptide (NTx) at the time of diagnosis to predict an increased risk of skeletal-related events (relative risk of 3.25 for prostate cancer, 1.79 for lung cancer and other tumors), disease progression (relative risk of 2.02 for prostate cancer, 1.91 for lung cancer and others), and death (relative risk of 4.59 for prostate cancer, 2.67 for lung cancer and others) as compared to patients with low NTx urinary levels (Brown et al. 2005). The authors concluded that high urinary NTx levels should prompt more aggressive treatment to prevent skeletal-related morbidity in patients with bone metastases from solid tumors (Brown et al. 2005). These data in patients with various malignant tumors suggest that bone markers such as urinary NTx are early surrogates for clinical outcome, and clinical studies on early prevention of skeletal events in cancer patients should stratify patients according to these markers. However, prospective validating studies are necessary if bone turnover markers are to be implemented into daily clinical practice. Below, clinical evidence on the prognostic value of various bone markers in breast-, prostate-, lung cancer and multiple myeloma is summarized.

Table 2 Markers of bone resorption and osteoclast regulators

Marker	Specimen	Normal range	Diagnostic use for bone metastases	Prognostic use for bone metastases
PYD	Urine	Adults: 19.5–25.1 nM/mM Cr (Coleman 2002)	High values associated with bone metastases in 153 cancer patients (Pecherstorfer et al. 1995) High values associated with bone metastases in prostate cancer patients (Ikeda et al. 1996)	
DPD	Urine	Adults: 1.8–15.5 μmol/mol (Pecherstorfer et al. 1997)	High values associated with bone metastases in 153 cancer patients (Pecherstorfer et al. 1995) High values associated with bone metastases in prostate cancer patients (Ikeda et al. 1996; Wymenga et al. 2001) High values associated with bone metastases in lung cancer patients (Dane et al. 2008)	
CTx	Urine	3.9–4.9 nM/mM Cr (Coleman 2002)	High values associated with bone metastases in breast cancer patients (Voorzanger-Rousselot et al. 2006)	
	Serum	PreM women: 0.29 ± 0.14 ng/mL (Souberbielle 2004) PostM women: 0.56 ± 0.23 ng/mL (Souberbielle 2004) Men: 0.30 ± 0.14 ng/mL (Souberbielle 2004)	High values associated with bone metastases in lung cancer patients (Kong et al. 2007)	

(continued)

Table 2 (continued)

Marker	Specimen	Normal range	Diagnostic use for bone metastases	Prognostic use for bone metastases
NTx	Urine	PreM women: 5–65 nM BCE/mM Cr (Osteomark 2008) Men: 3–63 nM BCE/mM Cr (Osteomark 2008)	High values associated with bone metastases in 276 cancer patients (Koizumi et al. 2003) High values associated with bone metastases in 97 cancer patients (Costa et al. 2002) High values associated with bone metastases in lung cancer patients (Chung et al. 2005)	High values predict SRE in 441 patients with predominantly prostate and lung cancer (Brown et al. 2005)
	Serum	Women: 6.2–19 nM BCE (Osteomark 2008) Men: 5.4–24.2 nM BCE (Osteomark 2008)		High values predict TTP and OS in 250 patients with metastatic breast cancer (Ali et al. 2004)
ICTP	Serum	Adults: 0.76–5.24 ng/mL (Shimozuma et al. 1999)	High values associated with bone metastases in 97 cancer patients (Costa et al. 2002) High values associated with bone metastases in breast cancer patients (Ulrich et al. 2001; Wada et al. 2004) High values associated with bone metastases in lung cancer patients (Aruga et al. 1997) High values associated with bone metastases in lung cancer patients (Kong et al. 2007)	High values predict OS in 141 patients with mainly early-stage NSCLC (Ylisirnio et al. 2001) High values predict OS in 313 patients with multiple myeloma (Fonseca et al. 2000)
TRAcP-5b	Plasma/serum	PreM. women: 0.5–3.8 U/L (Terpos et al. 2004) PostM. women: 0.5–4.8 U/L (Terpos et al. 2004)	High values associated with bone metastases in 276 cancer patients (Koizumi et al. 2003) High values associated with bone metastases in breast cancer patients (Voorzanger-Rousselot et al. 2006; Capeller et al. 2003; Chao et al. 2004; Korpela et al. 2006)	Low values predict relapse in bone in 79 patients with newly diagnosed NSCLC (Terpos et al. 2009)

(continued)

Diagnostic and Prognostic Use

Table 2 (continued)

Marker	Specimen	Normal range	Diagnostic use for bone metastases	Prognostic use for bone metastases
BSP	Serum	Men: 0.5–3.8 U/L (Coleman 2002) Adults: 8.0–9.4 ug/L (Coleman 2002)		High values predict relapse in bone in 388 early breast cancer patients (Diel et al. 1999) High values predict OS in 62 patients with multiple myeloma (Woitge et al. 2001)
	Tumor tissue			High tumor expression in 454 early breast cancer patients predicts relapse in bone and OS (Bellahcene et al. 1996) High tumor expression in 180 patients with prostate cancer predicts biochemical relapse (Waltregny et al. 1998) High expression predicts relapse in bone in 180 patients with resected NSCLC (Zhang et al. 2010)
RANKL	Plasma/serum	Adults: 0.80 ± 0.40 pmol/L (Morena et al. 2006)	High values associated with bone metastases in lung cancer patients (Karapanagiotou et al. 2010)	RANKL/OPG ratio in serum predicts OS in 121 patients with multiple myeloma (Terpos et al. 2009)
OPG	Plasma/serum	Adults: 2.42 ± 0.26 ng/L (Guang-da et al. 2005)	High values associated with bone metastases in prostate cancer patients (Jung et al. 2001; Narita et al. 2008; Aruga et al. 1997)	

Abbreviations PYD Pyridinoline, *DPD* Deoxypyridinoline, *CTx* C-telopeptide of type 1 collagen, *NTx* N-telopeptide of type 1 collagen, *ICTP* Carboxyterminal cross-linked telopeptide of type 1 collagen, *TRAcP-5b* Tartrate-resistant acid phosphatase type 5b, *BSP* bone sialoprotein, *RANKL* Receptor activator of nuclear factor-kB ligand, *OPG* Osteoprotegerin, *PreM* premenopausal, *PostM* postmenopausal

3.1 Prognostic Use of Bone Markers in Breast Cancer

Some interesting results have been published that assessed the prognostic value of various bone markers in patients with early or metastatic breast cancer. In 2001, Jukkola et al. assessed the prognostic value of PINP, PICP and ICTP in 373 patients with node-positive early breast cancer (Jukkola et al. 2001). Mean levels of PINP in serum were significantly elevated in patients who developed metastatic disease *in the follow-up* as compared to patients without tumor relapse in the bones. When patients with only bone metastases were compared with those not exhibiting bone metastases, PINP concentrations in serum were significantly higher in the group with recurrence in the bone, but there were no significant differences in serum PINP, PICP or ICTP values between patients with only bone metastases and those who developed soft or visceral metastases during the follow-up (Jukkola et al. 2001). These data were recently confirmed by a subgroup analysis of a randomized, double-blind placebo-controlled study in women with early breast cancer receiving either standard adjuvant therapy plus oral clodronate ($n = 419$) or placebo ($n = 432$) for 2 years (McCloskey et al. 2010). In the 230 women receiving oral clodronate and having paired measurements of PINP at baseline and after one year, there was a significant relationship between changes in serum PINP and the subsequent development of bone metastases. Women experiencing increasing serum PINP levels after one year of oral clodronate had a 20.8% risk of subsequent development of bone metastases (McCloskey et al. 2010). In 2004, Ali et al. found serum NTx levels to predict the time to progression (TTP) and overall survival (OS) in 250 patients with metastatic breast cancer (Ali et al. 2004). Time to progression was significantly shorter in patients with elevated serum NTx concentrations as compared to those with low NTx levels (139 as compared to 220 days, $p < 0.001$).

Recently, BSP has emerged as a new marker of bone resorption in breast cancer patients with bone metastases. Using a retrospective study design, Bellahcene et al. found that the amount of BSP expressed in breast cancer tissues (as assessed by semiquantitative immunohistochemistry) correlated with the propensity of the cancer to metastasize to the bones (Bellahcene et al. 1996). Some years later, Diel et al. performed a two-year prospective study, showing that serum BSP concentrations were highly predictive of future bone metastases in women with newly diagnosed, early breast cancer (Diel et al. 1999). Women with breast cancer and elevated serum BSP levels at baseline (i.e. before surgical tumorectomy) had a significantly increased risk of developing bone metastases as compared to patients with normal baseline BSP concentrations. Furthermore, these clinical data are supported by preclinical data, in that the expression of BSP has been demonstrated to be sufficient to promote skeletal metastasis in non-osteotropic cells (Zhang et al. 2004). A recent study by Tu et al. has demonstrated that the transgenic overexpression of BSP resulted in increased skeletal as well as systemic metastases in a murine breast cancer model (Tu et al. 2009). This evidence would strongly implicate BSP in promoting skeletal metastases in malignant tumors.

Finally, a large ongoing phase III clinical study assesses the value of "fixed" versus "marker-directed" dosing of zoledronic acid in 1400 patients with advanced breast cancer metastatic to bones, with SRE being the primary study endpoint (Coleman et al. 2008, BISMARK trial). In this study, zoledronic acid is given at 3–4 weekly intervals in patients with serum Ntx > 100 nM, at 8–9 weekly intervals in patients with serum Ntx between 50 and 100 nM, and in 15–16 weekly intervals in patients with serum Ntx < 50 nM. In the conventional study arm, zoledronic acid is given at 4 mg i.v. every 3–4 weeks.

3.2 Prognostic Use of Bone Markers in Prostate Cancer

Similar to studies in breast cancer (Bellahcene et al. 1996; Diel et al. 1999), tissue expression of BSP in prostate cancer might enable the identification of subgroups of patients who are at high risk for developing bone metastases or disease recurrence (De Pinieux et al. 2001). In 2001, Waltregny et al. analyzed immunohistochemical expression of BSP in 180 prostatectomy specimens for localized prostate cancer (Waltregny et al. 1998). Most of the prostate cancer lesions examined expressed BSP (78%), compared with no or low expression in the adjacent normal glandular tissue. Although a significant association was found between BSP expression and biochemical progression of prostate cancer, follow-up was too short to determine whether overexpression of BSP was also a predictor for the development of bone metastases (Waltregny et al. 1998). A recent study by Ramankulov et al. suggests that plasma concentrations of another non-collagenous bone protein, OPN, alone or in combination with other bone markers, may be useful as a diagnostic and prognostic marker in the detection of bone metastases in patients with prostate cancer (Ramankulov et al. 2007).

3.3 Prognostic Use of Bone Markers in Lung Cancer

In 2001, Ylisirnio et al. assessed serum concentrations of PINP, PICP and ICTP in 141 patients with mainly early-stage non small-cell lung cancer (NSCLC) (Ylisirnio et al. 2001). Patients with elevated serum concentrations of ICTP (>5ug/L) had a 64% higher risk of dying from lung cancer as compared to patients with low ICTP serum concentrations. However, the inclusion of patients with various stages of lung cancer makes interpretation of this study difficult. In a recent clinical study, Terpos et al. assessed the prognostic value of several bone markers in serum from 79 patients with newly diagnosed NSCLC (Terpos et al. 2009). Patients who later developed bone metastasis had decreased osteocalcin (Bauer et al. 2006) and TRAcP-5b concentrations as compared to those patients who never developed bone metastases (Terpos et al. 2009). In a case-control study, 30 patients with NSCLC who subsequently developed bone metastases were matched for clinicopathologic parameters to 30 control patients with resected NSCLC without any metastases and 26 patients with resected NSCLC and non-bone metastases, and the immunohistochemical expression of BSP in the primary cancer was reported to be associated with the progression of distant bone metastases (Papotti et al. 2006). This suggests that measuring BSP expression levels in lung cancers may be helpful in identifying patients at high risk to develop bone metastases (Papotti et al. 2006). However, this comes with the necessity of cross-laboratory validation of the immunohistochemical bioassay. This hypothesis is further supported by very recent data from Zhang et al., who showed BSP immunohistochemical expression in resected primary tumors from 180 Chinese NSCLC patients to be stronger in 40 out of the 180 patients who later developed bone metastases as compared to the other patients (Zhang et al. 2010). At the same time, tumor expression of OP was not a significant predictor of the development of bone metastases.

3.4 Prognostic Use of Bone Markers in Multiple Myeloma

In 2003, Tian et al. showed expression of dickkopf 1 (DKK1), an inhibitor of osteoblast differentiation, in myeloma cells from lytic tumors to inhibit osteoblasts (Tian et al. 2003). Additionally, myeloma cells express the receptor activator of nuclear factor κB ligand (RANKL), a major driver of osteoclastogenesis. Therefore, the simultaneous overexpression of RANKL and DKK1 by myeloma cells greatly increases bone resorption while inhibiting osteoblast differentiation and bone formation. In 1997, Pecherstorfer et al. published a study were they looked at urinary PYD in 50 patients with newly diagnosed and untreated MM, 40 patients with MGUS, 40 untreated patients with osteoporotic vertebral fractures, and 64 healthy adults (Pecherstorfer et al. 1997). Patients with MM had significantly higher levels of urinary DPD as compared to healthy adults, patients with monoclonal gammopathy of undetermined significance (MGUS) or patients with postmenopausal osteoporosis. In one of three patients progressing from initial MGUS into stage I MM, urinary DPD increased above the upper limit of the normal range, while it remained normal in 13 patients with stable MGUS. In general, urinary DPD had low sensitivities to predict the changes in monoclonal protein in stage I and II MM (<50%), but increased to 93% in stage III MM. Although urinary DPD correctly identified patients with advanced MM (stage III), the test did not discriminate between patients with MGUS, or with early (stage I) MM or osteoporosis, probably because bone resorption rates are similarly low in MGUS and early stage MM (Pecherstorfer et al. 1997).

There is a role for serum osteocalcin (Bauer et al. 2006) and BSP as prognostic markers in patients with MM, as suggested by some clinical studies. Back in 1990, Bataille et al. quantified OC in bone marrow tissue from crest biopsies and in serum from 19 patients with MM (Bataille et al. 1990). Reduced serum OC levels were shown to be associated with rapid disease progression and poor survival, probably as a consequence of impaired osteoblast activity (Bataille et al. 1990).

However, this association was not confirmed in other studies (Carlson et al. 1999; Mejjad et al. 1996), and more recent studies indicate that serum ICTP concentrations are a better prognostic marker in MM as compared to other biochemical indices (Abildgaard et al. 1998; Fonseca et al. 2000). Furthermore, Woitge et al. studied serum BSP in 62 patients with newly diagnosed MM followed over a period of four years, in 46 patients with monoclonal gammopathy of undetermined significance MGUS, in 71 patients with untreated benign vertebral osteoporosis and in 139 healthy controls (Woitge et al. 2001). Serum BSP concentrations increased with disease progression and higher serum concentrations of BSP distinguished between MM and benign osteoporosis, and were associated with shorter survival time in those patients suffering from MM (Woitge et al. 2001). Finally, Terpos et al. studied the prognostic value of serum RANKL and OPG in 121 patients with newly diagnosed MM to evaluate their role in bone disease and patient survival.

Serum levels of sRANKL were elevated in patients with MM and correlated with the extent of bone disease. Additionally, the RANKL/OPG ratio in serum, C-reactive protein (CRP), and β2-microglobulin were the final prognostic factors for overall survival within multivariate analysis. The authors generated a prognostic index based on these factors, categorizing patients into three risk groups (Terpos et al. 2003). These data suggest bone markers to be of distinct clinical value in predicting outcome in patients with multiple myeloma. Presently, a U.S. clinical study is assessing the optimal dosing schedule of bisphosphonates in patients with multiple myeloma according to urine NTx concentrations.

4 Diagnostic Use of Bone Markers

The early diagnosis of metastatic spread to the bones in patients with known malignant disease might be beneficial, as this allows the early initiation of bone-targeted treatment, which may avoid or delay secondary complications such as bone pain and immobility. We might call this secondary prophylaxis or prevention of skeletal-related events (SRE) due to malignant bone disease. Most studies in this area have compared biochemical markers of bone turnover between groups of cancer patients with or without established bone metastases. While this is a sensible and straightforward approach, its validity largely depends on a correct diagnosis in the "negative" group, that is the group of cancer patients declared to be free of skeletal disease. Given the different techniques used to prove the absence of malignant bone lesions, the assumption of a "negative status" might not always be correct. Additionally, many studies have included patients with various solid malignancies, and this might also lead to some bias. Lastly, the potential association between total tumor burden and the respective bone markers is usually not reported, although this would substantially support the rational for using bone turnover markers in the clinic. Not surprisingly, the available information on the diagnostic use of bone markers in metastatic bone disease is controversial. However, the picture becomes more consistent when comparisons are made between a marker of bone turnover and specific imaging techniques, in particular bone radioisotope scans in well-defined groups of patients (Ebert et al. 2004; Meijer et al. 2003).

4.1 Diagnostic Use of Bone Markers in Various Tumors

In 2003, Oremek et al. published a study that assessed the diagnostic value of serum BSAP and PICP in 200 patients with various newly-diagnosed or progressive solid tumors (Oremek et al. 2003). Both BSAP and PICP were elevated in patients with confirmed metastases to the bone, and the quantitative elevation of PICP and BSAP was correlated with tumor burden in the bones. Similarly, Koizumi et al. found serum NTx and TRAcP-5b to be of value for the diagnosis of bone metastatic disease in 75 cancer patients with as compared to 201 cancer patients without skeletal metastases (Koizumi et al. 2003). Pecherstorfer et al. performed a similar cross-sectional study of 153 patients with various solid tumors and an equal number of matched healthy controls, and analyzed serum levels of calcium, total AP, urinary excretion of calcium, PYD and DPD (Pecherstorfer et al. 1995). Within the total of cancer patients, individuals with skeletal metastases had higher serum concentrations of calcium, total AP, urinary PYD and DPD, as compared to patients without evidence of malignant bone disease. Urinary calcium however did not differ between cancer patients with or without bone metastases (Pecherstorfer et al. 1995). However, a significant proportion of cancer patients without any evidence of malignant bone involvement also had elevated urinary levels of DPD, and it remains unclear if these patients later developed overt metastatic disease of the bone (Pecherstorfer et al. 1995). Finally, Costa et al. studied serum bone-specific alkaline phophatase (BSAP), C-telopeptide of type-I collagen (ICTP) and urine levels of NTx in 97 cancer patients with either metastases to the bones or extraskeletal tissues (Costa et al. 2002). There was a marked and significant increase of urinary NTx by 152%, and serum ICTP of 144% in patients at the time of disease progression in the bones, and this was independent of bisphosphonate treatment. At the same time, extraskeletal disease had no effect on bone markers. The studies by Oremek and Costa suggest that there is a consistent rise of bone-specific alkaline phosphatase (BSAP) in patients with various malignant tumors and newly detected bone metastases (Oremek et al. 2003; Costa et al. 2002). However, this has not been confirmed in another study by Jung et al. (Jung et al. 2006). In the latter study, NTx, TRAcP-5b, OPG and RANKL were analyzed in the serum of 72 patients with renal-cell carcinoma and in 68 healthy controls. No bone marker led to the differentiation between patients with bone and those with non-bone metastases (Jung et al. 2006).

4.2 Diagnostic Use of Bone Markers in Breast Cancer

In 1991, Paterson et al. compared urinary PYD and DPD in 10 patients with bone metastases with 10 breast cancer patients without bone metastases, and found a non-significant difference for the bone markers between the groups (Paterson et al. 1991). Eight out of the 10 patients with metastases had above average urinary crosslinks, but sensitivity was low. Therefore, the analysis of urinary PYD/DPD is not recommended for diagnostic purposes in patients with breast cancer. In another clinical study, Keskikuru et al. analyzed preoperative serum levels of PINP, PICP and ICTP in 138 women with breast cancer and 94 women with benign breast disease, both before undergoing local tumorectomy, and 100 healthy controls (Keskikuru et al. 1999). While the sensitivity of these bone markers was low for discriminating breast cancer patients from non-cancer patients, a tendency toward higher serum levels of PINP and low PICP/PINP ratio was found in patients with advanced stage IV breast cancer (Keskikuru et al. 1999). Ulrich et al. compared urinary NTx, serum ICTP and serum BSAP in 106 breast cancer patients with ($n = 19$) and without ($n = 87$) bone metastases as diagnosed by bone scintigraphy (Ulrich et al. 2001). Serum ICTP best discriminated between patients with bone metastases compared to those without bone metastases, with a specificity of 91%, but a sensitivity of only 65%. The authors concluded that the sensitivity of these three markers did not seem to be sufficient enough for early identification of patients with subclinical bone metastases from breast cancer. Similar results were reported by Wada et al. who compared serum ICTP, TRAcP, urinary NTx and serum AP in 114 breast cancer patients without bone metastases, 23 patients with bone metastases and 19 patients with extraosseous metastases (Wada et al. 2004). Serum concentrations of ICTP and TRAcP were significantly higher in patients with bone metastases, and there was also a positive association between the amount of metastatic bone disease in bone scintigraphy and the concentrations of ICTP and TRAcP (Wada et al. 2004). In 2005, Lüftner et al. analyzed serum PINP as a potential marker of metastatic spread to the bones in 38 breast cancer patients with bone metastases and 24 patients without bone metastases (Luftner et al. 2005). The authors found a sensitivity of 50% for serum PINP to predict bone metastases at the threshold concentration of 95 ng/mL, and there was a positive association between elevated serum PINP and the amount of metastatic bone involved. The authors hypothesized that the low sensitivity for the diagnosis of bone metastases might be biologically related to ineffective bone repair in certain patients (Luftner et al. 2005). A further study compared various serum biochemical markers of angiogenesis, tumor invasion and bone turnover in 29 breast cancer patients without bone metastases, 28 patients with bone metastases and 15 healthy women (Voorzanger-Rousselot et al. 2006). Importantly, the authors were also able to assess these markers over a time of three years in 34 patients, of whom 15 patients developed bone metastases and 19 remained free of bone metastases. All bone markers were significantly higher in patients with bone metastases as compared to patients without bone metastases and healthy controls. The bone resorption markers TRAcP-5b, CTx and ICTP and the marker of angiogenesis VEGF were independently associated with bone metastases within multivariate analysis. These four markers correctly distinguished 85% of breast cancer patients with bone metastases from patients without bone metastases or healthy controls. Patients with primary breast cancer who developed bone metastases during follow-up had higher serum levels of TRAcP-5b (+95%,) at the time of primary diagnosis and higher increases of ICTP during follow-up as compared to patients who did not progress to bone metastases (Voorzanger-Rousselot et al. 2006). Overall, markers of bone resorption had the highest independent diagnostic value for detecting and potentially predicting bone metastases in breast cancer patients. Three studies in breast cancer patients assessed serum TRAcP-5b (Capeller et al. 2003; Chao et al. 2004; Korpela et al. 2006), a more specific marker as compared to TRAcP. In the studies by Chao et al., Capeller et al. and Korpela et al., serum TRAcP-5b was found to be a good surrogate for bone metastases in breast cancer patients when compared to patients without bone metastases and healthy controls (Capeller et al. 2003; Chao et al. 2004; Korpela et al. 2006). In the study by Chao et al., the sensitivity of TRAcP-5b to identify bone metastases in breast cancer was 73%, while specificity was 83% (Chao et al. 2004).

4.3 Diagnostic Use of Bone Markers in Prostate Cancer

In patients with prostate cancer, Ikeda et al. studied the diagnostic value of urinary pyridinoline (PYD) and deoxypyridinoline (DPD) for bone metastases in 15 patients with benign prostatic hypertrophy (BPH) versus 17 patients with carcinoma clinically confined to the prostate and 26 patients with overt bone metastatic disease (Ikeda et al. 1996). Urinary PYD and DPD clearly discriminated between patients with or without bone metastases, and patients receiving successful endocrine treatment for metastatic prostatic cancer had suppressed urinary PYD and DPD levels (Ikeda et al. 1996). Further studies in patients with prostate cancer showed that bone markers such as BSAP increased the diagnostic value of PSA for the diagnosis of bone metastases in patients with prostate cancer (Lorente et al. 1999; Wymenga et al. 2001). In the study by Lorente et al., serum BSAP showed a statistically significant association with the extent of malignant bone disease in 295 patients with newly diagnosed, untreated prostate cancer, 93 of whom had bone metastases on bone scan (Lorente et al. 1999). Interestingly, serum PSA concentrations did not show a significant association with the extent of bone metastases, but the combination of both serum BSAP and PSA was still the best predictor for malignant bone disease in multivariate logistic regression analysis, with a positive predictive value of 46.5% and a negative predictive value of 100% (Lorente et al. 1999). By adding BSAP to PSA for diagnosing metastatic spread to the bones, 32% of initial bone scans could be avoided. Similarly, Wymenga et al. showed that patients with newly diagnosed prostate cancer and bone metastasis had higher urinary DPD levels, and higher serum PSA and AP concentrations as compared to patients with localized prostate cancer (Wymenga et al. 2001). In the latter study, bone scans were taken as the "gold standard" for the diagnosis of bone metastases. Importantly, bone markers were more specific toward pathological bone processes as compared to PSA that is also dependent on extraosseous malignant disease, and is also subjected to hormonal manipulation. In 2001, Koizumi et al. analyzed various markers such as PINP, PICP, BSAP, OP, ICTP and PSA in 40 patients without and 25 untreated patients with bone metastases from prostate cancer (Koizumi et al. 2001). The levels of serum PINP correlated best with the extent of malignant bone disease, with a sensitivity of 72% and a specificity of 90%, using a threshold level of 47 ng/mL (Koizumi et al. 2001). Similar results were found in 36 patients with early or advanced prostate cancer, were PINP was a potent discriminator of bone metastases, with mean serum PINP concentrations being 18.3, 24.9 and 122.5 ng/mL in patients with negative ($n = 24$), equivocal ($n = 5$) or positive ($n = 7$) bone scans (Thurairaja et al. 2006). This is supported by a further study from Thurairaja et al., who assessed PINP in serum of prostate cancer patients with ($n = 12$) or without ($n = 24$) bone metastases (Thurairaja et al. 2006). The authors found patients with positive bone scans to have significantly higher serum concentrations of PINP as compared to those not having positive bone scans (112 ng/ml as compared to 18.3 ng/ml). This is further supported by the study of Koopmans et al., who assessed serum PINP concentrations in 64 patients with prostate cancer treated between 1999 and 2004 (Koopmans et al. 2007). While serum PINP was a good discriminator of bone metastatic disease, increased PINP levels in patients with bone metastases were detectable up to 8 months before the first positive bone scintigraphy (Koopmans et al. 2007). These data would support the use of PINP concentrations in serum as an early marker for the risk of developing bone metastases from prostate cancer.

In 2001, Brown et al. assessed the diagnostic value of serum OP concentrations in 24 patients with advanced prostate cancer as compared to 25 patients with recurrent prostate cancer, 25 patients with early prostate cancer, 25 patients with benign prostate hyperplasia and 6 healthy volunteers (Brown et al. 2001). Serum OP concentrations were significantly higher in patients with advanced prostate cancer as compared to the other groups, but there was no correlation between serum OP and PSA values (Brown et al. 2001). More explicit results for OP have been reported by Jung et al., who found a significant association between serum OP and bone metastatic spread in 93 patients with prostate cancer as compared to 35 patients with BPH and 36 male healthy controls (Jung et al. 2001). In the study by Jung et al., the diagnostic sensitivity of serum OP for bone metastases was 88%, while specificity was 93%. These results were later confirmed by the same group in 117 patients with prostate cancer, including 44 patients with bone metastases (Jung et al. 2003). Serum OP was increased in patients with bone metastases, with a sensitivity of 95% and a specificity of 89% at a threshold concentration of 2.86 pmol/L. Additionally to serum OP concentrations, Narita et al. also assessed the influence of the two germline genetic polymorphisms 149T/C and 950T/C in the promoter region of the OP gene in 161 patients with prostate cancer as compared to 195 healthy controls (Narita et al. 2008). While there was no significant difference in the genotype frequencies between prostate cancer patients and healthy controls, serum OP concentrations increased with age in both prostate cancer patients and healthy controls. Additionally, OP serum concentrations were significantly higher in age-matched patients with metastatic prostate cancer as compared to patients without metastatic disease and healthy controls. These results suggest that aging and bone metastasis have a major effect on OP serum concentrations (Narita et al. 2008).

An ongoing clinical study looks at changes in serum PINP, ICTP and PSA in roughly 100 men with early prostate cancer, receiving weekly zoledronic acid for 3 months. The primary study endpoint is to assess the relationship between changes in bone parameters, PSA and bone scans with respect to bone metastases. This study will give some insight on whether bone turnover markers may spare bone scans in patients with early prostate cancer, although the study does not answer the question whether any such effect is independent on the administration of bisphosphonates.

4.4 Diagnostic Use of Bone Markers in Lung Cancer

In 1997, Aruga published a study comparing 47 lung cancer patients with bone metastases with 44 patients without bone metastases (Aruga et al. 1997). The authors found serum ICTP to have the highest sensitivity (71%) for the diagnosis of bone metastases, with a specificity of 88% and a threshold for serum ICTP of 4.9 ng/mL (Aruga et al. 1997). A similar analysis compared the diagnostic value of urinary NTx, urinary DPD and total AP in serum from 33 lung cancer patients with bone metastases as compared to 118 patients without bone metastases (Chung et al. 2005). The authors found urinary NTx to have the highest sensitivity (73%) and specificity (84%) for the diagnosis of bone metastases, with a threshold level of 73 μmol/mol creatinine. Finally, Kong et al. analyzed serum ICTP, BSAP, CTx and osteocalcin (Bauer et al. 2006) in 96 male patients with NSCLC and 30 male patients with other pulmonary diseases (Kong et al. 2007). Serum concentrations of both CTx and ICTP were significantly higher in 61 lung cancer patients with bone metastases as compared to 35 lung cancer patients without bone metastases, and significantly correlated with the extent of bone disease. Although ICTP had a better sensitivity (75% versus 66%) and accuracy (73% versus 69%) as compared to CTx, they had a similar area under the receiver operating characteristic curve (0.85 vs. 0.83, respectively). In a Chinese study, Kong et al. analyzed CTx and ICTP, OC and BSAP in 96 male patients with NSCLC and 30 male patients with other pulmonary diseases (Kong et al. 2007). Serum concentrations of CTx and ICTP were significantly higher in 61 lung cancer patients with bone metastases as compared to 35 patients without bone metastases ($p < 0.001$), and significantly correlated with the extent of malignant bone disease. Sensitivity was 75% and 72% for ICTP and CTx, respectively; accuracy was 65% and 68% for ICTP and CTx, respectively. Obviously, sensitivity is too low to justify using these bone markers for diagnostic purposes. In 2008, Dane et al. measured urinary DPD, calcium, serum osteocalcin and total AP in 60 lung cancer patients (Dane et al. 2008). When bone scintigraphy was performed on all patients, 22 patients turned out to have bone metastases, and urinary DPD levels were significantly higher in patients with bone metastases as compared to those without bone metastases (Dane et al. 2008). As a note of caution, both small-cell and non small-cell histologies were included into the study of Dane et al.. In a recent study, Karapanagiotou et al. analyzed the diagnostic value of serum turnover markers OC, RANKL and OPG in 22 NSCLC patients with bone metastases, 18 NSCLC patients without bone metastases, 28 small-cell lung cancer (SCLC) patients and 29 healthy volunteers (Karapanagiotou et al. 2010). Decreased OC serum levels and increased osteopontin and RANKL serum levels were found in NSCLC patients with bone metastases (Karapanagiotou et al. 2010).

5 Conclusions

Available information on the prognostic and diagnostic use of bone turnover markers in cancer patients is from small retrospective studies, and this does not allow to recommend their use in daily clinical practice at present. Many bioassays for bone turnover markers have not been validated, and this makes inter-study comparison difficult. Additionally, circadian variability may also render the correct interpretation of clinical studies difficult. However, there are some promising retrospective data on the prognostic and diagnostic value of bone turnover markers that should be validated in future clinical studies.

5.1 Prognostic Use of Bone Turnover Markers

There is some limited evidence for bone turnover markers to predict the occurrence of metachronous bone metastases in patients with early-stage malignant tumors, with serum PINP and ICTP being the most promising candidates (Jukkola et al. 2001; Voorzanger-Rousselot et al. 2006; Koopmans et al. 2007). Another promising bone turnover marker is BSP that is expressed in primary cancer tissues of various tumors, and is excreted into serum. Accordingly, serum concentrations of PINP, ICTP or BSP should prospectively be evaluated at the time of tumorectomy in patients with early solid tumors, to define the sensitivity and specificity of these markers in predicting tumor relapse in the bones. If validated, specific bone turnover markers may be implemented into clinical practice to enable clinicians to tailor adjuvant treatment to avoid bone metastatic seeding in patients with early solid tumors. Immunohistochemical expression of BSP in tumor tissue may be a valid alternative to serum markers, but proper validation of the respective assays is mandatory before evaluation in prospective clinical studies.

5.2 Diagnostic Use of Bone Turnover Markers

While serum BSAP, PINP and OP were repeatedly shown to be associated with synchronous bone metastases in patients with breast or lung cancer, sensitivity of these markers usually was too low to suggest that these bone turnover marker might be preferred over conventional bone scans for the diagnosis of bone metastases. A somewhat higher sensitivity for the diagnosis of bone metastases was found for urinary NTx and serum ICTP in solid tumor patients, serum TRAcP-5b in patients with breast cancer and serum BSAP, PINP and OPG in prostate cancer patients. Available data suggest that the most promising application would be to add BSAP, ICTP, PINP or OPG to PSA in prostate cancer patients with suspected bone metastases to spare conventional bone scans. This should be validated in adequately powered prospective clinical studies.

References

Abildgaard N, Rungby J, Glerup H, Brixen K, Kassem M, Brincker H, Heickendorff L, Eriksen EF, Nielsen JL (1998) Long-term oral pamidronate treatment inhibits osteoclastic bone resorption and bone turnover without affecting osteoblastic function in multiple myeloma. Eur J Haematol 61:128–134

Ali SM, Demers LM, Leitzel K, Harvey HA, Clemens D, Mallinak N, Engle L, Chinchilli V, Costa L, Brady C, Seaman J, Lipton A (2004) Baseline serum NTx levels are prognostic in metastatic breast cancer patients with bone-only metastasis. Ann Oncol 15:455–459

Aruga A, Koizumi M, Hotta R, Takahashi S, Ogata E (1997) Usefulness of bone metabolic markers in the diagnosis and follow-up of bone metastasis from lung cancer. Br J Cancer 76:760–764

Bataille R, Delmas PD, Chappard D, Sany J (1990) Abnormal serum bone Gla protein levels in multiple myeloma. Crucial role of bone formation and prognostic implications. Cancer 66:167–172

Bauer DC, Garnero P, Hochberg MC, Santora A, Delmas P, Ewing SK, Black DM (2006) Pretreatment levels of bone turnover and the antifracture efficacy of alendronate: the fracture intervention trial. J Bone Miner Res 21:292–299

Bellahcene A, Menard S, Bufalino R, Moreau L, Castronovo V (1996) Expression of bone sialoprotein in primary human breast cancer is associated with poor survival. Int J Cancer 69:350–353

Bellahcene A, Maloujahmoum N, Fisher LW, Pastorino H, Tagliabue E, Menard S, Castronovo V (1997) Expression of bone sialoprotein in human lung cancer. Calcif Tissue Int 61:183–188

Brasso K, Christensen IJ, Johansen JS, Teisner B, Garnero P, Price PA, Iversen P (2006) Prognostic value of PINP, bone alkaline phosphatase, CTX-I, and YKL-40 in patients with metastatic prostate carcinoma. Prostate 66:503–513

Brown JM, Vessella RL, Kostenuik PJ, Dunstan CR, Lange PH, Corey E (2001) Serum osteoprotegerin levels are increased in patients with advanced prostate cancer. Clin Cancer Res 7:2977–2983

Brown JE, Cook RJ, Major P, Lipton A, Saad F, Smith M, Lee KA, Zheng M, Hei YJ, Coleman RE (2005) Bone turnover markers as predictors of skeletal complications in prostate cancer, lung cancer, and other solid tumors. J Natl Cancer Inst 97:59–69

Caillot-Augusseau A, Lafage-Proust MH, Soler C, Pernod J, Dubois F, Alexandre C (1998) Bone formation and resorption biological markers in cosmonauts during and after a 180-day space flight (Euromir 95). Clin Chem 44:578–585

Calvo MS, Eyre DR, Gundberg CM (1996) Molecular basis and clinical application of biological markers of bone turnover. Endocr Rev 17:333–368

Capeller B, Caffier H, Sutterlin MW, Dietl J (2003) Evaluation of tartrate-resistant acid phosphatase (TRAP) 5b as serum marker of bone metastases in human breast cancer. Anticancer Res 23:1011–1015

Carlson K, Larsson A, Simonsson B, Turesson I, Westin J, Ljunghall S (1999) Evaluation of bone disease in multiple myeloma: a comparison between the resorption markers urinary deoxypyridinoline/creatinine (DPD) and serum ICTP, and an evaluation of the DPD/osteocalcin and ICTP/osteocalcin ratios. Eur J Haematol 62:300–306

Chao TY, Ho CL, Lee SH, Chen MM, Janckila A, Yam LT (2004) Tartrate-resistant acid phosphatase 5b as a serum marker of bone metastasis in breast cancer patients. J Biomed Sci 11:511–516

Chung JH, Park MS, Kim YS, Chang J, Kim JH, Kim SK (2005) Usefulness of bone metabolic markers in the diagnosis of bone metastasis from lung cancer. Yonsei Med J 46:388–393

Coleman RE (2002) The clinical use of bone resorption markers in patients with malignant bone disease. Cancer 94:2521–2533

Coleman J, Brown E, Terpos A, Lipton MR, Smith R, Cook P (2008) Major, bone markers and their prognostic value in metastatic bone disease: clinical evidence and future directions. Cancer Treat Rev 34:629–639

Costa L, Demers LM, Gouveia-Oliveira A, Schaller J, Costa EB, de Moura MC, Lipton A (2002) Prospective evaluation of the peptide-bound collagen type I cross-links N-telopeptide and C-telopeptide in predicting bone metastases status. J Clin Oncol 20:850–856

Dane F, Turk HM, Sevinc A, Buyukberber S, Camci C, Tarakcioglu M (2008) Markers of bone turnover in patients with lung cancer. J Natl Med Assoc 100:425–428

De Pinieux G, Flam T, Zerbib M, Taupin P, Bellahcene A, Waltregny D, Vieillefond A, Poupon MF (2001) Bone sialoprotein, bone morphogenetic protein 6 and thymidine phosphorylase expression in localized human prostatic adenocarcinoma as predictors of clinical outcome: a clinicopathological and immunohistochemical study of 43 cases. J Urol 166:1924–1930

Diel IJ, Solomayer EF, Seibel MJ, Pfeilschifter J, Maisenbacher H, Gollan C, Pecherstorfer M, Conradi R, Kehr G, Boehm E, Armbruster FP, Bastert G (1999) Serum bone sialoprotein in patients with primary breast cancer is a prognostic marker for subsequent bone metastasis. Clin Cancer Res 5:3914–3919

Ebert W, Muley T, Herb KP, Schmidt-Gayk H (2004) Comparison of bone scintigraphy with bone markers in the diagnosis of bone metastasis in lung carcinoma patients. Anticancer Res 24:3193–3201

Ek-Rylander B, Flores M, Wendel M, Heinegard D, Andersson G (1994) Dephosphorylation of osteopontin and bone sialoprotein by osteoclastic tartrate-resistant acid phosphatase. Modulation of osteoclast adhesion in vitro. J Biol Chem 269:14853–14856

Fedarko NS, Jain A, Karadag A, Van Eman MR, Fisher LW (2001) Elevated serum bone sialoprotein and osteopontin in colon, breast, prostate, and lung cancer. Clin Cancer Res 7:4060–4066

Fisher LW, Fedarko NS (2003) Six genes expressed in bones and teeth encode the current members of the SIBLING family of proteins. Connect Tissue Res 44(Suppl 1):33–40

Fisher LW, Jain A, Tayback M, Fedarko NS (2004) Small integrin binding ligand N-linked glycoprotein gene family expression in different cancers. Clin Cancer Res 10:8501–8511

Fonseca R, Trendle MC, Leong T, Kyle RA, Oken MM, Kay NE, Van Ness B, Greipp PR (2000) Prognostic value of serum markers of bone metabolism in untreated multiple myeloma patients. Br J Haematol 109:24–29

Guang-da X, Hui-ling S, Zhi-song C, Lin-shuang Z (2005) Changes in plasma concentrations of osteoprotegerin before and after levothyroxine replacement therapy in hypothyroid patients. J Clin Endocrinol Metab 90:5765–5768

Heuck JC, Wolthers OD (1998) A placebo-controlled study of three osteocalcin assays for assessment of prednisolone-induced suppression of bone turnover. J Endocrinol 159:127–131

Ikeda I, Miura T, Kondo I (1996) Pyridinium cross-links as urinary markers of bone metastases in patients with prostate cancer. Br J Urol 77:102–106

Ivaska KK, Pettersson K, Nenonen A, Uusi-Rasi K, Heinonen A, Kannus P, Vaananen HK (2005) Urinary osteocalcin is a useful marker for monitoring the effect of alendronate therapy. Clin Chem 51:2362–2365

Jain A, Karadag A, Fohr B, Fisher LW, Fedarko NS (2002) Three SIBLINGs (small integrin-binding ligand, N-linked glycoproteins) enhance factor H's cofactor activity enabling MCP-like cellular evasion of complement-mediated attack. J Biol Chem 277:13700–13708

Jones DH, Nakashima T, Sanchez OH, Kozieradzki I, Komarova SV, Sarosi I, Morony S, Rubin E, Sarao R, Hojilla CV, Komnenovic V, Kong YY, Schreiber M, Dixon SJ, Sims SM, Khokha R, Wada T, Penninger JM (2006) Regulation of cancer cell migration and bone metastasis by RANKL. Nature 440:692–696

Jukkola A, Bloigu R, Holli K, Joensuu H, Valavaara R, Risteli J, Blanco G (2001) Postoperative PINP in serum reflects metastatic potential and poor survival in node-positive breast cancer. Anticancer Res 21:2873–2876

Jung K, Lein M, von Hosslin K, Brux B, Schnorr D, Loening SA, Sinha P (2001) Osteoprotegerin in serum as a novel marker of bone metastatic spread in prostate cancer. Clin Chem 47:2061–2063

Jung K, Stephan C, Semjonow A, Lein M, Schnorr D, Loening SA (2003) Serum osteoprotegerin and receptor activator of nuclear factor-kappa B ligand as indicators of disturbed osteoclastogenesis in patients with prostate cancer. J Urol 170:2302–2305

Jung K, Lein M, Stephan C, Von Hosslin K, Semjonow A, Sinha P, Loening SA, Schnorr D (2004) Comparison of 10 serum bone turnover markers in prostate carcinoma patients with bone metastatic spread: diagnostic and prognostic implications. Int J Cancer 111:783–791

Jung K, Lein M, Ringsdorf M, Roigas J, Schnorr D, Loening SA, Staack A (2006) Diagnostic and prognostic validity of serum bone turnover markers in metastatic renal cell carcinoma. J Urol 176:1326–1331

Karadag A, Ogbureke KU, Fedarko NS, Fisher LW (2004) Bone sialoprotein, matrix metalloproteinase 2, and alpha(v)beta3 integrin in osteotropic cancer cell invasion. J Natl Cancer Inst 96:956–965

Karapanagiotou EM, Terpos E, Dilana KD, Alamara C, Gkiozos I, Polyzos A, Syrigos KN (2010) Serum bone turnover markers may be involved in the metastatic potential of lung cancer patients. Med Oncol 27:332–338

Keskikuru R, Kataja V, Kosma VM, Eskelinen M, Uusitupa M, Johansson R, Risteli L, Risteli J, Jukkola A (1999) Preoperative high type I collagen degradation marker ICTP reflects advanced breast cancer. Anticancer Res 19:4481–4484

Koizumi M, Yonese J, Fukui I, Ogata E (2001) The serum level of the amino-terminal propeptide of type I procollagen is a sensitive marker for prostate cancer metastasis to bone. BJU Int 87:348–351

Koizumi M, Takahashi S, Ogata E (2003) Comparison of serum bone resorption markers in the diagnosis of skeletal metastasis. Anticancer Res 23:4095–4099

Kong QQ, Sun TW, Dou QY, Li F, Tang Q, Pei FX, Tu CQ, Chen ZQ (2007) Beta-CTX and ICTP act as indicators of skeletal metastasis status in male patients with non-small cell lung cancer. Int J Biol Markers 22:214–220

Koopmans N, de Jong IJ, Breeuwsma AJ, van der Veer E (2007) Serum bone turnover markers (PINP and ICTP) for the early detection of bone metastases in patients with prostate cancer: a longitudinal approach. J Urol 178:849–853 discussion 853; quiz 1129

Korpela J, Tiitinen SL, Hiekkanen H, Halleen JM, Selander KS, Vaananen HK, Suominen P, Helenius H, Salminen E (2006) Serum TRACP 5b and ICTP as markers of bone metastases in breast cancer. Anticancer Res 26:3127–3132

Leeming DJ, Koizumi M, Byrjalsen I, Li B, Qvist P, Tanko LB (2006) The relative use of eight collagenous and noncollagenous markers for diagnosis of skeletal metastases in breast, prostate, or lung cancer patients. Cancer Epidemiol Biomarkers Prev 15:32–38

Lorente JA, Valenzuela H, Morote J, Gelabert A (1999) Serum bone alkaline phosphatase levels enhance the clinical utility of prostate specific antigen in the staging of newly diagnosed prostate cancer patients. Eur J Nucl Med 26:625–632

Luftner D, Jozereau D, Schildhauer S, Geppert R, Muller C, Fiolka G, Wernecke KD, Possinger K (2005) PINP as serum marker of metastatic spread to the bone in breast cancer patients. Anticancer Res 25:1491–1499

McCloskey E, Paterson A, Kanis J, Tahtela R, Powles T (2010) Effect of oral clodronate on bone mass, bone turnover and subsequent metastases in women with primary breast cancer. Eur J Cancer 46:558–565

Meijer WG, van der Veer E, Jager PL, van der Jagt EJ, Piers BA, Kema IP, de Vries EG, Willemse PH (2003) Bone metastases in carcinoid tumors: clinical features, imaging characteristics, and markers of bone metabolism. J Nucl Med 44:184–191

Mejjad O, Le Loet X, Basuyau JP, Menard JF, Jego P, Grisot C, Daragon A, Grosbois B, Euller-Ziegler L, Monconduit M (1996) Osteocalcin is not a marker of progress in multiple myeloma. Le Groupe d'Etude et de Recherche sur le Myelome (GERM). Eur J Haematol 56:30–34

Morena M, Terrier N, Jaussent I, Leray-Moragues H, Chalabi L, Rivory JP, Maurice F, Delcourt C, Cristol JP, Canaud B, Dupuy AM (2006) Plasma osteoprotegerin is associated with mortality in hemodialysis patients. J Am Soc Nephrol 17:262–270

Mori K, Ando K, Heymann D, Redini F (2009) Receptor activator of nuclear factor-kappa B ligand (RANKL) stimulates bone-associated tumors through functional RANK expressed on bone-associated cancer cells? Histol Histopathol 24:235–242

Narita N, Yuasa T, Tsuchiya N, Kumazawa T, Narita S, Inoue T, Ma Z, Saito M, Horikawa Y, Satoh S, Ogawa O, Habuchi T (2008) A genetic polymorphism of the osteoprotegerin gene is associated with an increased risk of advanced prostate cancer. BMC Cancer 8:224

Nguyen TV, Meier C, Center JR, Eisman JA, Seibel MJ (2007) Bone turnover in elderly men: relationships to change in bone mineral density. BMC Musculoskelet Disord 8:13

Oremek GM, Weis A, Sapoutzis N, Sauer-Eppel H (2003) Diagnostic value of bone and tumour markers in patients with malignant diseases. Anticancer Res 23:987–990

Osteomark NTX (2008) Accurate answers for osteoporosis patient management: urine ELISA, serum ELISA. http://www.osteomark.com/UEPerformance.cfm

Papotti M, Kalebic T, Volante M, Chiusa L, Bacillo E, Cappia S, Lausi P, Novello S, Borasio P, Scagliotti GV (2006) Bone sialoprotein is predictive of bone metastases in resectable non-small-cell lung cancer: a retrospective case-control study. J Clin Oncol 24:4818–4824

Paterson CR, Robins SP, Horobin JM, Preece PE, Cuschieri A (1991) Pyridinium crosslinks as markers of bone resorption in patients with breast cancer. Br J Cancer 64:884–886

Pecherstorfer M, Zimmer-Roth I, Schilling T, Woitge HW, Schmidt H, Baumgartner G, Thiebaud D, Ludwig H, Seibel MJ (1995) The diagnostic value of urinary pyridinium cross-links of collagen, serum total alkaline phosphatase, and urinary calcium excretion in neoplastic bone disease. J Clin Endocrinol Metab 80:97–103

Pecherstorfer M, Seibel MJ, Woitge HW, Horn E, Schuster J, Neuda J, Sagaster P, Kohn H, Bayer P, Thiebaud D, Ludwig H (1997) Bone resorption in multiple myeloma and in monoclonal gammopathy of undetermined significance: quantification by urinary pyridinium cross-links of collagen. Blood 90:3743–3750

Puistola U, Risteli L, Kauppila A, Knip M, Risteli J (1993) Markers of type I and type III collagen synthesis in serum as indicators of tissue growth during pregnancy. J Clin Endocrinol Metab 77:178–182

Ramankulov A, Lein M, Kristiansen G, Loening SA, Jung K (2007) Plasma osteopontin in comparison with bone markers as indicator of bone metastasis and survival outcome in patients with prostate cancer. Prostate 67:330–340

Santini D, Perrone G, Roato I, Godio L, Pantano F, Grasso D, Russo A, Vincenzi B, Fratto ME, Sabbatini R, Della Pepa C, Porta C, Del Conte A, Schiavon G, Berruti A, Tomasino RM, Papotti M, Papapietro N, Onetti Muda A, Denaro V, Tonini G (2011) Expression pattern of receptor activator of NFkappaB (RANK) in a series of primary solid tumors and related bone metastases. J Cell Physiol 226:780–784

Sassi ML, Eriksen H, Risteli L, Niemi S, Mansell J, Gowen M, Risteli J (2000) Immunochemical characterization of assay for carboxyterminal telopeptide of human type I collagen: loss of antigenicity by treatment with cathepsin K. Bone 26:367–373

Seibel MJ, Woitge HW, Pecherstorfer M, Karmatschek M, Horn E, Ludwig H, Armbruster FP, Ziegler R (1996) Serum immunoreactive bone sialoprotein as a new marker of bone turnover in metabolic and malignant bone disease. J Clin Endocrinol Metab 81:3289–3294

Shimozuma K, Sonoo H, Fukunaga M, Ichihara K, Aoyama T, Tanaka K (1999) Biochemical markers of bone turnover in breast cancer patients with bone metastases: a preliminary report. Jpn J Clin Oncol 29:16–22

Souberbielle JC (2004) Exploration biologique des osteoporoses. Medicine Nucleaire - Imagerie fonctionelle et metabolique 28(2):77–84

Teitelbaum SL (2000) Bone resorption by osteoclasts. Science 289:1504–1508

Terpos E, Szydlo R, Apperley JF, Hatjiharissi E, Politou M, Meletis J, Viniou N, Yataganas X, Goldman JM, Rahemtulla A (2003) Soluble receptor activator of nuclear factor kappaB ligand-osteoprotegerin ratio predicts survival in multiple myeloma: proposal for a novel prognostic index. Blood 102:1064–1069

Terpos E, Politou M, Szydlo R, Nadal E, Avery S, Olavarria E, Kanfer E, Goldman JM, Apperley JF, Rahemtulla A (2004) Autologous stem cell transplantation normalizes abnormal bone remodeling and sRANKL/osteoprotegerin ratio in patients with multiple myeloma. Leukemia 18:1420–1426

Terpos E, Kiagia M, Karapanagiotou EM, Charpidou A, Dilana KD, Nasothimiou E, Harrington KJ, Polyzos A, Syrigos KN (2009) The clinical significance of serum markers of bone turnover in NSCLC patients: surveillance, management and prognostic implications. Anticancer Res 29:1651–1657

Thurairaja R, Iles RK, Jefferson K, McFarlane JP, Persad RA (2006) Serum amino-terminal propeptide of type 1 procollagen (P1NP) in prostate cancer: a potential predictor of bone metastases and prognosticator for disease progression and survival. Urol Int 76:67–71

Tian E, Zhan F, Walker R, Rasmussen E, Ma Y, Barlogie B, Shaughnessy JD Jr (2003) The role of the Wnt-signaling antagonist DKK1 in the development of osteolytic lesions in multiple myeloma. N Engl J Med 349:2483–2494

Tu Q, Zhang S, Fix A, Brewer E, Li YP, Zhang ZY, Chen J (2009) Targeted overexpression of BSP in osteoclasts promotes bone metastasis of breast cancer cells. J Cell Physiol 218:135–145

Ulrich U, Rhiem K, Schmolling J, Flaskamp C, Paffenholz I, Salzer H, Bauknecht T, Schlebusch H (2001) Cross-linked type I collagen C- and N-telopeptides in women with bone metastases from breast cancer. Arch Gynecol Obstet 264:186–190

Valverde P, Tu Q, Chen J (2005) BSP and RANKL induce osteoclastogenesis and bone resorption synergistically. J Bone Miner Res 20:1669–1679

Voorzanger-Rousselot N, Juillet F, Mareau E, Zimmermann J, Kalebic T, Garnero P (2006) Association of 12 serum biochemical markers of angiogenesis, tumour invasion and bone turnover with bone metastases from breast cancer: a crossectional and longitudinal evaluation. Br J Cancer 95:506–514

Wada N, Ishii S, Ikeda T, Kitajima M (2004) Inhibition of bone metastasis from breast cancer with pamidronate resulting in reduction of urinary pyridinoline and deoxypyridinoline in a rat model. Breast Cancer 11:282–287

Waltregny D, Bellahcene A, Van Riet I, Fisher LW, Young M, Fernandez P, Dewe W, de Leval J, Castronovo V (1998) Prognostic value of bone sialoprotein expression in clinically localized human prostate cancer. J Natl Cancer Inst 90:1000–1008

Waltregny D, Bellahcene A, de Leval X, Florkin B, Weidle U, Castronovo V (2000) Increased expression of bone sialoprotein in bone metastases compared with visceral metastases in human breast and prostate cancers. J Bone Miner Res 15:834–843

Woitge HW, Pecherstorfer M, Horn E, Keck AV, Diel IJ, Bayer P, Ludwig H, Ziegler R, Seibel MJ (2001) Serum bone sialoprotein as a marker of tumour burden and neoplastic bone involvement and as a prognostic factor in multiple myeloma. Br J Cancer 84:344–351

Wymenga LF, Groenier K, Schuurman J, Boomsma JH, Elferink RO, Mensink HJ (2001) Pretreatment levels of urinary deoxypyridinoline as a potential marker in patients with prostate cancer with or without bone metastasis. BJU Int 88:231–235

Ylisirnio S, Hoyhtya M, Makitaro R, Paaakko P, Risteli J, Kinnula VL, Turpeenniemi-Hujanen T, Jukkola A (2001) Elevated serum levels of type I collagen degradation marker ICTP and tissue inhibitor of metalloproteinase (TIMP) 1 are associated with poor prognosis in lung cancer. Clin Cancer Res 7:1633–1637

Zhang JH, Wang J, Tang J, Barnett B, Dickson J, Hahsimoto N, Williams P, Ma W, Zheng W, Yoneda T, Pageau S, Chen J (2004) Bone sialoprotein promotes bone metastasis of a non-bone-seeking clone of human breast cancer cells. Anticancer Res 24:1361–1368

Zhang L, Hou X, Lu S, Rao H, Hou J, Luo R, Huang H, Zhao H, Jian H, Chen Z, Liao M, Wang X (2010) Predictive significance of bone sialoprotein and osteopontin for bone metastases in resected Chinese non-small-cell lung cancer patients: a large cohort retrospective study. Lung Cancer 67:114–119

Osteolytic and Osteoblastic Bone Metastases: Two Extremes of the Same Spectrum?

Angelica Ortiz and Sue-Hwa Lin

Abstract

Normal bone development and maintenance are sustained through a balanced communication between osteoclasts and osteoblasts. Invasion of the bone compartment by cancer cells causes an imbalance in their activities and results in predominantly bone lysing or bone forming phenotypes depending on the origin of the cancer. Tumor-induced bone lesions usually exhibit disturbances of both cell types. Thus, osteoclast activity is activated in a predominantly osteoblastic lesion and vice versa. These cancer-induced bone responses favor the survival and growth of cancer cells in their new environment. Therapies that can restore the balance may limit the growth of cancer cells in the bone. The recent development of agents that target the osteolytic components of bone metastasis, including bisphosphonates and denosumab, showed promising results in osteolytic bone diseases such as multiple myeloma but were less effective in improving the osteoblastic bone disease found in prostate cancer. Thus, while osteolytic components are present in both osteoblastic and osteolytic bone lesions, inhibition of the osteolytic component is not sufficient to alter the vicious cycle leading to tumors with an osteoblastic phenotype. These observations suggest that osteolytic and osteoblastic bone metastases are not the same and tumor-induced osteoblastic and osteolytic activity play different roles in supporting their growth and survival.

A. Ortiz · S.-H. Lin (✉)
Department of Molecular Pathology, Unit 89,
The University of Texas M. D. Anderson Cancer Center,
1515 Holcombe Blvd., Houston, TX 77030, USA
e-mail: slin@mdanderson.org

S.-H. Lin
Department of Genitourinary Medical Oncology,
The University of Texas M. D. Anderson Cancer Center,
Houston, TX 77030, USA

Keywords

PCa · Bone metastasis · Osteoblast · Osteoclast

Contents

1 Skeletal Responses to Tumor Invasion.. 226
2 Bone Remodeling in Physiological Conditions... 227
3 Osteoblast-Induced Vicious Cycle: Bone Remodeling in Prostate Cancer Bone Metastasis.. 227
4 Uncoupling of Bone Turnover by Invasion of Prostate Cancer Cells 229
5 Osteoclast-Induced Vicious Cycle: Bone Remodeling in Multiple Myeloma.................. 229
6 Osteolytic and Osteoblastic Bone Metastases: Are They Two Extremes of the Same Spectrum? 229
References.. 231

1 Skeletal Responses to Tumor Invasion

Bone metastasis commonly occurs in a majority of patients with advanced lung, breast, and prostate cancer, and with less frequency in patients with carcinoma of other organ origins. Bone metastases are classified as osteolytic (bone resorbing) or osteoblastic (bone forming). The processes of bone resorption and bone formation are normally coupled. In a disease state, such as cancer, this coupling is distorted toward either the osteolytic or osteoblastic phenotype. These terms mainly describe the overall phenotype of the disease-induced bone responses; mixed lesions containing both elements are also present. For example, prostate cancer predominantly yields bone forming lesions (Logothetis and Lin 2005), however, high osteoclast activity is also present, as indicated by elevated serum and urinary markers of bone resorption (Clarke et al. 1991; Sano et al. 1994; Takeuchi et al. 1996). Breast cancer patients predominantly present with osteolytic lesions, though a few cases show osteoblastic activity (Roodman 2004). Multiple myeloma is the cancer that mainly develops lytic bone lesions, though myeloma is not commonly identified as a metastatic cancer (Roodman 2004). Together, this suggests a spectrum of skeletal responses to tumor invasion (Mundy 2002). We will focus on the mechanisms that govern the two extreme phenotypes, i.e. osteoblastic lesion of prostate cancer bone metastasis and osteolytic lesion of multiple myeloma, and discuss whether inhibition of osteoclast activity by bisphosphonates and denosumab is sufficient to alter the progression of these diseases.

2 Bone Remodeling in Physiological Conditions

Normal bone development and maintenance are sustained through a balanced communication between osteoclasts and osteoblasts, cells which aid in bone destruction and bone formation, respectively, in accordance with mechanical demands to keep the shape and strength of bone within strict limits (Seeman and Delmas 2006). These events are coordinated through cell–cell contact and/or diffusible paracrine factors (Matsuo and Irie 2008). These intercellular communications act in concert to initiate the bone remodeling cycle. In the normal condition, the bone remodeling cycle begins in response to stimuli, such as loss of mechanical loading, low blood calcium, or alterations in hormones/cytokines (Matsuo and Irie 2008). In response to these changes in the bone environment, osteocytes secrete regulatory factors to activate osteoclast differentiation (Matsuo and Irie 2008), which mediates bone resorption. Bone resorption releases growth factors from the bone matrix, including TGFβ and bone morphogenetic proteins (BMPs) that are abundant in bone (Ott 2002). These molecules then stimulate osteoblast precursors to begin bone formation. Thus, in normal bone formation, osteoclast and osteoblast activities are tightly coupled, with bone resorption (osteoclast) preceding bone formation (Ott 2002). Osteolytic or osteoblastic bone responses to tumor invasion are due to the imbalance of these two opposing activities. These cancer-induced bone changes likely in favor of tumor cell growth and survival in the bone microenvironment.

3 Osteoblast-Induced Vicious Cycle: Bone Remodeling in Prostate Cancer Bone Metastasis

Prostate cancer metastasis is generally characterized as osteoblastic. Radiographically, prostate cancer bone metastasis showed increased uptake of Tc-99 m MDP in bone scan (Noguchi et al. 2003). Histologically, the tumor cells are surrounded with irregular woven bone (Roudier et al. 2003, 2008). Patients with osteoblastic patterns of bone metastasis not only present with elevated bone-specific alkaline phosphatase but also bone resorption markers such as urine N-telopeptide (NTx) (Clarke et al. 1991; Sano et al. 1994; Takeuchi et al. 1996), suggesting the presence of osteoclastic activity in the predominantly osteoblastic bone lesions (Clarke et al. 1991; Charhon et al. 1983; Percival et al. 1987; Urwin et al. 1985). The woven bone found in the bone metastases is structurally weak and prone to fracture (Roudier et al. 2003). The frailty observed in the skeleton of patients with osteoblastic lesions may be due to the heterogeneity of lesions with both osteopenic and osteodense lesions within individuals as determined by histomorphometric analysis of metastatic biopsies (Roudier et al. 2008).

Prostate cancer growth in bone uniquely favors bone formation. Prostate cancer patients are generally older males who would normally suffer from osteoporosis, but instead present with osteosclerotic growths in radiological examinations. This suggests a close interaction between prostate cancer cells and bone forming cells. The mechanism by which this occurs is likely mediated by interactions between the prostate cancer cells and the different components of the bone microenvironment (Logothetis and Lin 2005; Choueiri et al. 2006). Many studies suggest that prostate cancer cells secrete factors that benefit osteoblast proliferation or differentiation (Dai et al. 2004, 2005; Lee et al. 2011; Li et al. 2008; Lin et al. 2008). Analyses of the conditioned medium from prostate cancer cell lines identified tumor growth factor-β (Marquardt et al. 1987), endothelin-1 (Nelson et al. 1995, 2003), urokinase-type plasminogen activator (uPA) (Rabbani et al. 1990), FGF9 (Li et al. 2008), and BMP4 (Lee et al. 2011) that exhibit effects on osteoblast proliferation and/or differentiation. Samples of osteoblastic bone lesions from patients with prostate cancer were also studied to determine factors secreted by the prostate cancer cells that would affect bone formation. These clinical samples identified BMPs, platelet-derived growth factor (PDGF), fibroblast growth factor (FGF), vascular endothelial growth factor (VEGF), and uPA (Choueiri et al. 2006). Additionally, isolation of protein factors from the bone marrow aspirates of men with prostate cancer and bone metastasis has also identified proteins that are involved in osteogenesis (Lin et al. 2008).

Increased osteoblast activity likely favors prostate cancer cell growth in bone. Factors such as osteonectin, osteopontin, osteocalcin, and bone sialoprotein secreted by osteoblasts have been shown to affect different prostate cancer cell functions (Chen et al. 2007; Gordon et al. 2009; Jacob et al. 1999; Khodavirdi et al. 2006). Bone sialoprotein, for example, increases the activation of the FAK-associated pathway that leads to increased cancer cell invasion in a Matrigel-coated Boyden-chamber assay and increased cell survival upon withdrawal of serum (Gordon et al. 2009). Osteopontin affects prostate cancer cell proliferation, invasion, and intravasation potential (Khodavirdi et al. 2006).

As osteoblasts secrete factors to increase prostate cancer cell proliferation and invasion in bone, increased osteoblast activity also leads to an increase in calcium-phosphate deposition. This results in hypocalcemia-induced secretion of parathyroid hormone (PTH) (Murray et al. 2001), which induces RANK ligand (RANKL) expression in bone marrow stromal cells and osteoblasts. RANKL functions to promote osteoclast differentiation and activation, leading to bone matrix degradation. This results in the release of growth factor from the matrix, which further promotes tumor cell proliferation. In addition, it was reported that some prostate cancer cells secrete RANKL, which could directly activate osteoclasts (Chen et al. 2006; Penno et al. 2009). Thus, the osteoclast activity observed may be due to both osteoblast hyperactivity and prostate cancer cell involvement. Together, these osteoblast-induced events may enhance the proliferation and survival of prostate cancer cells in bone. Thus, we refer to this as the "osteoblast-induced vicious cycle".

4 Uncoupling of Bone Turnover by Invasion of Prostate Cancer Cells

In the normal bone regulation process, bone resorption (osteoclast) precedes bone formation (Ott 2002). However, in metastatic development of prostate cancer, the osteoclast–osteoblast coupling is disrupted. This phenomenon was examined by Lee et al. (2002) using the osteoblastic xenograft LAPC-9 and zoledronate, which limits the osteoclast activity. The study concluded that osteoclast activity may not be critical for the development of osteoblastic lesions associated with prostate tumor cells (Lee et al. 2002). This observation is consistent with the histopathological analysis of human bone metastasis specimens, which showed variable association of bone formation and bone resorption independent of bone volumes (Roudier et al. 2008). Together, these observations indicate that prostate cancer invasion completely uncoupled the normal process of bone turnover.

5 Osteoclast-Induced Vicious Cycle: Bone Remodeling in Multiple Myeloma

Multiple myeloma promotes osteoclast activation while actively suppressing osteoblastic bone forming functions, resulting in predominantly osteolytic lesions. Multiple myeloma is clinically characterized through histomorphometric studies as having a lower number of osteoblasts and decreased bone formation, suggesting that osteoblasts are affected in this disease. The mechanism of bone disease in myeloma is described in Chap. 6. In contrast to prostate cancer, multiple myeloma bone disease can be described as osteoclast-induced vicious cycle in that myeloma cells produce or induce other cells in the bone marrow to secrete osteoclast activating factors to increase osteoclasts. Increased osteoclast activity leads to bone resorption, which results in the release of growth factors and cytokines from bone matrix, and these factors further increase the growth and survival of the myeloma cells. In contrast to prostate cancer, osteoblast activity is suppressed in multiple myeloma (see Chap. 6). Thus, multiple myeloma and prostate cancer bone disease represent two ends of a spectrum.

6 Osteolytic and Osteoblastic Bone Metastases: Are They Two Extremes of the Same Spectrum?

Because an increase in osteoclast activity is involved in both osteolytic and osteoblastic bone metastasis and growth factors are being released from the bone matrix during bone degradation, it seems that inhibition of osteolytic activity should be able to interfere with both osteoclast- or osteoblast-induced vicious cycles that support tumor growth. Strategies that were developed and applied in the clinical setting to affect osteolytic events include the use of bisphosphonates and targeting the biological regulators of osteoclast activation, e.g. RANKL. Bisphosphonates are synthetic analogs of pyrophosphate, which act as powerful inhibitors of osteoclast function and are used to treat osteolytic diseases (Rogers 2003; Roudier et al. 2003). The molecular mechanisms of action of bisphosphonates have been extensively reviewed in the other chapters and will not be repeated here. The nitrogen-containing bisphosphonates, such as zoledronate, affect not only osteoclasts but also tumor cell apoptosis (Rogers 2003).

The clinical data on the effects of bisphosphonates on prostate, breast, multiple myeloma, and lung cancers are discussed in detail in several chapters. In multiple myeloma, clinical data seem to suggest that bisphosphonates, especially the highly potent zolendronic acid, are able to reduce osteolytic markers, skeletal related events, and improve overall survival (see Chap. 6). Several bisphosphonates have been used to treat patients with prostate cancer bone metastases, such as clodronate, ibandronate, pamidronate, and zoledronic acid (Dearnaley et al. 2009; Heidenreich et al. 2002; Saad et al. 2002; Small et al. 2003). While they are all able to ameliorate bone pain due to tumor burden, only zoledronic acid has shown a long-term reduction and delay in skeletal related events (Saad 2008). In clinical analyses of 648 patients undergoing various treatments, 77% of prostate cancer patients with vertebral metastasis that were treated with zoledronic acid experienced a reduction in pain and some improved motor function (Cereceda et al. 2003). When overall survival was used as an endpoint, zoledronic acid was shown to benefit patients with elevated levels of bone turnover markers (Lipton et al. 2008). Because prostate cancer bone metastasis is heterogeneous with a spectrum of predominantly osteoblastic to predominantly osteolytic phenotypes, the question remains whether zoledronic acid is also helpful for those prostate cancer bone metastasis with predominantly osteoblastic components. In a preclinical study, Thudi et al. (2008) demonstrated that nude mice injected with Ace-1 and treated with zoledronic acid showed an inhibition of bone resorption but no significant difference in osteoblastic lesion. In human specimens, histopathological assessment of osteoblastic metastases from prostate cancer by Roudier et al. (2008) showed that bisphosphonates do not appear to modify the overall architecture of bone in prostate cancer bone metastasis. Together, these results suggest that interfering with the osteolytic components of prostate cancer bone metastasis by zoledronic acid is not sufficient to change the biology of the osteoblast-induced vicious cycle.

Denosumab is a human monoclonal IgG2 antibody against RANKL, which binds and neutralizes RANKL in order to decrease bone resorption. Unlike zoledronic acid, there is no evidence that denosumab directly affects cancer cell apoptosis. In multiple myeloma, both bisphosphonates and denosumab can effectively reduce skeletal related events, and denosumab treatment shared similar survival benefits as zoledronic acid (Henry et al. 2011). In prostate cancer bone metastasis, a recent randomized, double-blind study comparing denosumab versus zoledronic acid for the treatment of bone metastases in men with castration-resistant prostate cancer showed that denosumab was better than zoledronic acid in delaying first on-study skeletal-related event by a difference in the median time of

3.6 months (18%) (Fizazi et al. 2011). However, the overall survival was similar between the two groups (Fizazi et al. 2011). Thus, the denosumab study seems to further support our hypothesis that interfering with the osteolytic components of prostate cancer bone metastasis is not sufficient to alter the biology of the osteoblast-induced vicious cycle.

Together, the clinical trial results from using agents that inhibit osteolytic activity seem to suggest that osteolytic and osteoblastic bone metastases are not the same. Thus, treatment strategies that target the prostate cancer-induced osteoblastic responses in addition to the osteolytic responses might be needed for treatment of bone metastases in men with castration-resistant prostate cancer.

References

Cereceda LE, Flechon A, Droz JP (2003) Management of vertebral metastases in prostate cancer: a retrospective analysis in 119 patients. Clin Prostate Cancer 2:34–40

Charhon SA, Chapuy MC, Delvin EE, Valentin-Opran A, Edouard CM, Meunier PJ (1983) Histomorphometric analysis of sclerotic bone metastases from prostatic carcinoma with special reference to osteomalacia. Cancer 51:918–924

Chen G, Sircar K, Aprikian A, Potti A, Goltzman D, Rabbani SA (2006) Expression of RANKL/RANK/OPG in primary and metastatic human prostate cancer as markers of disease stage and functional regulation. Cancer 107:289–298

Chen N, Ye XC, Chu K, Navone NM, Sage EH, Yu-Lee LY et al (2007) A secreted isoform of ErbB3 promotes osteonectin expression in bone and enhances the invasiveness of prostate cancer cells. Cancer Res 67:6544–6548

Choueiri M, Tu S-M, Yu-Lee LY, Lin SH (2006) The central role of osteoblasts in the metastasis of prostate cancer. Cancer Metastasis Rev 25:601–609

Clarke NW, McClure J, George NJ (1991) Morphometric evidence for bone resorption and replacement in prostate cancer. Br J Urol 68:74–80

Dai J, Kitagawa Y, Zhang J, Yao Z, Mizokami A, Cheng S et al (2004) Vascular endothelial growth factor contributes to the prostate cancer-induced osteoblast differentiation mediated by bone morphogenetic protein. Cancer Res 64:994–999

Dai J, Keller J, Zhang J, Lu Y, Yao Z, Keller ET (2005) Bone morphogenetic protein-6 promotes osteoblastic prostate cancer bone metastases through a dual mechanism. Cancer Res 65: 8274–8285

Dearnaley DP, Mason MD, Parmar MK, Sanders K, Sydes MR (2009) Adjuvant therapy with oral sodium clodronate in locally advanced and metastatic prostate cancer: long-term overall survival results from the MRC PR04 and PR05 randomised controlled trials. Lancet Oncol 10:872–876

Fizazi K, Carducci M, Smith M, Damião R, Brown J, Karsh L et al (2011) Denosumab versus zoledronic acid for treatment of bone metastases in men with castration-resistant prostate cancer: a randomised, double-blind study. Lancet 377:813–822

Gordon JA, Sodek J, Hunter GK, Goldberg HA (2009) Bone sialoprotein stimulates focal adhesion-related signaling pathways: role in migration and survival of breast and prostate cancer cells. J Cell Biochem 107:1118–1128

Heidenreich A, Elert A, Hofmann R (2002) Ibandronate in the treatment of prostate cancer associated painful osseous metastases. Prostate Cancer Prostatic Dis 5:231–235

Henry DH, Costa L, Goldwasser F, Hirsh V, Hungria V, Prausova J, et al. (2011) Randomized, double-blind study of denosumab versus zoledronic acid in the treatment of bone metastases in patients with advanced cancer (excluding breast and prostate cancer) or multiple myeloma. J Clin Oncol 29:1125–1132

Jacob K, Webber M, Benayahu D, Kleinman HK (1999) Osteonectin promotes prostate cancer cell migration and invasion: a possible mechanism for metastasis to bone. Cancer Res 59:4453–4457

Khodavirdi AC, Song Z, Yang S, Zhong C, Wang S, Wu H et al (2006) Increased expression of osteopontin contributes to the progression of prostate cancer. Cancer Res 66:883–888

Lee YP, Schwarz EM, Davies M, Jo M, Gates J, Zhang X et al (2002) Use of zoledronate to treat osteoblastic versus osteolytic lesions in a severe-combined-immunodeficient mouse model. Cancer Res 62:5564–5570

Lee YC, Cheng CJ, Bilen MA, Lu JF, Satcher RL, Yu-Lee LY et al (2011) BMP4 promotes prostate tumor growth in bone through osteogenesis. Cancer Res 71:5194–5203

Li Z, Mathew P, Yang J, Starbuck M-W, Zurita AJ, Liu J et al (2008) Androgen receptor-negative human prostate cancer cells induce osteogenesis through FGF9-mediated mechanisms. J Clin Invest 118:2697–2710

Lin S-H, Cheng CJ, Lee Y-C, Ye X, Tsai W-W, Kim J et al (2008) A 45 kDa ErbB3 secreted by prostate cancer cells promotes bone formation. Oncogene 27:5195–5203

Lipton A, Cook R, Saad F, Major P, Garnero P, Terpos E et al (2008) Normalization of bone markers is associated with improved survival in patients with bone metastases from solid tumors and elevated bone resorption receiving zoledronic acid. Cancer 113:193–201

Logothetis C, Lin S-H (2005) Osteoblasts in prostate cancer metastasis to bone. Nat Rev Cancer 5:21–28

Marquardt H, Lioubin MN, Ikeda T (1987) Complete amino acid sequence of human transforming growth factor type b2. J Biol Chem 262:12127–12131

Matsuo K, Irie N (2008) Osteoclast–osteoblast communication. Arch Biochem Biophys 473: 201–209

Mundy GR (2002) Metastasis to bone: causes, consequences and therapeutic opportunities. Nat Rev Cancer 2:584–593

Murray RM, Grill V, Crinis N, Ho PW, Davison J, Pitt P (2001) Hypocalcemic and normocalcemic hyperparathyroidism in patients with advanced prostatic cancer. J Clin Endocrinol Metab 86:4133–4138

Nelson JB, Hedican SP, George AH, Reddi AH, Piantadosi S, Eisenberger MA et al (1995) Identification of endothelin-1 in the pathophysiology of metastatic adenocarcinoma of the prostate. Nature Med 1:944–949

Nelson JB, Nabulsi AA, Vogelzang NJ, Breul J, Zonnenberg BA, Daliani DD et al (2003) Suppression of prostate cancer induced bone remodeling by the endothelin receptor A antagonist atrasentan. J Urol 169:1143–1149

Noguchi M, Kikuchi H, Ishibashi M, Noda S (2003) Percentage of the positive area of bone metastasis is an independent predictor of disease death in advanced prostate cancer. Br J Cancer 88:195–201

Ott SM (2002) Histomorphometric analysis of bone remodeling. In: Bilezikian JP, Raisz LG, Rodan GA (eds) The principles of bone biology. Academic Press, San Diego, pp 303–319

Penno H, Nilsson O, Brändström H, Winqvist O, Ljunggren O (2009) Expression of RANK-ligand in prostate cancer cell lines. Scand J Clin Lab Invest 69:151–155

Percival RC, Urwin GH, Harris S, Yates AJP, Williams JL, Beneton M et al (1987) Biochemical and histological evidence that carcinoma of the prostate is associated with increased bone resorption. Eur J Surg Oncol 13:41–49

Rabbani SA, Desjardins J, Bell AW, Banville D, Mazar A, Henkin J et al (1990) An amino-terminal fragment of urokinase isolated from a prostate cancer cell line (PC-3) is mitogenic for osteoblast-like cells. Biochem Biophys Res Commun 173:1058–1064

Rogers MJ (2003) New insights into the molecular mechanisms of action of bisphosphonates. Curr Pharm Des 9:2643–2658

Roodman GD (2004) Mechanisms of bone metastasis. N Engl J Med 350:1655–1664

Roudier MP, Vesselle H, True LD, Higano CS, Ott SM, King SH et al (2003) Bone histology at autopsy and matched bone scintigraphy findings in patients with hormone refractory prostate cancer: the effect of bisphosphonate therapy on bone scintigraphy results. Clin Exp Metastasis 20:171–180

Roudier MP, Morrissey C, True LD, Higano CS, Vessella RL, Ott SM (2008) Histopathological assessment of prostate cancer bone osteoblastic metastases. J Urol 180:1154–1160

Saad F (2008) New research findings on zoledronic acid: survival, pain, and anti-tumour effects. Cancer Treat Rev 34:183–192

Saad F, Gleason DM, Murray R, Tchekmedyian S, Venner P, Lacombe L et al (2002) A randomized, placebo-controlled trial of Zoledronic acid in patients with hormone-refractory metastatic prostate carcinoma. J Natl Cancer Inst 94:1458–1468

Sano M, Kushida K, Takahashi M, Ohishi T, Kawana K, Okada M et al (1994) Urinary pyridinoline and deoxypyridinoline in prostate carcinoma patients with bone metastasis. Br J Cancer 70:701–703

Seeman E, Delmas PD (2006) Bone quality—the material and structural basis of bone strength and fragility. N Engl J Med 354:2250–2261

Small EJ, Smith MR, Seaman JJ, Petrone S, Kowalski MO (2003) Combined analysis of two multicenter, randomized, placebo-controlled studies of pamidronate disodium for the palliation of bone pain in men with metastatic prostate cancer. J Clin Oncol 21:4277–4284

Takeuchi S, Arai K, Saitoh H, Yoshida K, Miura M (1996) Urinary pyridinoline and deoxypyridinoline as potential markers of bone metastasis in patients with prostate cancer. J Urol 156:1691–1695

Thudi NK, Martin CK, Nadella MV, Fernandez SA, Werbeck JL, Pinzone JJ et al (2008) Zoledronic acid decreased osteolysis but not bone metastasis in a nude mouse model of canine prostate cancer with mixed bone lesions. Prostate 68:1116–1125

Urwin GH, Percival RC, Harris S, Beneton MNC, Williams JL, Kanis JA (1985) Generalised increase in bone resorption in carcinoma of the prostate. Br J Urol 57:721–723